Handbook of
Communication
in Anaesthesia, Pain
Management, and
Intensive Care

Handbook of Communication in Anaesthesia, Pain Management, and Intensive Care

A practical guide to exploring the art

SECOND EDITION

Edited by

Allan M. Cyna
Suyin G.M. Tan
Marion I. Andrew
Laura L. Burgoyne
Scott W. Simmons

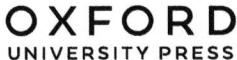
OXFORD
UNIVERSITY PRESS

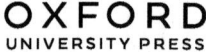

OXFORD
UNIVERSITY PRESS

Great Clarendon Street, Oxford, OX2 6DP,
United Kingdom

Oxford University Press is a department of the University of Oxford.
It furthers the University's objective of excellence in research, scholarship,
and education by publishing worldwide. Oxford is a registered trade mark of
Oxford University Press in the UK and in certain other countries

First Edition published in 2011
Second Edition published in 2024

Published in the United States of America by Oxford University Press
198 Madison Avenue, New York, NY 10016, United States of America

British Library Cataloguing in Publication Data
Data available

Library of Congress Control Number: 2024936325

ISBN 978–0–19–885866–9

DOI: 10.1093/med/9780198858669.001.0001

Printed in the UK by
Ashford Colour Press Ltd, Gosport, Hampshire

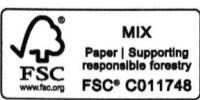

Ayesha, Sophia and Benjamin
Oban, Lewis, Arran, Todd, Ailsa, ZaZa,
Solomoni and Sally
Doris, Mary and Louise
Rob
Sally

Foreword

One of the great myths of anaesthesia is that anaesthetists are doctors that don't like talking to people. Yet every anaesthetist will have personal examples of where communication—good and bad—has had a profound influence on a patient, colleagues, or the anaesthetist themselves.

Communication is fundamental to what we as anaesthetists do. As the technical aspects of anaesthesia have become more science (and perhaps) less art, so the importance of good communication has become more and more visible. It is common parlance to refer to communication as part of non-technical skills, but as Stavros Prineas highlights, perhaps it is time to reframe these as paratechnical—alongside, not instead of or in contradistinction to, the technical aspects of the anaesthetist's role.

This book should make the reader uncomfortable. Yes, the traditional 'basics' of good communication are covered—listening, the importance of non-verbal signals—but there is so much more. And that *more* may be difficult reading. In part this may be because communication is personal. It is fundamentally about you or me. A cannula not going in first time doesn't reflect on me as an individual, but poor communication does. And therein lies a trap—we can believe that cannulation skills can be taught but are less willing to admit that good communication is also a teachable skill.

Anaesthetists have been brought up in a medical model, but the science—and it is a science—of communication requires us to step outside that model, particularly the benign paternalism that it frequently evokes. Good communication means stepping into the reality of the patient, which may be far removed from our medical reality. That becomes uncomfortable—the control is shifting away from the anaesthetist and towards the patient.

Anaesthetists are very comfortable with the concept of placebo—especially when applied to drugs and procedures. Most have probably seen the positive effect of good communication. But the nocebo effect—the ability of communication to cause harm or adverse effects is less well known. The ethics and praxis of how to be honest with patients without making things worse with what we say and do are not straightforward. We are rightly required to provide material information to our patients—for practical, humanitarian, ethical, and legal reasons—but this book contains a wealth of material suggesting that how we do so could often be better.

Anaesthetists probably spend more time communicating with other members of the healthcare team than directly with patients. A lot of energy has been devoted across the globe to the implementation of checklists and handover tools to improve information transfer in the perioperative period. This handbook goes beyond the tools and explores the times when this is difficult. The senior colleague who may be doing something unsafe, times of conflict, the director who doesn't seem to understand the realities of work on the ground.

The contents of this handbook may make the reader uncomfortable, but not despondent. The book is above all practical. There are tools, tips, and exemplars in abundance, offering the reader a guide to improve their communication, and that of their colleagues.

Our patients deserve the best care possible and that demands excellent communication. This handbook is a wonderful combination of theory, science, and practical tools and tips. Now, to put it into practice.

Iain Moppett
Professor of Anaesthesia and Perioperative Medicine
University of Nottingham

Preface

'Whether you think you can or whether you think you can't—you are probably right!'
Adapted from Henry Ford

Communication with patients and colleagues frequently goes well, yet few anaesthetists consciously appreciate how they achieve this, or how to teach what they do. Such intuitive skills are usually gained through many years of experience, rather than via a specific structure. We encourage the reader to continue with their current modes of communication when these are working well. This book is primarily concerned with providing a resource that offers ways of improving communication when the usual strategies are not working, or where the situation is unfamiliar. Strategies are suggested that can allow anyone working in critical care or pain medicine to understand the language structures involved, and facilitate the teaching of such skills.

The concepts and tools used in this book draw on a wide range of ideas and constitute a blend of models of clinical practice, teaching, and research. We also invite the reader to consider the use of two novel frameworks, 'GREAT' and 'LAURS' discussed in detail in the first section of the book and then referred to throughout. The structured approach of 'GREAT' is a simple tool for working through an interaction, while 'LAURS' has an underlying philosophy of the need to respect the perspective of others to create the opportunity for shared understanding. The listening, acceptance, utilizing, reframing, and suggesting elements are invoked repeatedly throughout the book and have applicability in a wide range of clinical settings, as well as contexts such as informed consent, use of social media, and working with managers. Clinicians will be very familiar with the use of story-telling and metaphor in their professional and day-to-day lives. 'LAURS' reminds us of the need to consider the diversity of languages and cultural backgrounds of others, for whom seemingly simple language, let alone colloquialisms may mean little or even the exact opposite of what we intend.

This book also discusses aspects of communication that can greatly enhance patients' well-being. The first of these is to optimize the patient's perception of control over what is happening to them. Secondly, to appreciate that the way we communicate can increase the choices available to both patients and anaesthetists. Thirdly, to recognize that patients have both the ability and desire to assist and cooperate with their care wherever possible. To achieve this end, hospital experiences should be perceived by both patient and anaesthetist in the most positive mindset possible in any particular situation or context.

Although written with a view to be of interest primarily to anaesthetists, much of what is proposed would easily benefit other professional groups. We hope that paramedical, nursing, and midwifery professional groups benefit from reading it, as many of the concepts could be readily adapted to these disciplines.

Finally, the reviewers of our original proposal universally recognized the need for a book on communication in anaesthesia. We are grateful for the considerable feedback from colleagues that we have received during its development and writing. We have all learned a lot, and enjoyed ourselves along the way. The structure of the book is self-explanatory and, as a group, anaesthetists are impatient. We have therefore cut a rather wordy draft preface so that you can just get on with it . . .

AMC
SGMT
MIA
LLB
SWS

Acknowledgements

We thank:

Evelyn M Hood for her invaluable assistance copyediting and proofreading the draft manuscript

&

Stavros Prineas for all the cartoon illustrations

Additional video content

Discover additional video content by searching for this book's title or ISBN (9780198858669) at academic.oup.com/oxford-medicine-online. If you would like access to the whole book, or are interested in accessing other titles, you can recommend it to your librarian.

Contents

Abbreviations

ACE	Adverse childhood experiences		ICU	Intensive care unit
ADE	Adverse developmental experience		LA	Local anaesthetic
AHPRA	Australian Health Practitioners Regulation Agency		LAURS	Listening, Acceptance, Utilization, Reframing, and Suggestion
ANTS	Anaesthetists' non-technical skills		LMA	Laryngeal mask airway
ANZCA	Australian and New Zealand College of Anaesthetists		MET	Medical emergency team
			MI	Motivational interviewing
ASA	American Society of Anesthesiologists		MI	Myocardial infarction
			PACU	Post-anaesthetic care unit
ASD	Autism spectrum disorder		PCA	Patient-controlled analgesia
BCC	Basal cell carcinoma		PDPH	Post-dural puncture headache
BIS	Bispectral index		PECS	Picture exchange communication system
CSE	Combined spinal-epidural			
CVC	Central venous catheter		PONV	Postoperative nausea and vomiting
DNR	Do-not-resuscitate		POST	Pain-oriented sensory testing
ECG	Electrocardiograph		PTSD	Post-traumatic stress disorder
GA	General anaesthesia		SARS	Severe acute respiratory syndrome
GrA	Graded assertiveness		SBAR	Situation, Background, Assessment, and Recommendation
GREAT	Greeting, Rapport, Expectations, Addressing concerns, and Tacit Agreement			
			SOP	Standardized operating procedures
			TIVA	Total intravenous anaesthesia
HEAPS	Human Error and Patient Safety			
ICMJE	International Committee of Medical Journal Editors			

Contributors to the second edition

Marion I. Andrew
Consultant Anaesthetist, Women's and
Children's Hospital, Adelaide, Australia

Christel J. Bejenke
Retired Anesthesiologist; active practice
Medical Counseling; Santa Barbara,
CA, USA

Laura L. Burgoyne
Senior Consultant Paediatric
Anaesthetist, Department of Children's
Anaesthesia, Women's and Children's
Hospital, Adelaide, Australia

Meredith J. Craigie
Retired, previously at: Specialist Pain
Medicine Physician, Clinical Associate
Professor, University of Adelaide
CALHN Pain Management Unit, The
Queen Elizabeth Hospital, Woodville
SA, Australia

Allan M. Cyna
University of Adelaide; Consultant
Anaesthetist, Women's and Children's
Hospital, Adelaide, Australia

Marie-Elisabeth Faymonville
Professor, ArsèneBurny Cancerology
Institute, University Hospital of Liège,
Belgium and Sensation and Perception
Research Group, GIGA Consciousness,
University of Liège, Belgium

Kirsty Forrest
Professor, Dean of Medicine Bond
University, Consultant Anaesthetist,
Queensland, Australia

Ernil Hansen
Professor, Department of
Anesthesiology, University Regensburg
Medical Center, Regensburg, Germany

Maurice Hennessy
Learning and Development Facilitator,
Australian and New Zealand College of
Anaesthetists, Melbourne, Australia

Gillian M. Hood
Consultant Anaesthetist, Glen Osmond,
SA, Australia

Mark P. Jensen
Professor, Department of Rehabilitation
Medicine, University of Washington,
Seattle, WA, USA

Elvira V. Lang
Founder and President of Comfort Talk,
157 Ivy Street, Brookline, MA, USA

Daniel Nethercott
Consultant in Critical Care, Department
of Critical Care, Bolton NHS Foundation
Trust, Bolton, UK

Catherine Olweny
Paediatric Anaesthetist, Royal Children's
Hospital, Melbourne, Australia;
Registered Counsellor and Clinical
Hypnotherapist

Stavros Prineas
Head of Anaesthesia, Blue Mountains
Hospital, Sydney, Australia

Sancha C. Robinson
Staff Specialist Anaesthetist, Department of Anaesthesia, John Hunter Hospital, Newcastle, NSW, Australia; Staff Specialist Anaesthetist, Department of Anaesthesia, Calvary Mater Newcastle, Newcastle, NSW, Australia; Professional Coach, Associate Certified Coach credential, International Coaching Federation

Tanya Selak
Consultant Anaesthetist, Department of Anaesthesia, Wollongong Hospital, New South Wales, Australia

Audrey Shafer
Professor Emeritum of Anesthesiology, Perioperative and Pain Medicine, Stanford University School of Medicine; Staff Anesthesiologist, Veterans Affairs Palo Alto Health Care System, Palo Alto, CA, USA

Maire Shelley
Adult Intensive Care Unit, Wythenshawe Hospital, Manchester, UK

Scott W. Simmons
Retired, previously at: Department of Anaesthesia, Mercy Hospital for Women, Heidelberg, Victoria, Australia

Andrew F. Smith
Honorary Professor of Anaesthesia and Perioperative Medicine, Consultant Anaesthetist, Director, Lancaster Patient Safety Research Unit, Royal Lancaster Infirmary, Ashton Road, Lancaster UK

Diana C. Strange Khursandi
Retired Anaesthetist, Queensland, Australia

Suyin G.M. Tan
VMO Anaesthetist/Pain Physician, South East Regional Hospital, Bega NSW, Australia

Audrey Vanhaudenhuyse
Professor, Sensation and Perception Research Group, GIGA Consciousness, University of Liège, Belgium; and Algology Interdisciplinary Center, University Hospital of Liège, Belgium

Andrew Watson
Director of Anaesthesia, Pain and Perioperative Medicine, Calvary, Public Hospital, Canberra, Australia

Contributors to the first edition

Dr Marion I. Andrew
Department of Women's Anaesthesia,
Women's and Children's Hospital,
Adelaide, SA 5006, Australia

Dr Christel J. Bejenke
Anesthesiologist, Santa Barbara,
California, USA

Dr Allan M. Cyna
Department of Women's Anaesthesia,
Women's and Children's Hospital,
Adelaide, SA 5006, Australia

Professor Marie-Elisabeth Faymonville
Department of Algology and Palliative
Care, Domaine Universitaire du Sart
Tilman, CHU Liège-B 35, Belgium

Professor Ernil Hansen
Department of Anesthesiology,
University Regensburg Medical Center,
D-93042 Regensburg, Germany

Dr Gillian M. Hood
Southern Group of Anaesthetic
Specialists, Flinders Private Hospital,
Bedford Park, South Australia, Australia

Dr Vincent J. Kopp
Associate Professor, Department of
Anesthesiology, School of Medicine,
University of North Carolina at Chapel
Hill, Chapel Hill, NC 27599, USA

Dr Elvira V. Lang
Department of Radiology, Beth Israel
Deaconess Medical Center, Harvard
Medical School, 330 Brookline Ave,
Boston, MA 02115, USA

Dr Andrew McWilliam
Department of Anaesthesia, Royal
Lancaster Infirmary, Lancaster LA1
4RP, UK

Professor Alan F. Merry
Department of Anaesthesiology,
University of Auckland, Private Bag
92019, Auckland, New Zealand

Dr Sally N. Merry
Werry Centre for Child and Adolescent
Mental Health, Department of
Psychological Medicine, Faculty of
Medical and Health Sciences, University
of Auckland, Private Bag 92019,
Auckland, New Zealand

Dr Daniel Nethercott
Adult Intensive Care Unit, Wythenshawe
Hospital, Southmoor Road, Manchester
M23 9LT, UK

Dr Stavros Prineas
Bathurst Base Hospital, NSW Australia,
Clinical Lecturer, Notre Dame
University, Sydney, Australia

Dr Susanna Richmond
Department of Anaesthesia, Royal
Lancaster Infirmary, Ashton Road,
Lancaster LA1 4RP, UK

Dr David Sainsbury
Department of Children's Anaesthesia,
Women's and Children's Hospital, 72
King William Rd, Adelaide, SA 5006,
Australia

Professor Audrey Shafer
Stanford University School of Medicine,
Veterans Affairs Palo Alto Health Care
System, 3801 Miranda Avenue, Palo
Alto, CA 94304, USA

Dr Maire Shelly
Adult Intensive Care Unit, Wythenshawe
Hospital, Southmoor Road, Manchester
M23 9LT, UK

Dr Scott W. Simmons
Department of Anaesthesia, Mercy
Hospital for Women, 163 Studley Road,
Heidelberg, Victoria 3084, Australia

Dr Andrew F. Smith
Department of Anaesthesia and
Lancaster Patient Safety Research Unit,
Royal Lancaster Infirmary, Ashton Road,
Lancaster, LA1 4RP, UK

Dr Diana C. Strange Khursandi
Deputy Director of Clinical Training,
Medical Education Unit, Caboolture
Hospital, Caboolture, Queensland 4510,
Australia

Dr Suyin G.M. Tan
Specialist Anaesthetist and Pain
Physician, South East Regional Hospital
NSW Australia

Section 1

Principles of communication

Chapter 1

Introduction

Stavros Prineas, Andrew F. Smith,
and Suyin G.M. Tan

'A journey of a thousand miles begins with a single step.'
Confucius

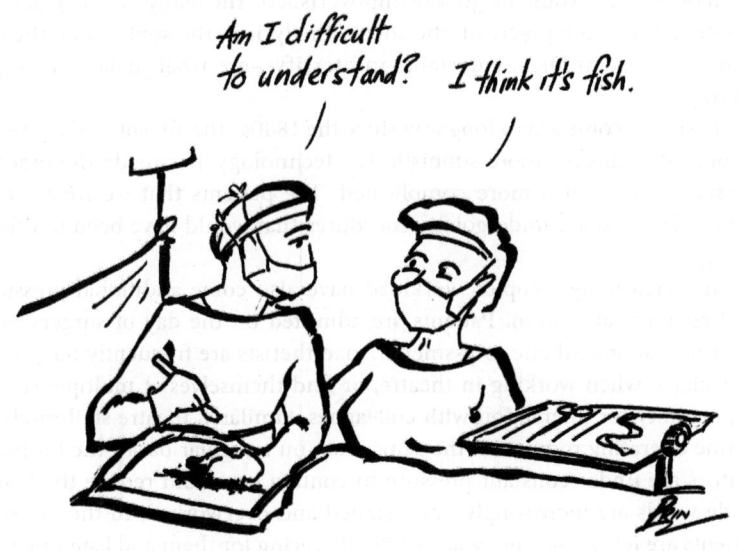

What this chapter is about

The importance of communication in anaesthetic practice

Communication is a fascinating and, on occasions, mysterious topic. At its heart, it is the means of expressing how we perceive and influence the world around us. It is a *sociotechnical* activity—a way to exchange information and meaning, and to connect. While a means to an end, it is also an end in itself. Without the ability to share with others, life would be greatly impoverished. The many human dimensions of communication—the practical, the social, the lyrical, the subliminal, the ability to soothe, to injure, inform, entertain, and terrify—are what makes this topic so challenging.

Anaesthesia has come a very long way since the 1840s. The advent of more selective drugs, coupled with ever more sophisticated technology, has made the practice of anaesthesia safer, yet also more complicated. The patients that we treat are often older and sicker, and are undergoing procedures that would have been unthinkable 20 years ago.

With an increasingly complex workload have also come additional pressures of time and resource allocation. Patients are admitted on the day of surgery, leaving minimal time for anaesthetic assessment. Anaesthetists are frequently busy, isolated and unavailable when working in theatre, or find themselves at multiple sites with little opportunity for interaction with colleagues. Similarly, theatre staff rarely work in the same operating room with the same team on a regular basis. The hospital ad-ministrators are under constant pressure to contain costs and reduce the length of stay, while wards are increasingly understaffed and overworked. In the midst of all this, patients are left wondering who is actually caring for them and listening to their concerns.

Anaesthetists play a crucial role in multi-professional teams in a wide variety of clinical settings, of which theatre is only one. There is the high dependency unit, the labour suite, paediatrics, the chronic pain clinic—to name but a few. In almost every aspect of anaesthetic clinical practice the ability to communicate effectively is a vital component of patient care. Many anaesthetists voice more concerns regarding communication challenges than about technical skills, which they are generally well-equipped to handle.[1] A recent survey of anaesthetists showed that over 90% believed poor communication caused procedural delay and that further work is required to improve communication in the stressful operating theatre environment, particularly at the surgeon–anaesthetist interface.[2]

Anaesthetists frequently communicate using highly technical language.[3] This can be off-putting to some patients, is likely to cause misunderstandings and, in some contexts, adversely affect patient safety.

When communication breaks down

There is growing recognition that many of the problems that beset modern healthcare stem from deficiencies in communication. Studies of adverse events show that communication failure is a root cause in about 50% of cases. Similarly, a substantial proportion of patient complaints and litigation result from communication breakdown between patients and their carers.[4] Consider the following cases:

A 'broken routine'

Communication around the time of induction is designed to reassure the patient while also signalling to others that anaesthetic induction is taking place (see Chapter 8). The following interview with an anaesthetic assistant shows what happens when the usual communication routine is absent and how the smooth, predictable sequence of events can be disrupted:

> 'There have been a couple of other cases where I've felt uneasy really. In one particular instance, the anaesthetist gave the anaesthetic without warning the patient and the patient panicked. I felt uneasy then, I felt very uneasy because the patient sat bolt upright and started grabbing hold of her throat and I felt bad because I hadn't warned the patient. I thought the anaesthetist was going to do it . . . the patient was scared stiff . . . If that was me, I would have quite a phobia about coming into theatres now.'
> (Interview with an anaesthetic assistant conducted during communication research.)[5]

This vignette illustrates how carefully anaesthetists need to ensure that the patient's journey into unconsciousness is made not only in safety but also with appropriate psychological preparation and communication. It also shows how closely individuals within the anaesthesia team work together. It is, fortunately, rare for another member of the team not to supplement communication left by another.

Power relationships in complex hierarchical organizations, such as a teaching hospital, can often determine how and whether staff are willing to speak up and escalate concern, particularly when confronted with a deteriorating patient or an obvious error by a colleague. The concept of *authority gradients* and their impact is discussed in Chapter 17.

A disoriented team

This report comes from an Australian coroner's case.[6] The medical emergency team (MET) is called to a 44-year-old patient in respiratory distress and haemodynamic collapse. The patient is rapidly deteriorating, and the early response on the ward is hectic. An intensive care unit (ICU) registrar and a senior ICU resident, both experienced in intubation, arrive, followed by the MET nurse and trolley. As the most senior medical officer present, the ICU registrar is presumed by others to be the team leader. He instructs those present to prepare for intubation. While they are pre-oxygenating, the anaesthetic registrar arrives and is directed to take the airway and intubate. She is a brand-new recruit, has never performed an emergency intubation before but does not declare this, and the other MET members do not ask if she is happy to perform the task. She inadvertently intubates the oesophagus, and this initially goes undetected. The patient continues to deteriorate and arrests. The team start CPR. Oesophageal intubation is diagnosed and corrected. Spontaneous cardiac output returns but there is extensive hypoxic brain damage and the patient dies 10 days later in ICU.

Failure of handover with fatal consequences

A 68-year-old man was admitted to hospital for a craniotomy to remove a large pituitary adenoma. Immediately prior to induction, the anaesthetist was called to take care of an emergency craniotomy in a trauma patient. He gave only a brief report to the anaesthetist who took over the case, and did not mention that two weeks previously the tumour had been partially debulked via a transnasal, trans-sphenoidal approach. The second anaesthetist decided to intubate the patient via the nasal route. and attempted to advance the nasotracheal tube through the left nostril. After meeting slight resistance, the tube was passed through the freshly granulating hole made from the previous operation and into the brainstem, leading to immediate circulatory collapse and, ultimately, demise four days later. What was remarkable about this case report was that while over two pages of discussion was devoted to the anatomy and pathophysiology of the injury, only one sentence was given to the lack of handover.[7] This observation is not made to disparage the team in question, but rather to make the more general assertion that frequently in the analyses of clinical events, poor communication is not examined with the same due diligence as other technical aspects of care.

Right advice; wrong manner and timing

In a case reported from the archives of a medical defence organization,[8] an anaesthetist at a private clinic gave a lumbar epidural to a patient in preparation for elective caesarean section. The patient was in her twenties and a heavy smoker. During the procedure, the patient appeared to have a satisfactory block for surgical anaesthesia. The anaesthetist had been concerned that the patient's absence from the ward for a cigarette had disrupted the operating list, and that her coughing perioperatively had made the surgical procedure much more difficult. He had expressed his views about smoking, 'You've seen your daughter born; if you give up smoking you might see her get married too'.

She began a legal claim for pain and psychological distress, alleging that the anaesthetist had failed to provide the proper pre-anaesthetic care, failed to ensure adequate surgical anaesthesia, and failed to ensure that she did not suffer unnecessary pain and distress after the delivery. The claimant also alleged that the anaesthetist had 'harassed' her and his manner towards her had contributed to her postnatal depression.

The experts consulted felt that while the technical aspects of the anaesthetic had been carried out appropriately, the anaesthetist's manner and poor communication had indeed contributed to the patient's psychological condition. The case was settled for a five-figure sum.

Well-intentioned health promotion advice here led to an unsatisfactory outcome. While it is without doubt correct that smoking reduces life expectancy, this was neither the time nor the manner in which to communicate this.

Benefits of improved communication

In contrast to the problems caused when communication breaks down, many benefits can be expected from improved clinical communication. The literature on patient benefits has been carefully reviewed for a number of outcomes in a variety of healthcare settings.[9,10] Little of this work has been carried out within the domain of the anaesthetist, though there are some notable exceptions.[11,12] More recently, training in communication skills for the preoperative visit was found to increase patient satisfaction.[12] The perception that clinicians are more effective can only enhance personal and professional self-esteem and work satisfaction, and general improvement in interaction with other human beings should extend also to relationships with colleagues.[13] Hospitals can benefit too. If it is perceived that more effective care is being provided for patients, the reputation of the institution will be enhanced amongst patients, referring doctors and the community in general. One might also expect a decrease in litigation by patients.[4] In a UK review of 21 years of litigation against obstetric anaesthetists, 'good communication'—along with early provision of information and diligent record-keeping—were cited as the best safeguards to minimize 'the frustration of patients that can then lead them to seek a legal route to redress if they suffer an injury following central neuraxial blockade.'[14]

Models of communication

Communication is a complex human activity which has been studied from several perspectives[15]: *semiotic* (communication as the transfer of *meaning*, however that is defined); *cybernetic* (communication as the exchange of packets of information between a transmitter and receiver); *rhetorical* (communication as a means of persuasion); *phenomenological* (communication as a way of showing ourselves to others, walking in another person's shoes, and sharing experiences); *psychosocial* (communication reflecting how we think and behave in groups e.g. how/why we follow orders, or escalate concern); *sociocultural* (how communication reflects wider social and cultural trends e.g. manners, memes and 'netiquette'); and *critical* (communication as a way of verifying facts or beliefs, reflecting on events and performance, and seeing things clearly).

The various models of communication differ largely in the language used to describe what are fundamentally similar or, even identical, concepts. Communication theory informs us that there are many conceptual patterns of communication, such as the Calgary–Cambridge model[16] for conducting medical consultations or team communication models.[17] Until recently, training in communication skills has focused on content and process whereas many aspects of communication are implied. Explicit or conscious aspects, and implicit, tacit, or subconscious aspects, all need consideration

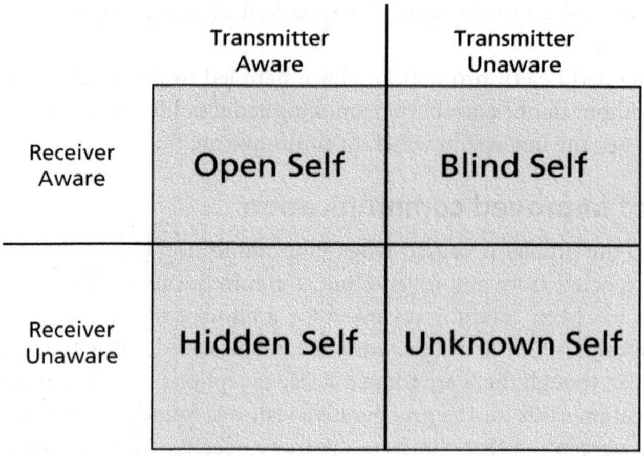

	Transmitter Aware	Transmitter Unaware
Receiver Aware	Open Self	Blind Self
Receiver Unaware	Hidden Self	Unknown Self

Fig. 1.1 The 'Johari window'. Derived from Luft and Ingham (1955).[18]

when learning and teaching effective communication. (See Chapters 2 and 4.) This concept underpins much of the content of this book.

One of the early representations of this idea was the 'Johari window' named after the two psychologists who formulated it (Figure 1.1).[18] They proposed that at any given moment in time, individuals are receiving and transmitting information from four distinct sources: the 'open self', where both transmitter and receiver consciously share information; the 'hidden self', where the transmitter attempts to communicate around issues or agendas of which the receiver is unaware; the 'blind self', where the transmitter is sending verbal or non-verbal signals without being consciously aware of them; and the 'unknown self', from which signals are being sent and received without the conscious awareness of either party.

Mehrabian's classic study[19] suggests that over 90% of the emotional meaning of an interaction between any two people is carried non-verbally (by body language, tone of voice, etc.). The hypnosis literature is explicit in its use of conscious-subconscious communication which has an established role in clinical psychology (see Chapters 2–4 and 23). We explicitly discuss suggestibility in influencing subconscious responses—in particular, how this increases with mounting stress, be this of patients, anaesthetists themselves, or their colleagues.

The practical import of this concept for anaesthetists is to emphasize that when two people such as an anaesthetist and a patient interact, communication is naturally occurring at several levels—verbal and non-verbal, explicit and implicit, and that all levels of communication are amenable to influence both positive and negative. Influential communication can be learned, used therapeutically, and readily taught to most people, including most anaesthetists.

A number of the communication paradigms discussed in this book may appear unfamiliar, yet they are evidence-based and have structures which can be learned and taught. It is hoped this approach will provide anaesthetists with a range of strategies to deal successfully with challenges in practice that were previously deemed almost impossible to overcome.

Communication skills training in anaesthesia

Anaesthetists are taught vast amounts on the molecular structure of drugs and the physical principles of the equipment they use, but few will have had any training on how to talk to a distressed patient, deal with an angry surgeon or a frightened child. Nevertheless, these are scenarios which confront anaesthetists daily.

Although much has been written about communication and doctors in general, there are almost no writings on useful communication skills of relevance to the anaesthetist in their various roles within and outside the theatre environment. Training in communication seeks to address these issues.

Current communication skills training is explicitly emphasized by the anaesthesia colleges in the UK, USA, and Australia. The CanMEDS model[20] proposes some key communication competencies such as: gaining rapport and trust; eliciting relevant information; conveying relevant information and explanations; developing a common understanding with patients and families, colleagues, and other professionals; and conveying effective oral and written information about a medical encounter.

Similarly, key communication evidence-based strategies have been advocated by the Calgary–Cambridge group in the context of the medical consultation.[16] Although some of these are of relevance and value to anaesthetists particularly in the context of the Pre-Anaesthetic Clinic, there are many areas of anaesthetic practice that require supplemental approaches. The acute contexts of much of anaesthetic practice means that other strategies must be considered.

Much of the knowledge required for anaesthetic practice—drug doses, physiological mechanisms—is taught explicitly. Such teaching is readily implemented, accessible to conscious awareness and quantifiable and therefore easily translated into evidence-based guidelines. The intuitive nature of many of the professional skills required of a consultant anaesthetist has led to the erroneous belief that they cannot be taught explicitly. Indeed, most teaching of such skills relies on the subconscious learning obtained through the modelling of mentors or peers.

Being aware of the subconscious aspects of our lives facilitates an engagement in moment-to-moment self-monitoring that brings into conscious awareness personal knowledge and deeply held values that are usually 'below the radar'.[21] These aspects of anaesthetic care are receiving increasing attention and are being recognized as an essential component of patient care.[22]

There is a wealth of knowledge from the fields of psychology, neuroscience, safety, and human factors that can enable us to better understand how we communicate, especially in the time-pressured stressful environment of the operating theatre. This information has been slow to percolate into anaesthetic practice. A survey of delegates at a neuroanaesthesia conference showed that 89% claimed to have had no formal training to improve their communication skills in either their undergraduate or postgraduate training, and that 82% felt such training should be mandatory.[23] While there are now abundant data suggesting healthcare workers enjoy communication skills training[24] and feel it beneficially changes their practice,[25] (corresponding to Kirkpatrick levels[26] I and II, respectively) data linking specific communication techniques to a reduction in adverse patient outcomes (Kirkpatrick level IV) remain elusive. This is noteworthy given how often 'poor communication' is quoted as a major, if not *the* major, contributor to clinical adverse events (see earlier). So, for the time being, in terms of the technical aspects of patient safety, communication skills training resides more within the province of medical philosophy than in medical science.

Addressing patient needs

Communication is maximally effective when it is seen as a tool directed to the patient's needs as well as to those of the anaesthetist. The consultation model proposed by Tate is useful here[27] (see Figure 1.2). It is based on the assumption that patients and doctors bring quite different agendas to any consultation.

These agendas may not align and may even conflict. For instance, the anaesthetist's first priority may be to gather information and collect facts, with the sharing of understanding further down the agenda. The patient, on the other hand, may be concerned with hopes, fears, and hidden or perceived problems, with the exact detail of previous anaesthetic issues being of lesser importance.

It is useful to keep in mind the goals of the patient–anaesthetist encounter. The first two of these goals are usually foremost in every patient–anaesthetist interaction: viz. to ensure that patient *safety* is maximized; and to optimize patient *comfort* before, during, and after the procedure. The third goal is often neither recognized nor considered a priority—to allow the patient *to feel a sense of control* in, what is frequently for them, an out-of-control situation where they become dependent on the anaesthetist's

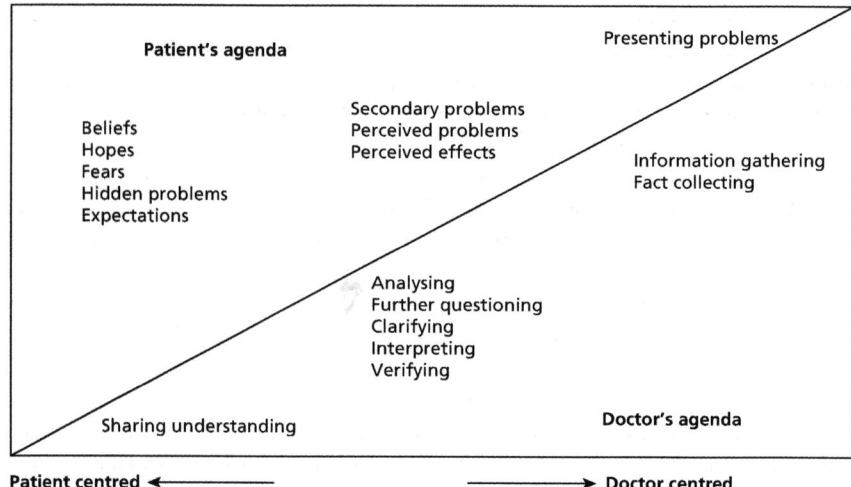

Fig. 1.2 A power-shift model of the consultation. Copyright © 1997 From *The Doctor's Communication Handbook*, Second Edition, by P. Tate, Abingdon: Radcliffe Medical Press. Reproduced by permission of Taylor and Francis Group, LLC, a division of Informa Plc.

skill and care. Patients frequently consider themselves victims of their illness or help-less in the face of incomprehensible technology.[28] The way in which anaesthetists com-municate can change the patient's perception from being a passive bystander, to being allowed to participate in that care. This can be empowering for both parties. The final goal to consider is how to respect the choices available to both patient and anaesthe-tist in any particular context. Exactly which path is optimal will not only depend on the patient's wishes but also the anaesthetist's level of comfort and skill for any par-ticular path.

A 'one size fits all' approach to communication is frequently inappropriate as communication must be tailored to the individual needs and responses of the pa-tient. For example, in some situations good communication will be facilitated by frequent eye contact, while in others it may be optimized by avoiding any eye con-tact whatsoever.

Although communication must be individualized, there are generic patterns and tools such as utilization, reframing, and the use of suggestion. There is a growing body of evidence supporting the view that *the how* and *the way* anaesthetists communicate can affect patient experience and be therapeutic in its own right.[29]

Some communication tools—'LAURS' and 'GREAT'—are detailed in Chapter 2. They function as a framework from which an individualized approach can be generated.

What can anaesthetists learn about communication from other disciplines?

Social psychology tells us that clinicians will influence patients whether communica-tions are verbalized or not. How this occurs will depend on how the interaction takes place, its context, the patients' perceptions, and past experiences. Advances in commu-nication reflect the influence of the positive psychology movement as researched by Seligman.[30] This concept is a focus on what the patient does well without overempha-sizing their difficulties. Noticing and amplifying what is right with the patient, rather than what is wrong, is an approach that is unfamiliar to many anaesthetists.

Recent efforts in understanding the neurobiology underpinning nocebo hyperalgesia and placebo analgesia emphasize the importance of expectation in affecting patient behavioural and perceptual responses. Indeed, expectation may be the driver for pla-cebo and nocebo in equal measure.[31] Current clinical research evidence suggests that warning a patient of a perceptual experience using language with negative emotional content, such as '*This will hurt!*' or sympathizing in a way that refers to negative experi-ences, is unhelpful[32] (see Chapter 3).

The patient's state of consciousness will determine the type of communication that is likely to be most effective or therapeutic. During the conduct of general anaesthesia, the states of consciousness can be categorized for the purpose of this discussion as three states. The conscious and unconscious states are familiar to all anaesthetists, rea-sonably well understood, and usually easily recognizable. Anaesthetists are the experts in managing the unconscious state of patients when in a coma or under general anaesthesia. However, it is frequently unappreciated that many patients in an 'unconscious' state will be fluctuating between an unconscious state and a third state of conscious awareness—the subconscious state. This is further elaborated in Chapters 2, 4, and 23.[33]

Amongst the general public, at least until a few years ago, doctors were, and still are to a degree, seen as the equivalent of the magicians and sorcerers of old. They have access to, and knowledge of, wondrous potions and magical procedures that cure leukaemia, infection, treat injuries, relieve pain, treat diabetes, and effectively contain chronic disease.

For doctors, however, anaesthetists are the magicians and sorcerers of today. They enable even the most debilitated patients to survive their surgical procedures. They place intravenous access or central lines when all others have failed. They 'miraculously' manage preoperative anxiety, relieve postoperative pain, have a detailed understanding of the mysterious anaesthetic machine, and somehow effectively manage any deviation from normal physiology. Such intricacies of anaesthetic clinical practice are but some of a range of complexities that few non-anaesthetic peers, and even fewer patients, understand. However, true mastery is demonstrated not only through technical prowess but through the effectiveness of anaesthetic communications with patients and colleagues.

Summary

The more that is learned about 'useful communication' the more it is realized that there are common specific processes involved that have structure, can be readily understood, and therefore can be taught. Problem areas that regularly occur in communication, and which require to be recognized and addressed include:

- alternative viewpoints, perceptions, misinformation and misperceptions;
- individual anxieties and concerns;
- variation in response to direction (being told what to do);
- the issue of control is critical for many patients and colleagues;
- the anaesthetist is in a unique and powerful position and must recognize at all times the patient's vulnerability.

Possible solutions that facilitate problem resolution include:

- recognizing that the way anaesthetists communicate will inevitably change perceptions, feelings, and behaviour of patients, colleagues, and ourselves;
- increasing or allowing patients some control over what is happening to them is essential if anxiety is not to escalate;
- a cooperative relationship should be engendered wherever possible.

A power struggle between the anaesthetist, patients, and other colleagues, be they nurses or surgeons, should be avoided at all costs as this is invariably counterproductive.

Key points

1. Reflective listening and observing are key aspects of a patient-centred approach to communication relevant to anaesthetists.

2. Good communication brings considerable benefits to all concerned.

3. A common theme within communication models is the idea that there are both conscious (explicit) and subconscious (implicit) aspects. This implies that communication is occurring at multiple levels of conscious awareness.

4. Anaesthetists and patients may bring very different expectations and agendas to their encounters.

5. The nature of anaesthesia means that patients may be in varying states of consciousness. This will determine the type of communication most likely to be therapeutic.

References

1. Smith AF, Shelly MP (1999). Communication skills for anesthesiologists. *Can J Anaesth*, **46**(11), 1082–8.

2. Elks KN, Riley RH (2009). A survey of anaesthetists' perspectives of communication in the operating suite. *Anaesth Intensive Care*, **37**(1), 108–11.

3. Babitu UQ, Cyna AM (2010). Patients' understanding of technical terms used during the pre-anaesthetic consultation. *Anaesth Intensive Care*, **38**(2), 349–53.

4. Levinson W, Chaumeton N (1999). Communication between surgeons and patients in routine office visits. *Surgery*, **125**(2), 127–34.

5. Smith AF, Pope C, Goodwin D, Mort M (2005). Communication between anesthesiologists, patients and the anesthesia team: a descriptive study of induction and emergence. *Can J Anesth*, **52**(9), 915–20.

6. Walker LA (2014). Findings into the death of Sukanya Thurairajah. Coroner's Court of the ACT. Available at: https://courts.act.gov.au/__data/assets/pdf_file/0003/961824/thurairajah_.pdf (Accessed 4 July 2023)

7. Paul M, Dueck M, Kampe S, Petzke F, Ladra A (2003). Intracranial placement of a nasotracheal tube after transnasal trans-sphenoidal surgery. *Br J Anaesth*, **91**(4), 601–4.

8. Evening Standard (UK) (2012). Doctor's smoking jibe wins mother £44,000 payout. Available at:https://www.standard.co.uk/hp/front/doctor-s-smoking-jibe-wins-mother-ps44-000-payout-7220778.html (Accessed 15 April 2024).

9. Ong LML, deHaes CJM, Hoos AM, Lammes FB (1995). Doctor–patient communication: a review of the literature. *Soc Sci Med*, **40**(7), 903–18.

10. Stewart MA (1995). Effective physician–patient communication and health outcomes: a review. *Can Med Assoc J*, **152**(9), 1423–33.

11. Egbert LD, Battit GE, Welch CE, Bartlett MK (1964). Reduction of postoperative pain by encouragement and instruction of patients—a study of doctor-patient rapport. *N Engl J Med*, **270**, 825–7.

12. Anderson EA (1987). Preoperative preparation for cardiac surgery facilitates recovery, reduces psychological distress and reduces the incidence of acute postoperative hypertension. *J Cons Clin Psychology*, **55**(4), 513–20.

13. Harms C, Young JR, Amsler F, Zettler C, Scheidegger D, Kindler CH (2004). Improving anaesthetists' communication skills. *Anaesthesia*, **59**(2), 166–72.

14. McCombe K, Bogod D (2020). Learning from the law. A review of 21 years of litigation for nerve injury following central neuraxial blockade in obstetrics. *Anaesthesia*, **75**(4), 541–8.

15. Craig RT, Muller HL (2007). *Theorizing communication: readings across traditions*. Los Angeles, CA: Sage Publications Inc.

16. Kurtz S, Silverman J, Benson J, Draper J (2003). Marrying content and process in clinical method teaching: enhancing the Calgary–Cambridge guides. *Acad Med*, **78**(8), 802–9.

17. AHRQ (no date). Available at: http://teamstepps.ahrq.gov/ (Accessed 23 February 2023).

18. Luft J, Ingham H. (1955). The Johari window, a graphic model of interpersonal awareness. *Proceedings of the Western training laboratory in group development*. Los Angeles: UCLA.

19. Mehrabian A, Ferris SR (1967). Inference of attitudes from nonverbal communication in two channels. *J Cons Psychology*, **31**(3), 248–58.

20. Frank JR (2005). *The CanMEDS 2005 physician competency framework. Better standards. Better physicians. Better care.* Ottawa: Royal College of Physicians and Surgeons of Canada.

21. Epstein RM (1999). Mindful practice. *J Am Med Assoc*, **282**(9), 833–9.

22. Kumar M, Chalwa R (2018). Communication skills and anaesthsiologists—editorial. *Anaesth Essays Res*, **7**(2), 145–6.

23. Kumar A, Sokhal N, Aggarwal R, et al. (2021). Communication skills training through 'role-play' in an acute critical care course. *Natl Med J India*, **34**(2), 92–4.

24. Salgaonkar SV, Kulkarni AD, Chapane SP (2021). Assessment of communication skill during process of preoperative visit and informed consent by anesthesiology residents. *J Anesthesiol Clin Pharm*, **37**(4), 548–53.

25. Kirkpatrick J, Kirkpatrick WK (2021) An introduction to the New World Kirkpatrick Model. Available at: https://www.cpedv.org/sites/main/files/file-attachments/introduction_to_the_kirkpatrick_new_world_model_-eval_002.pdf (Accessed 1 January, 2023).

26. Hool A, Smith AF (2009). Communication between anaesthesiologists and patients: how are we doing it now and how can we improve? *Curr Opin Anaesthesiol*, **22**(3), 431–5.

27. Tate P (1997). *The doctor's communication handbook*. Abingdon: Radcliffe Medical Press, 2nd edition.

28. Bejenke CJ (1996). Painful medical procedures. In: Barber J (ed). *Hypnosis and suggestion in the treatment of pain: a clinical guide*, pp. 209–61. London: WW Norton.

29. Lang EV, Hatsiopoulou O, Koch T, et al. (2005). Can words hurt? Patient-provider interactions during invasive procedures. *Pain*, **114**(1–2), 303–9.

30. Seligman M, Csikszentmihalyi M (2000). Positive psychology: an introduction. *Am Psychol*, **55**(1), 5–14.

31. Colloca L, Sigaudo M, Benedetti F (2008). The role of learning in nocebo and placebo effects. *Pain*, **136**(1–2), 211–18.

32. Varelmann D, Pancaro C, Cappiello EC, Camman WR (2010). Nocebo-induced hyperalgesia during local anesthetic injection. *Anesth Analg*, **110**(3), 868–70.

33. Slater P, Van-Manen A, Cyna AM (2024). Clinical hypnosis and the anaesthetist: a practical approach. BJA Educ, **24**(4), 121–8.

Chapter 2

Structures

Allan M. Cyna, Marion I. Andrew,
and Suyin G.M. Tan

'Too often we underestimate the power of a touch,
a smile, a kind word, a listening ear ...'
Leo Buscaglia, Love (1972)

What this chapter is about

Communication concepts of relevance to the practice of anaesthesia

Anaesthetic culture tends to view patients as physiological specimens to which pharmacological and technical procedures are applied and utilized to optimize various measurable parameters. However, this aspect is only one small part of a patient's anaesthetic care.

The medical model to which many anaesthetists still cling is very much a paternalistic one. Although terms such as patient 'autonomy' and 'choice' are frequently used, achieving these laudable aims in clinical practice remains elusive. Promoting patient autonomy and fostering a therapeutic relationship are areas of practice that have traditionally not been of direct concern to anaesthetists. The communication skills required to achieve this are centred on listening to what patients are really saying, and accepting the patients' alternative, but sometimes radically different, view of the world. In addition, anaesthetists can use their understanding of this alternative view to communicate in a way that is likely to engender cooperation and trust. Language affects our patients, our colleagues, and our own perceptions with profound implications in the practice of anaesthesia.

The anatomy of communication

Dissecting the anatomy of communication begins with a message between two or more people. This message can take many forms—for example, as a request for assistance or information, a command, advice, clarification, addressing a concern or the provision of reassurance (see Chapter 1). The message, superficially, is contained only in words.[1] However, the meaning of the communication carried in the message is invariably far more complex. Spoken words are accompanied by pitch, volume, and intonation, facial expression, and body posture. For example, take the six words 'He anaesthetized that patient last Tuesday'. Box 2.1 shows six different meanings of this sentence. Each one is dependent on just one change in emphasis.

This demonstrates that with just one small change of emphasis on one word the entire meaning of the phrase can change. One can begin to imagine how many hundreds of pieces of information—probably thousands—are being conveyed implicitly in any one interpersonal interaction or communication. It is, of course, impossible to dissect each nuance, but we can begin to understand some aspects of language and non-verbal cues in a way that will help ensure the accuracy of our communications.

Box 2.1 Words and their meaning

'**He** anaesthetized that patient last Tuesday.'

i.e. He, not one of the other registrars, anaesthetized the patient.

'He **anaesthetized** that patient last Tuesday.'

i.e. He anaesthetized the patient rather than just using sedation.

'He anaesthetized **that** patient last Tuesday.'

i.e. Definitely that patient, rather than another patient.

'He anaesthetized that **patient** last Tuesday?'

i.e. The person is unsure whether he anaesthetized that patient, or another one.

'He anaesthetized that patient **last** Tuesday.'

i.e. He anaesthetized that patient last Tuesday, and not the Tuesday 3 weeks ago.

'He anaesthetized that patient last **Tuesday**?'

i.e. He anaesthetized that patient last Tuesday, and not last Wednesday.

Conscious (explicit) and subconscious (tacit) communication

As anaesthetists we are familiar with the terms 'implicit', 'tacit' and 'explicit'. These terms are usually used in discussions concerning memory or awareness. In the context of this and several other chapters, explicit communications are interpreted consciously, while implicit or tacit aspects of communication are interpreted subconsciously. No matter how conscious the message appears to be, there are always subconscious components which have the potential to influence meaning and function as a suggestion.[2] Usually, the content or intent of the communication is obvious—for example, '*Pass me the bougie*'. Although this statement seems a simple request, the implicit message may be that the anaesthetist is experiencing a degree of difficulty which may be recognized by an experienced skilled assistant yet go completely unnoticed by other members of the theatre team. All statements will contain additional, complex meanings and, when listened to carefully, can provide valuable insights that facilitate useful responses.

The tone, pitch, volume, pacing and body language all combine to give information regarding the person's cognitive and emotional state, indicating their confidence, comfort, sense of well-being, pain, fear, guilt, depression, or anxiety. In short, paraphrasing the song, '*It's not* (only) *what you say it's the way that you say it!*' and the implicit intent of the words used that largely determines how they are perceived by the listener. The way we communicate will inevitably change perceptions, feelings, and behaviour of patients, our colleagues, and ourselves.

Human interaction: the patient and anaesthetist

As much of the anaesthetist's interaction with patients is when they are unconscious, a paternalistic model of care is, to some extent, inevitable. The anaesthetist is then in loco parentis, for the patient. The anaesthetist's responsibility for the safety of the patient, conscious or unconscious, is always present. However, the authoritative model of the paternalistic role, while necessary at times, has the potential to erode the patient's perception of control, and limits the therapeutic opportunities available to both parties.

In the management of emergency and complex intraoperative situations, subconscious processes may kick in, resulting in the anaesthetist dissociating from the patient as a fellow human being. Anaesthetists do not choose consciously to dehumanize patients. This state of mind serves as a protective mechanism to maintain an emotional distance that allows the clinician to function optimally in technically difficult and emergency situations (see Chapter 5). Examples of dehumanizing language are when we think of the patient as a procedure—for example, '*a difficult intubation*', an extension of our anaesthetic equipment such as, '*connect him to the drip*' or the body as a container, '*fill him up with fluids*'. This representation of a person as object may appear dehumanizing and is not exclusive to anaesthetists. However, understanding why some dehumanizing behaviours occur allows us to recognize how it might inadvertently creep into everyday practice. Recognition allows insight, preventing or limiting objectification of the patient, and minimizing misunderstandings and offence which may lead to patient complaint. This recognition also facilitates re-engaging with the patient as a person as soon as possible after such mechanisms are no longer required.

Similarly, highly technical language can be off-putting to some patients and is likely to promote miscommunication and, in some contexts, can adversely affect patient safety.[4]

Patient rapport and advocacy

Trust is the foundation of any doctor-patient relationship. Enhancing rapport is one way of building trust in our clinical interactions.[5] Trust develops when a commonality of purpose is communicated: being as the person with whom one is talking.

Rapport in anaesthesia is the harmonious relationship engendered between anaesthetist and patient in establishing a common goal. The development of patient rapport will inevitably facilitate all other anaesthetic interactions. We all have our own mechanisms of establishing rapport, such as the use of humour, authority, confidence, and empathy. A fundamental theme and strategy running throughout the book is the importance of listening to those with whom we are interacting, be they patient or colleague. Rapport allows patients to develop confidence in the anaesthetist's abilities and, conversely, facilitates developing the anaesthetist's confidence in patients' abilities to cooperate and assist with their care.

Many patients have the skills to cope with potentially painful or distressing surgical procedures. They may feel out of control and fail to realize they have psychological resources that have been useful and readily available to them in other aspects of their lives. These could be utilized successfully in the anaesthetic context. For example, there's the patient who is frightened of pain after surgery yet has previously fractured a fibula during a rugby match or while skiing without any pharmacological pain relief for a period of time after the injury.

Patient autonomy and the perception of control

The first step in enhancing autonomy is to give patients a perception of control. Whether this be real or imagined is immaterial. An example of how to do this is to ask the patient for permission prior to examining them.

'Is it okay to examine your back?'

There is a fine balance between recognizing and respecting a patient's autonomy and fulfilling our ethical duty to care for them in the most effective and safest manner possible.

Our perception of the risks and benefits may be radically different from that of the patient (see Chapter 7). It is our acceptance of the patient's alternative reality that enables us to communicate in a way that maximizes the patient's understanding of the issues and enables a solution to be found.

Accepting different realities

We experience the world in our own individual way through different perceptual filters depending on context. We often assume that everybody sees what we see, values what we value, and believes as true what we believe is so. Nevertheless, there are an infinite number of realities and truths.[3] Contrary to the saying; 'Seeing is believing', the concept of realities being discussed in many of the chapters is one of 'Believing is seeing'. This concept becomes obvious when one shows the needle-phobic patient a 24G neonatal intravenous (IV) cannula. If the first premise were true, the patient would not subsequently describe the cannula as a 'molten hot poker piercing their body', a 'knitting needle', or a 'horse needle' (see Chapter 15).

For the purposes of improving and teaching anaesthetic communication skills, just three realities need to be considered. The first reality is that of the anaesthetist (the listener, i.e. the person whose goal it is to communicate therapeutically). The second reality is that of the other person, be it patient or colleague, with whom the anaesthetist is communicating. This reality may or may not overlap (see the aforementioned needle-phobic example) to a variable degree with the first, dependent on topic and context.

For example, during IV cannulation:

1st Reality—Anaesthetist: 'Just a little sting with a needle.'
2nd Reality—Patient (hiding and going along with the anaesthetist's reality of a sting): 'Is it going to hurt?'
Or
1st Reality—Anaesthetist: 'Is it okay to finish positioning your drip' (avoids antici-patory anxiety that is induced when communicating the start of a procedure by focusing on the procedure being completed) 'so we ensure your safety by keeping you rehydrated and comfortable?' The therapeutic meaning of drip placement as comfort and safety as a possible reality is stated rather than a perception of what it might feel like.
2nd Reality—Patient: 'Is it going to hurt?'
Anaesthetist: 'Each patient experiences things differently, some tell me it hurts (validating and accepting the patient's concern as real), but most patients are sur-prised to discover it to be a lot easier than they thought. One thing I can tell you with certainty is that you will feel what you feel!'

Finally, there is a third reality that encompasses an infinite number of alternative ways of communicating. This reality is useful to appreciate when you hear yourself thinking, 'I've tried everything'. It is always available, even when there seems no other choice to consider during an interaction between two individuals or groups. This concept implies that there is a wavelength at which communication could successfully take place, it just hasn't been found yet.

This third reality can be thought of as a collective subconscious that is available to us when it is recognized as a possibility. In practice, the third reality comes in to play when we have a challenging patient where it is believed everything has been tried and the clinician is at a loss as to what to do next or how to move forward in a thera-peutic way. If one then thinks of the third reality when confronted with a challenging situation, interesting and surprising thoughts come to the clinician's mind that can then be used therapeutically.

For example, a 21-year-old patient with chronic pain was referred following being under the care of the chronic pain team, several psychologists, and psychiatrists over a 4-year period. She walked in dishevelled, crying, unable to speak above a whisper, barefoot, with loose shorts and a cold compress on her face. The clinician didn't know where to start and referred to the third reality. Some interesting thoughts came to mind. Firstly, the patient turned up for her appointment and, she had arrived on time! This recognition allowed the clinician to welcome the patient and communicate how this fact showed how determined she was to start feeling better having overcome numerous difficulties and challenges getting to the appointment on time. It could be also suggested indirectly that, *'patients who show such determination are usually more than halfway to achieving their therapeutic goals'.*

When less is more

Physical examination is usually performed more easily from both the clinician's and patient's perspective when conducted formally.[4] In an observational study investigating how doctors get consent for examination, when the doctor turned away and became occupied elsewhere while the patient was getting ready, there were both fewer difficulties in terms of patient cooperation and less embarrassment than when the doctor maintained verbal and visual contact with the patient and engaged in small talk. It was concluded that the doctor's behaviour was crucial, in this context, to patient rapport and that good practice depends on both non-verbal and verbal skills.

Patient advocacy

Patient advocacy is a core role of all doctors and other healthcare workers. The most effective form of advocacy is when patients are empowered to be their own advocate. Unlike a medication or technical intervention that tends to disempower patients, effective communication can generate a sense of mastery over what is happening to them.

When patients are rendered unconscious, there is an implicit onus transferred to the anaesthetist to advocate for them temporarily. One sometimes hears the words, *'I am the patient advocate'*. Unfortunately, the implication here is that everybody else in the vicinity—usually theatre—is **not** the patient's advocate. This may impair team communication and achieve the opposite of what is intended.

Being a patient advocate requires the anaesthetist to establish rapport with the patient, have some understanding of their core values, wishes and concerns, and to act and behave *'below the radar'*. Paradoxically, an essential component of being a patient advocate is not drawing attention to the anaesthetist's advocacy and professionalism. The **'LAURS'** concept will facilitate understanding and working with both patients and the surgical team.[5]

The 'LAURS' of communication and a 'GREAT' way to structure an interaction

There are two major concepts used in many of the chapters that follow. The first of these can be used in part or whole, as a means of developing and maintaining rapport during an interaction—the 'LAURS' concept: Listening reflectively; Acceptance; Utilization; Reframing; Suggestion. The second of these concepts provides a learnable template that can be used to structure any interaction—the 'GREAT' template: Greeting; Rapport (using 'LAURS'); Expectations; Addressing concerns; Tacit agreement.

These acronyms provide a common structure and framework, both implicitly and explicitly, throughout the book in a whole range of interactions and contexts. Whether patients are 2 or 92, these underlying communication structures can be utilized to underpin any therapeutic interaction.

The 'LAURS' concept

The 'LAURS' concept uses a structured approach as an easy way to remember key concepts of effective therapeutic communication when our usual strategies or words are either not working or not coming to mind easily. The application of the 'LAURS' concept may occur as individual components or as a conceptual whole.[5]

The first part of the 'LAURS' concept is to *Listen*.[6–8] *The three essential steps to improving communication skills are:*

Step 1: Listen

Step 2: Listen

Step 3: Listen

Listening reflectively

The steps for effective listening:

- observe yourself and recognize your role as a listener;
- beware thinking about your response rather than listening to what is being said;
- resist the temptation to interrupt or second-guess what patients are thinking;
- recognize that silence can be useful to both clinicians and patients, and a pause does not always mean that patients have said all they want to say.

It is essential to, check-in to seek clarification regarding the anaesthetist's understanding of what patients mean, and the patient's understanding of what the anaesthetist means (see next).

As doctors, we are used to telling patients what we need them to do, rather than listening to them and responding to their needs. Listening to what patients or colleagues are saying involves more than hearing what one thinks has been said. Listening while observing is one of the most important aspects of communication. It consists of a series of observations—looking at the patient's demeanour and posture while noting tone, pace, volume, and pitch of the voice, as well as the words used. It is not just about being silent while the patient is talking.

There are four questions to ask when listening reflectively. First, did you hear what was said? Second, did you understand what was meant? Third, does the patient know that he/she has been heard? Finally, does the patient know he/she has been understood? A 'checking-in' process that allows for reflective listening takes seconds rather than minutes.

How not to listen:

> **Patient:** '*I don't want to feel anything during the caesarean.*'
> **Anaesthetist:** '*Look you'll be alright … there is nothing to worry about—you'll be fine.*'

Alternatively …

> **Patient:** '*I don't want to feel anything during the caesarean.*'
> **Anaesthetist:** '*Well, you may feel something.*'
> **Patient:** '*Will I feel any pain?*'
> **Anaesthetist:** '*I don't know! But what I do know is that* your *block is working beautifully so we are expecting you to be nice and comfortable but if anything bothers you, let me know.*'

Listening for content

This concept involves listening for the overall content on hearing the words used. For example, a woman came for elective caesarean section—for grade IV placenta praevia—with a list of demands, as she had desperately wanted 'natural childbirth'. Her demands included: '*I want three support people in the room during my operation*', having been told that it was hospital policy only to have one person in the operating theatre during a caesarean; '*I want the drapes down for the entire procedure*', having been told that this was not sterile and wouldn't be allowed for safety reasons. She wanted her partner '*to video the procedure and birth*' despite video being prohibited. These statements were interpreted by the anaesthetic registrar as having to meet these demands literally or else … !

Listening for meaning

How could these words be reconciled with hospital policy and safe clinical practice? The answer began by listening not only to the actual words but for the underlying meaning and wishes in terms of the patient's core values. Patients frequently express underlying wishes as demands to be met, in an attempt to establish some sense of control and choice over what is happening.

Listening and 'checking-in'

For this woman, the meaning of the various statements began to be understood by gaining patient rapport. The first step was accepting the importance to her of having any concerns and wishes addressed as fully as possible in the context of her and her baby's safety.

> '*I want three support people in the room during my operation.*'

When the woman was asked what the role of each person was, she said that she wanted her partner, to '*see the baby being born*', and her two best friends to be with her to '*provide support*' through the operation. These requests were addressed by asking, '*Would it be okay if one friend was with you for part of the operation and the other could take over at a time you decided was best for you?*' It transpired that the partner did not want to be in the operating room and the woman was informed that, '*he could still be there to see the baby being born*' as there was a glass partition where he could observe the baby's birth.

When asked why she wished the drapes to be down she replied that she wanted this in order '*to see the baby being born*'—a request that was easily addressed as this is standard practice and she was informed that as soon as the baby was about to be delivered, '*we will lower the drapes for you so that you can see the baby being born*'.

Finally, she was informed that as many still pictures as she liked could be taken by her partner or support person. There was no further mention of video. The vast majority of patients are willing to be flexible if they feel listened to and understood. Building rapport in this way and addressing even one request usually allows the patient to feel they have some control over what is happening.

The second part of the '*LAURS*' concept is to *Accept*.

Acceptance

Acceptance of another person's alternative reality is sometimes a difficult concept for anaesthetists to grasp. It is the concept of being open-minded and having a non-judgemental attitude towards other people. This can be a hard philosophical issue, especially if the patient's beliefs seem illogical or not in the patient's best interests. There is little point in arguing with patients logically if they are stressed or distressed, as their responses are primarily subconscious.

For example, patients with easily visible veins on the dorsum of the hands who have an 'irrational fear' that IV insertion will be '*like a molten sword piercing my skin*' and that they will experience excruciating pain when a 22G cannula is inserted. Acceptance of alternative realities is a fundamental prerequisite for communicating effectively and is a core communication skill when attempting to gain patient rapport. In this example, the anaesthetist might be tempted to dismiss the patient's concern by saying something like, '*Don't worry, you'll be fine*', or, '*There is nothing to worry about—it's only a little needle*'. Such statements are unhelpful as there is disparity between the anaesthetist's and the patient's perception of the experience. A statement of Acceptance might look like, '*Of course it seems like a molten sword. This is very common in patients suffering with needle phobia*'. For further details on how to manage such disparities, see Chapters 4, 10, 11, 15, and 23.

Engendering empathy is harder when there is discord between the differing realities of the patient and anaesthetist, or the surgeon and anaesthetist, as this frequently leads to miscommunication and conflict. Especially when there is a strong emotional attachment to a belief. Anger is usually a demand for recognition of emotions or views, and the patient or a colleague may be indirectly expressing that they do not feel listened to, or their viewpoint appreciated. When appropriate, venting of the patient's emotions can be encouraged. This involves accepting the emotion, be it crying or anger, in a non-judgemental way and utilizing it.

> '*It's okay to cry* (Acceptance and Utilization) ... *It's the body's way of allowing you to relax and feel more comfortable* (Utilization and Reframe) ... *Please feel free to cry until **you are** as **relaxed and comfortable*** (Suggestion) *as you can be for just now.*'

Anaesthetists may also need to recognize that their own anger or frustration or guilt may emerge as subconscious responses. Once recognized consciously, subconscious, knee-jerk responses can be interrupted. This pattern-break of one's own subconscious behaviour allows logical consideration of some other more useful communication strategy to optimize patient care.

A temporary acceptance of the patient's beliefs or emotions, no matter how strange they may appear, allows the anaesthetist to gain rapport and then move on to a situation that is more therapeutic for the patient. For example, a patient in established labour was shouting at the anaesthetist as he entered the room. She stated that there was no way she could sit up to allow epidural catheter placement for analgesia. The dialogue continued:

> **Woman:** '*I can't sit up. It's too painful!*'
> **Anaesthetist:** '*That's okay, you don't have to sit up during this contraction but in a moment when you are ready for the epidural to be placed as comfortably and as quickly as possible, you will find **you can do this.***'
> **Woman:** '*I can't, I can't, I can't!*'
> **Anaesthetist:** '*I know you can't just now* (Acceptance), *but during the next rest or the one after, you will find you can **sit up comfortably** (Suggestion) and **stay still** (Suggestion) without even thinking about it.*'

The anaesthetist acknowledges the reality of the patient's inability to sit still and, has utilized an alternative reality. That the patient can do more than she thinks she can in the very near future, within one or two contractions and without her necessarily appreciating consciously this future reality herself until she finds herself doing it (see also Chapter 10). In this way, the anaesthetist is able to engage with the patient in a more cooperative and constructive manner.

Another example is the patient who is severely distressed and expressing pain, despite having no obvious organic basis or diagnosis for being in pain. Unless the patient's reality of being in pain is accepted and believed as true, an opportunity is missed to engage with patients in a way that facilitates the treatment of their problem.

The third part of the '*LAURS*' concept is to *Utilize*.

Utilization

Our perceptions are frequently communicated in the form of sensory perceptual language, usually of the three main senses: visual; kinaesthetic; and auditory. Visual language incorporates phrases such as '*I'm not **looking** forward to my surgery*' or '*I **see** what you mean*'. Kinaesthetic phrases include '*It doesn't **feel** right*' or '*It's like a **weight*** *off my shoulders'*. Examples of auditory language are '*I **hear** what you say*' or '*That **sounds** clear to me*'. Gustatory or olfactory language is much less commonly utilized, such as in '*It leaves a bad **taste** in my mouth*' or '*It doesn't **smell** right*'.

Utilizing the patient's perceptual world is likely to increase rapport and allow the anaesthetist to reframe negative perceptions and experiences.

For example, a patient might say, '*I am not **looking** forward to the anaesthetic. I'm a bit worried I won't wake up*'. Rather than respond with a platitude such as, '*Of course you will wake up*' or '*It's very unlikely that will happen*', the anaesthetist can use the patient's perceptual language and reframe it into something useful such as, '*You may not be **looking forward** to the anaesthetic but perhaps you can **see yourself waking up** in recovery surprised that it was a little easier than you had thought*'.

Developing an ear for patients' or colleagues' preferred communication mode and style can lead to engagement with other people in a way that increases rapport and the chances of being heard and understood. Almost anything a patient or colleague says or does can be utilized therapeutically. The only limiting factor here is the anaesthetist's imagination—for example, when the anxious patient asks whether the anaesthetist will be in theatre there all the time or asks, '*How will you know if I'm asleep?*' These concerns can be dealt with by explaining all the different types of monitors in some detail and then utilizing the experience. For example,

> **Patient:** '*How will you **know** I'm okay?*'
> **Anaesthetist:** '*When you are in the operating room we will position a number of monitors to ensure you are as **safe and comfortable** as possible throughout the procedure, and for when you wake up in the recovery room. For instance, we will place some ECG stickers on your chest and a blood pressure cuff on your arm to monitor your heart, a pulse monitor on the finger to check the oxygen level in the blood. **Knowing** how closely you are being looked after **will help you relax**.'*

All patients have strengths and abilities, qualities, and experiences used effectively in other contexts such as at work, at school or playing sports, and these can be utilized to meet the challenge anaesthesia and surgery represent. If patients have had good or successful experiences while in hospital previously, these can be focused upon. For example, the patient who has managed to mobilize effectively on the day of previous similar surgery can be encouraged by saying that now the patient knows what to do for this success to be repeated.

The fourth part of the 'LAURS' concept is to **Reframe**.

Reframing

The reframe is a concept whereby a patient's concern that is generating a thought, perception, or behaviour that is unhelpful such as, anxiety—is reframed in a way that generates a thought, perception, or behaviour that is helpful or therapeutic, such as relaxation. If an anxious patient states that he is very stressed and that he doesn't want '*too many people*' in the operating room, the anaesthetist can reframe this concern by utilizing this perception. A reframe can be communicated that '*Every person in the operating room will have a job to do helping you feel as safe and comfortable as possible*'. Then, no matter how many people there are in the room, the patient can be reassured that there will be only enough people to do their job and no more.

The fifth part of the '*LAURS*' concept is to **Suggest**.

Suggestion

Suggestions are verbal or non-verbal communications that can lead to subconscious, non-volitional responses in mood, perception, or behaviour.[8,9] Patients and people generally are in large part subconscious beings. This is the basis of how the consumer society is targeted by the advertising industry. It is also the '*raison d'être*' for poetry, art, and prose.

At times, the ability of people to respond to communications in a subconscious way is termed suggestibility. Suggestibility increases when patients are highly anxious, distressed, or when in pain. It also increases in pregnancy[10] and is higher in the paediatric population.[11] We tend to focus on, and associate with, what is being suggested. This is highly relevant in the recovery room after surgery, when the patient is repeatedly asked for their pain scores. This encourages an association of the surgery with injury, rather than the healing process of recovery.[12] See also Chapters 3, 4, 8, and 23.

Positive expectancy can enhance the anaesthetic experience and is a highly relevant communication tool in the practice of anaesthesia. A positive suggestion is a communication that has the potential to elicit a positive therapeutic response. For example, '*Most people find it is more comfortable than they thought*' is an indirect positive suggestion to elicit the perception of comfort.

Negative suggestions and nocebo—see Chapters 3, 15, and 23.

Lang et al. have shown that the ubiquitous use of language with negative emotional content is likely to increase patients' anxiety, pain, and distress.[2,13] Negative suggestions have been recognized in the context of medicine in general, and anaesthesia in particular, as giving rise to nocebo effects.[2] See Chapters 3 and 23.

A 'GREAT' structure for an interaction

Many anaesthetists will already have implicit templates for many aspects of their clinical practice and almost universally these can be incorporated within or supplemented by 'GREAT'.[6]

Greeting

The 'greeting' confirms the identity of persons in the interaction. Introducing yourself is an opportunity to provide the patient with information on how those in the interaction would like to be addressed and build rapport. For example, '*What would you like me to call you?*' Some patients may say '*Just call me George*', others prefer more formality, '*Mr Sullivan is fine*'. Similarly, the clinician might prefer being called '*Dr ...*' or have the patient use their first name. This simple interaction can be the starting point of generating patient rapport by means of a *Yes set* (see Chapter 4). *'So it's okay if I call you George?'*

Some patients, if very nervous, may say, *'Just call me whatever you like'*. The doctor could then ask patients what their friends call them and if they respond with a name, the doctor can then ask, *'Is it okay if I call you that?'* This invariably generates another *'Yes'* with the implication of the interaction being that between friends.

Rapport

The 'How to' of developing rapport, whether it be with colleagues or patients can be greatly enhanced by using the '**LAURS**' concept. This concept can be used throughout the interaction as a means of maintaining and improving rapport. Although to communicate effectively does not necessarily require the people involved to like or respect each other, it does require listening and an acceptance of the other's reality, and recognizes that cooperation is required to achieve a common goal. Any therapeutic process or complex interaction can reasonably be seen as a journey in which there are 'potholes in the road'. A good relationship involving trust copes better with such obstacles, minimizes unnecessary delays, and can prevent complete derailment.

Expectations

If not already clarified during the greeting phase, expectations should be explicitly addressed at this stage. Following examination, explanation of management choices such as therapy or procedure recommendations can occur.

Addressing concerns

The issue here is to address matters both explicitly and implicitly while being aware of many patients' perception of a loss of control and vulnerability. It is during this stage that something highly relevant usually surfaces. For example, a patient in the pre-anaesthetic clinic having a minor procedure was asked after the informed consent process if he had any questions or concerns. He stated that he did have one concern that he didn't want to end up in the intensive care unit (ICU) again after his anaesthetic following his *'out of control sugars'* postoperatively. He had forgotten to mention he was an insulin-dependent diabetic.

Tacit agreement

The end of most interactions frequently involves a tacit agreement that a trusting relationship has been formed and an agreement reached on where to go from here. In recognition of the trust established, termination of the interview can be followed by thanking the patient.

Key points

1. Therapeutic communication involves common specific processes that have structure, can be readily understood, and therefore, taught.

2. 'LAURS' can facilitate the anaesthetist's communications, in ways that are likely to optimize patient care.

3. The anaesthetist is in a unique and powerful position and needs to recognize the patient's vulnerability.

4. Listening increases patient rapport, allows concerns to be responded to and helps prevent misinformation and misperceptions.

5. Integrating 'GREAT' and 'LAURS' in clinical interactions can allow patients to: cooperate more fully with their anaesthetic care; feel a sense of control; decrease anxiety; and increase patient autonomy.

References

1. Silverman J, Kurtz, S, Draper, J. (2013). *Skills for communicating with patients*. CRC Press.

2. Arrow K, Burgoyne LL, Cyna AM (2022). Implications of nocebo in anaesthesia care. *Anaesthesia*, **77 Suppl 1**, 11–20.

3. Krauss BS (2015). 'This may hurt': predictions in procedural disclosure may do harm. *BMJ (Clinical research ed)*, **350**, h649.

4. Heath C (1987). What is a good GP? *BMJ (Clinical research ed)*, **294**(6569), 415–16.

5. Cyna AM (2019). The LAURS of hypnotic communication and the 'lived in imagination' technique in medical practice. *Int J Clin Exp Hypn*, **67**(3), 247–61.

6. Cyna AM (2018). A GREAT interaction and the LAURS of communication in anesthesia. *Acta Anæsthesiologica Belgica*, **66**(3), 131–5.

7. Cyna AM, Simmons SW (2017). Enhancing communication in obstetric anaesthesia - listen, listen, listen. *Int J Obstet Anesth*, **32**, 87–8.

8. Cyna AM, Andrew MI, Tan SG (2009). Communication skills for the anaesthetist. *Anaesthesia*, **64**(6), 658–65.

9. Pulling BW, Braithwaite FA, Moseley GL, et al. (2022). Suggestions in hypnosis to aid pain education (SHAPE) in people with chronic low-back pain: a pilot feasibility randomized, controlled trial. *Int J Clin Exp Hypn*, **70**(3), 251–76.

10. Alexander B, Turnbull D, Cyna A (2009). The effect of pregnancy on hypnotizability. *Am J Clin Hypn*, **52**(1), 13–22.

11. Cyna AM, Hewson DW, Hardman JG (2023). Clinical hypnosis: implications in anaesthesia and perioperative care. *Br J Anaesth*, **130**(6), 647–50.

12. Chooi CS, White AM, Tan SG, Dowling K, Cyna AM (2013). Pain vs comfort scores after Caesarean section: a randomized trial. *Br J Anaesth*, **110**(5), 780–7.

13. Lang EV, Hatsiopoulou O, Koch T, et al. (2005). Can words hurt? Patient-provider interactions during invasive procedures. *Pain*, **114**(1–2), 303–9.

Chapter 3

How words hurt

Elvira V. Lang, Laura L. Burgoyne,
and Allan M. Cyna

'If you assume there is no hope, you guarantee there will
be no hope.'
Noam Chomsky

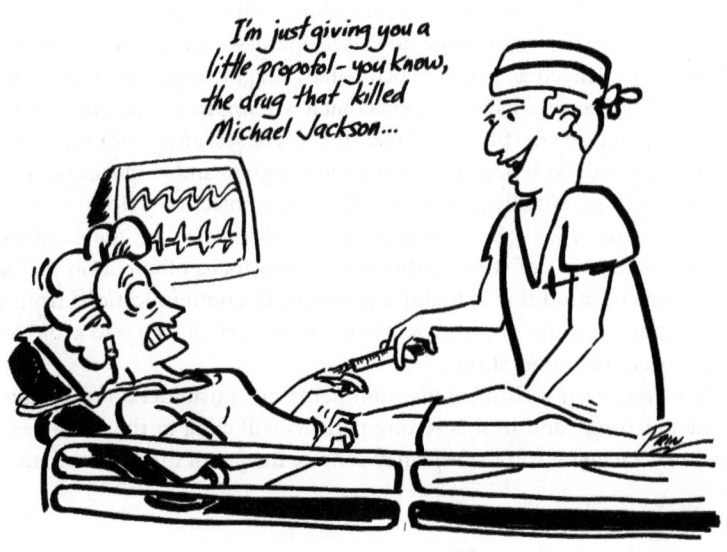

What this chapter is about

Negative suggestions and how to look out for them

Suggestions are statements that evoke an image in the listener's mind. They may be positive, conjuring up an image of peace and hope or a desirable mood and behaviour, or they may be negative, eliciting thoughts of pain and doom. Once mentioned, the suggestion is front and centre: '*You probably didn't think of an endotracheal tube before we mentioned it right now—even if we reminded you that there is absolutely no need to think of it.*'

When anaesthetists tell patients that a procedure such as intravenous or arterial line placement '*will hurt*', the communication itself increases the likelihood of this perception being experienced as pain.[1-3] Fortunately, suggestibility can also be used in a positive way[4]—for example, telling patients that it will improve their comfort to cough during IV cannulation[5] or practice breathing exercises after abdominal surgery.[6] Simply avoiding words with negative connotations significantly reduces pain and anxiety associated with potentially painful stimuli such as injection of local anaesthetic.[3,7]

Remaining factual, '*I will give you the local anaesthetic now*', or '*the numbing medicine*' will suffice. In times of stress, patients assume a focus of attention that leads to a hypnotic frame of mind that is highly suggestible to communications from the anaesthetist, whether negative or positive.[8] Hence an important step is to avoid words or phrases with negative connotations.

Often, however, even well-meaning comments are misunderstood. Many words have double meanings, and in this setting patients will cling to the more pessimistic interpretation.[9] '*I will put you to sleep*' may conjure images of the veterinarian euthanizing a pet.

Placebo and nocebo effects

The effects of suggestion are evident in the widely recognized phenomenon of placebo. Placebo analgesia occurs when the administration of a substance known to be inert produces an analgesic response if the subject is told it will make them comfortable. Interestingly, this type of suggestion-concordant response can also be analgesic, and when the suggestion elicits a negative response the phenomenon is called the nocebo effect.[10,11] Such effects following negative verbal or non-verbal cues lead to negative patient perceptions, mood (affect), or behaviour. For example, offering the patient a sick bowl (emesis basin) can result in the patient feeling nauseous or even vomiting. More than two-thirds of an unselected sample of 34 college students reported mild head-aches when told that a non-existent electric current was passing through their heads. Reports such as these are consistent with a view that clinical focusing on pain may in itself be a cause of pain.[12] Negative reactions to placebo medications (drugs without an active ingredient) are well documented, and similar responses can be induced in patients presenting for anaesthesia, where the use of negative language tends to increase patients' stress, negative expectations, and perceptions. For example, asking patients for pain scores may increase requests for analgesia postoperatively[13] and warning patients about pain can completely reverse the analgesic effect of local anaesthetic cream.[14] Several common 'language traps' have been examined with a view to formulating alternative ways to communicate with patients.[11,15]

For example, the side effects of propofol can be exaggerated if patients are advised during the injection that the propofol '*will sting*' or '*hurt*' during injection. Alternative communications could be that propofol gives, '*a warm or a cool feeling*' during its administration. Some anaesthetists suggest that propofol '*sparkles*' as it is injected—a sensation frequently appreciated by patients as pleasant. If one is concerned about describing the perception of propofol as positive, a more neutral alternative could be that it is: '*a powerful anaesthetic that may or may not be noticed as it begins to have an effect*'. Even more neutral could be '*I am starting the propofol now*', and leaving the patient the right to his or her own experience and description. Some anaesthetists may feel the need to warn everyone regarding injection pain despite the fact that the incidence is under 40%.[16] If the types of communications given prior to injection are not controlled for, it is likely that the very act of suggesting pain may have an effect on the results of research on this topic.[7]

Nocebo communication is also common during insertion of epidural catheters[17] and awareness and avoidance of such language is likely to improve the subjective experience for the patient.[3] In an obstetric study, patients were randomized to a reassuring placebo script, '*We are going to give you a local anaesthetic which will numb the area*' or a standard, nocebo script, '*You are going to feel a big bee sting; this is the worst part of the procedure*'. Patients who received the placebo script reported lower pain ratings during local anaesthetic injection.[3]

The underlying neurobiology and clinical effects of nocebo communications when interacting with patients has generated increasing interest in recent years.[11] A diagrammatic representation of the neurobiology of nocebo can be seen in Figure 3.1.

Tables 3.1 and 3.2 show examples of nocebo communications commonly used in hospital practice when interacting with patients and their possible therapeutic reframes.[11]

Minimizing and negating words

Minimizing words such as '*a bit*', '*a little*', '*tiny*', '*just*', or '*only*' do not mitigate the patient's response to negative suggestions. The image is already created in the mind, and modifiers do not displace its adverse effects. For example, '*Just a tiny **sting** that will only **hurt** for a bit*' already sets the stage for stinging and hurting.[7,18,19] Negating words like '*don't worry*' mean there is '*something to worry about!*' and usually fail to

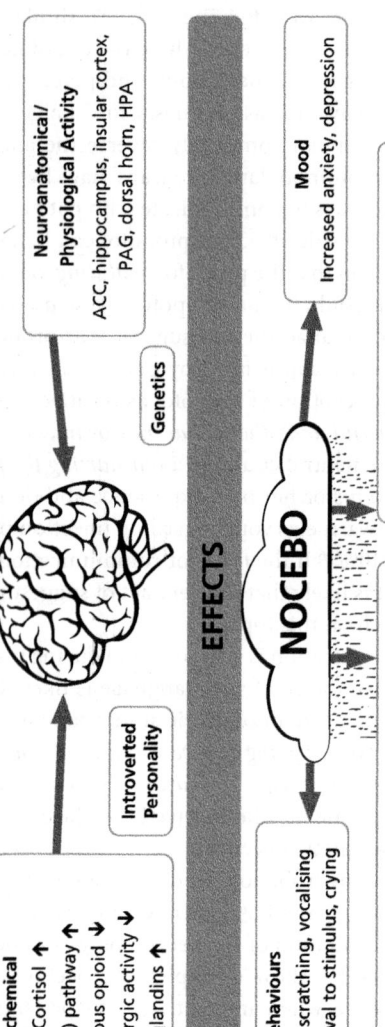

Fig. 3.1 Overview of the neurobiology of the nocebo effect. ACC, anterior cingulate cortex; ACTH, adrenocorticotrophic hormone; CCK, cholecystokinin; HPA, hypothalamic–pituitary–adrenal axis; PAG, peri-aqueductal grey; PFC, prefrontal cortex; PONV, postoperative nausea and vomiting.

Reproduced from Arrow K et al., 'Implications of nocebo in anaesthesia care', *Anaesthesia*, 77 Suppl 1, 11–20, with permission from Wiley. Copyright 2022, Association of Anaesthetists.

Table 3.1 Nocebo in anaesthesia and possible therapeutic reframe

Nocebo communication	Nocebo meaning	Therapeutic alternative	Therapeutic meaning
Prior to propofol *This may sting*	Suggests *sting*	*Propofol is a **powerful** anaesthetic*	Effective anaesthesia
Bee sting coming (prior to LA injection)	Suggests *bee sting*	*Let me know when it **feels comfortable***	Comfort is the goal
*This may/may not **hurt***	Suggests *hurt*	*You will feel what you feel* *You may or may not feel something*	Leaves the interpretation with the patient
*We'll give you some **painkillers** after surgery*	Suggests *postoperative pain* will occur and require medication	*If required, we'll give you some medication to help things **heal and recover** as **comfortably** as possible*	Medication is available to improve comfort if required to help with recovery
*Let me know if you feel **sick***	Suggests patient will be *sick*	*Most people find they can **eat and drink** as soon as they feel like it*	Suggests eating and drinking postoperatively
*I'm just inserting the epidural **needle**—you may feel some **pain***	Induces anticipatory anxiety	*Is it ok to **finish** your epidural to get you **comfortable** as **quickly** and **safely as possible**?*	Goal directs the mind to the end of the procedure focusing on comfort and safety
*There's nothing to **worry** about*	Suggests there is something to worry about!	*We're **here to help***	Therapeutic information
*This is **the worst** part, I am sorry*	Suggests there is something the anaesthetist needs to apologize for	*Most people find **this is** a little **easier** than they thought/anticipated*	Indirect suggestion for changing expectations to a more positive experience
*Don't be **frightened** of all the people in the operating room, it can be a bit **scary***	Be frightened and scared	*All the people in the room have a job to do helping keep you **safe** and **comfortable***	Suggests patient comfort and safety
*Epidural analgesia is the most effective form of **pain** relief when contractions get really **painful** as labour progresses*	It will be necessary to have an epidural to have the most effective pain relief	*As labour progresses contractions get stronger. **The stronger the contraction, the more effective** they are in getting you closer and **closer to seeing and holding your baby***	The meaning behind a contraction is goal focused—to see and hold the baby
Prior to giving sodium citrate before a caesarean *antacid tastes **disgusting/horrible/salty***	Suggests a negative perception	*This antacid will settle the stomach and allow for a **safer** anaesthetic*	Informs patient of the therapeutic goal—anaesthesia safety

Adapted from Arrow K et al., 'Implications of nocebo in anaesthesia care', *Anaesthesia*, **77 Suppl 1**, 11–20, with permission from Wiley. Copyright 2022, Association of Anaesthetists.

Table 3.2 Nocebo in anaesthesia suggesting death and possible therapeutic reframe

Nocebo communication	Nocebo meaning	Therapeutic alternative	Therapeutic meaning
In the context of anaesthesia induction. *Would you like to **kiss your child goodbye**?*	Suggests death	*We will **look after your child** and **you will see him /her soon***	Child will be returned safely
*One **final check***	Suggests death	*Just a **safety check** before we start*	Suggests goal is safety
*The anaesthetist will **put you to sleep***	Patients may have had a pet 'put to sleep'—suggests death	*The anaesthetist will **keep you safe and comfortable for when you wake up in recovery***	Implies patient will not wake up during surgery and will wake up at the end of surgery comfortably and safely
*We're just **putting you under***	Implies drowning	*You can **find yourself** waking up in the recovery room (PACU) soon*	Suggests recovery

PACU, post-anaesthetic care unit.

Reproduced from Arrow K et al., 'Implications of nocebo in anaesthesia care', *Anaesthesia*, **77 Suppl 1**, 11–20, with permission from Wiley. Copyright 2022, Association of Anaesthetists.

mitigate negative effects. Saying '*This won't hurt*' is double jeopardy. The suggestion in itself brings attention to hurting and, if it does hurt, the anaesthetist has lost credibility. Similarly, asking a patient '*Not to move*', rather than, '*Stay still like a statue*', will probably lead to a subconscious response *to move*.

Try—the failure word

'**Try**' is a word that anticipates failure. For example, '*Try to ignore the sound of the drill*' is likely to focus the patient's attention on the drill—just as being asked, '*Try not to think of an ampoule of propofol!*' (see also Chapters 4 and 22).

Therapeutic communication

Anaesthetists can provide positive meaning to interventions that patients may otherwise experience as uncomfortable. For example, therapeutic communications could be, '*This local anaesthetic will numb the skin*', rather than '*sting*', or '*The anaesthetist is there to ensure your comfort and safety during the surgery and until you wake up in recovery*' rather than '*… put you to sleep*'. This implies that comfort is one way to interpret a sensation. Similarly, patients are reassured that they will be anaesthetized throughout the procedure, and that they will wake up at the end! Alternatively, the anaesthetist could say, '*We will keep you under general anaesthesia for as long as is necessary, so that you can wake refreshed*', or '*Modern anaesthetics can allow us to tailor the* *effects to your needs'.* Such suggestions allow patients to experience procedures in a way that facilitates a neutral or positive behavioural response.[20] See also Tables 3.1 and 3.2.

Negative suggestions and the nocebo effect— case examples

Case study 1—negative suggestions have no effect?

An 8-year-old boy was asked in the pre-anaesthetic consultation two hours prior to surgery whether he wanted an intravenous (IV) or inhalational induction. His father stated that he should have the gas as this would help him vomit less. The boy insisted that he didn't want a mask and that he wanted *'the needle'* to go to sleep. The anaesthetist asked the parent whether it would be okay to go along with the boy's wishes, as there was no evidence that an IV induction would increase the risk of postoperative nausea and vomiting.

The father reluctantly agreed but stated to the boy, *'As long as you know that you **will vomit in recovery when you wake up**, if you have the needle'.* The boy had a smooth induction and an uneventful procedure but woke up in recovery crying and vomiting. His first words were, *'I should have listened to my dad!'* Children are more suggestible than adults, particularly when stressed.[21] Parents are powerful authority figures and this parent had made a powerful suggestion for the child to vomit in recovery.

Case study 2—negative suggestions have no effect?

A surgeon chatted with a 21-year-old patient during pre-oxygenation. He told the patient, who was scheduled for a circumcision, that it would *'hurt like hell in recovery'.* When questioned by the anaesthetist, the surgeon said, *'It always does hurt'.* Despite a penile nerve block and IV fentanyl, the patient woke up distressed, in pain, and needing a prolonged stay in recovery while an analgesia protocol regime was administered. Surgeons are powerful authority figures and there is a high response rate among patients to their expectations and suggestions. Over the last ten years the same surgeon started telling patients that they *'can wake up comfortably as the wound heals and everything gets better'.*

Case study 3—negative suggestions have no effect?

Antacid was administered prior to a caesarean section and the patient was instructed, *'You need to take this. It tastes disgusting and will probably make you feel sick'.* The woman hesitated for a moment and then drank the antacid only to grimace and exclaim, *'My god! That tastes disgusting!'* A few minutes later she vomited on the way to theatre. The patient used the same words as the anaesthetist, and the negative suggestion led to a negative experience and the behavioural response of vomiting.

An alternative communication could have been, *'We would like you to take this. It is an antacid which pleasantly coats the stomach and helps you stay safe if you need a sleeping anaesthetic'.*

The editors' anecdotal experience is that women who are told the purpose for the antacid, rather than a description of how bad it tastes, frequently make no comment on the taste. This is the subject of future research. If there are still any with doubts about the effects of negative suggestion, excerpts from a transcript of a taped recording of one of the author's (EV) colleagues injecting local anaesthetic prior to a procedure[19] illustrates the point most effectively.

Case study 4—negative suggestions have no effect?

The patient is draped and the doctor is about to inject local anaesthetic prior to large core breast biopsy.

Dr A: 'OK, you are going to feel a **pinch** and a lot of **burning** and **stinging**. This is a **pinch** ... a **pinch** ... okay? **Burning** and **stinging**. How are you doing? Doing okay? **Pinch** and **sting**. Do you feel that? More **stinging**.' **Patient:** 'I can still feel a needle in there.' **Dr A:** 'You feel a **needle** but do you feel any sharp pain?'
Patient: 'I am okay, I just feel a needle.'
Dr A: 'You feel a something moving but nothing **painful**, nothing **sharp** right?'
Patient: 'Oh ... I feel prickly ... Yeah.'
Dr A: 'What was that? **Sharp**? ... Sorry.'
Patient: 'That hurts!'
Dr A: '**Sorry.**'
[The doctor removes the needle].
Patient: 'That kills, it hurts, it hurts, it hurts.'
Dr A: 'There is nothing there.'
[The doctor places a gauze on the puncture site]
Dr A: 'Does it **sting**?'
Patient: 'It didn't sting before . . . weren't you doing it before? Wait, wait, wait. What did you just do? The last three times you injected me it didn't hurt. It stung a little but this time it feels like you are cutting the flesh out of my chest.'
Dr A: 'Sorry about that, is it **burning** now?'

(Case study 4 is reprinted with permission Lang EV (2009). Avoiding negative suggestions. In: Lang EV, Laser E (eds) *Patient sedation without medication*, pp. 56–63. Oxford: Trafford.)

The ethics of communication

It is just as inadvisable to say something '*will hurt*' as it is to say it '*will be comfortable*' when there is a possibility that it will be neither. The anaesthetist is left wondering what to say when the patient asks, '*Will this hurt?*'

Since the patient's response to stimulation cannot be known beforehand, there is no honest answer. If the anaesthetist responds by saying, '*It is quite variable. Some people experience discomfort, others tell me how surprised they are to feel more comfortable than they might have thought*' is entirely honest, with the added benefit of giving an indirect positive suggestion[20] (see Chapters 2 and 23). Similarly, if a patient asks, '*Will I have much pain after my operation?*' the anaesthetist can and should always respond honestly, and yet, wherever possible, avoid the use of negative suggestions. Adding a measure of control is also helpful. Thus, a response might be, '*The healing response is highly individual. Some patients may experience discomfort* (instead of '*pain*'), *while others are surprised that the sensation of the wound healing is more comforting than they had expected. If there should be some discomfort, there is no need to fight it, just admit it, and most importantly, let doctors know right away. You can have as much medication as you wish within the limits of safety, to recover as quickly and comfortably as possible*'.

Choosing the word *'discomfort'* rather than *'pain'* and reframing *'pain'* as *'a healing sensation'* changes the meaning of the sensation from one of disability, to one of recovery. Addressing the patient's concerns is always paramount and these need to be dealt with.

Note the use of the indirect suggestion *'some patients . . . '* This implies indirectly that the patient too may feel more comfortable than expected. There sometimes is concern regarding the ethics of not telling patients something will hurt when the anaesthetist thinks that it might. However, the best available evidence suggests that the patient's and the anaesthetist's expectations, in some part, determine the experience. Nocebo terms such as *'pain', 'tissue damage', 'surgical trauma',* and *'injury'* can be reframed to the therapeutic, placebo-enhanced meaningful experience of *'surgical success', 'healing',* and *'recovery'.* Such reframes have been shown to reduce requests for analgesia postoperatively.[11]

Anaesthetists are in the privileged position of influencing their patients' perceptions, moods, and behaviours in powerful and subtle ways. There is an increasing recognition that patients who believe they will get better tend to realize this prophecy, while the nocebo effect causes patients to feel worse. An understanding of how communications function as suggestions can minimize the sabotage and harm caused by negative language.[11,22] Reframing negative language in a way that leads to therapeutic, rather than nocebo effects is a valuable tool for the anaesthetist's armamentarium.[11]

Key points

1. Negative suggestions are ubiquitous in hospital practice in general, and in anaesthesia in particular.

2. There is now clear evidence from both observational and randomized controlled studies that negative suggestions increase pain perception and anxiety.

3. 'Try' is a failure word and should be used with caution.

4. Using positive language and suggestions can help generate positive outcomes.

5. Anaesthetists need to be aware of nocebo effects on outcomes such as pain, anxiety, and PONV.

Additional video content

Dr Elvira Lang has produced a great training video for her company Comfort Talk, that demonstrates how the use of words can affect communication (Video 3.1). Find this video and discover additional video content by searching for this book's title or ISBN (9780198858669) at academic.oup.com/oxford-medicine-online. If you would like access to the whole book, or are interested in accessing other titles, you can recommend it to your librarian.

References

1. Dutt-Gupta J, Bown T, Cyna AM (2007). Effect of communication on pain during intravenous cannulation: a randomized controlled trial. *Br J Anaesth*, **99**(6), 871–5.

2. Lang EV (2005). Response to Cyna and Andrew. *Pain*, **117**(1), 239–40.

3. Varelmann D, Pancaro C, Cappiello EC, Camann WR (2010). Nocebo-induced hyperalgesia during local anesthetic injection. *Anesth Analg*, **110**(3), 868–70.

4. Bjenke CJ (1996). Painful medical procedures. In: Barber J (ed.) *Hypnosis and suggestion in the treatment of pain; a clinical guide*, pp. 209–61. London: WW Norton.

5. Usichenko TI, Pavlovic D, Foellner S, Wendt M (2004). Reducing venipuncture pain by a cough trick: a randomized crossover volunteer study. *Anesth Analg*, **98**(2), 343–5.

6. Egbert LD (1986). Preoperative anxiety: the adult patient. *Int Anesthesiol Clin*, **24**(4), 17–37.

7. Lang EV, Hatsiopoulou O, Koch T, Berbaum K, Lutgendorf S, Kettenmann E, et al. (2005). Can words hurt? Patient-provider interactions during invasive procedures. *Pain*, **114**(1–2), 303–9.

8. Spiegel H (1963). Current Perspectives on Hypnosis in Obstetrics. *N Y State J Med*, **63**(Oct 15), 2933–41.

9. Ewin D, Eimer B (2006). *Ideomotor signals for rapid hypnoanalysis*. Springfield, IL: Charles C. Thomas Publishers.

10. Benedetti F, Lanotte M, Lopiano L, Colloca L (2007). When words are painful: unraveling the mechanisms of the nocebo effect. *Neuroscience*, **147**(2), 260–71.

11. Arrow K, Burgoyne LL, Cyna AM (2022). Implications of nocebo in anaesthesia care. *Anaesthesia*, 77 **Suppl 1**, 11–20.

12. Schweiger A, Parducci A (1981). Nocebo: the psychologic induction of pain. *Pavlov J Biol Sci*, **16**(3), 140–3.

13. Chooi CS, White AM, Tan SG, Dowling K, Cyna AM (2013). Pain vs comfort scores after Caesarean section: a randomized trial. *Br J Anaesth*, **110**(5), 780–7.

14. Aslaksen PM, Lyby PS (2015). Fear of pain potentiates nocebo hyperalgesia. *J Pain Res*, **8**, 703–10.

15. Schenk PW (2008). 'Just breathe normally': word choices that trigger nocebo responses in patients. *Am J Nurs*, **108**(3), 52–7.

16. Kam E, Abdul-Latif MS, McCluskey A (2004). Comparison of Propofol-Lipuro with propofol mixed with lidocaine 10 mg on propofol injection pain. *Anaesthesia*, **59**(12), 1167–9.

17. Sellors JE, Cyna AM, Simmons SW (2002). Aseptic precautions for inserting an epidural catheter: a survey of obstetric anaesthetists. *Anaesthesia*, **57**(6), 593–6.

18. Corydon Hammond D (1998). Formulating hypnotic and post-hypnotic suggestions. In: Corydon Hammond D (ed.) *Handbook of hypnotic suggestions and metaphors*, pp. 11–44. Chicago, IL: American Society of Clinical Hypnosis.

19. Lang EV (2009). Avoiding negative suggestions. In: Lang EV, Laser E (ed.) *Patient sedation without medication*, pp. 56–63. Bloomington, IN: Trafford.

20. Cyna AM, Andrew MI, Tan SG (2009). Communication skills for the anaesthetist. *Anaesthesia*, **64**(6), 658–65.

21. Olness K, Gardner GG (1978). Some guidelines for uses of hypnotherapy in pediatrics. *Pediatrics*, **62**(2), 228–33.

22. Lang EV, Benotsch EG, Fick LJ, et al. (2000). Adjunctive non-pharmacological analgesia for invasive medical procedures: a randomised trial. *Lancet*, **355**(9214), 1486–90.

Chapter 4

Language and the subconscious

Allan M. Cyna, Marion I. Andrew,
and Suyin G.M. Tan

'This chapter is so subconscious that you don't even
know that you know it!'
AMC, MIA, SGMT

What this chapter is about

Many of the communications commonly encountered in anaesthetic practice elicit subconscious responses, and thus they frequently go unrecognized.[1] This form of communication involves verbal and non-verbal cues (also known as suggestions) that can elicit automatic changes in perception or behaviour. Much of this chapter is about language structures that are known to elicit subconscious changes in perception, mood, or behaviour, both with patients and anaesthetists.[2] Recognizing subconscious responses facilitates communication. As is discussed later, anaesthetists can communicate with patients and colleagues in ways that utilize subconscious functioning. To all intents and purposes this looks like intuitive communication, which in fact, has structure and therefore can be learned and taught.

The conscious and the subconscious

The conscious and unconscious states are familiar to all anaesthetists. However, it is infrequently appreciated that all patients, whether in a conscious or unconscious state, will also be functioning subconsciously (see Chapters 2, 3, 15, and 23).[3] In the unconscious patient it is well recognized that subconscious activities occur.[3] The first step in perceiving subconscious responses is to be aware that all human behaviours and communications have subconscious aspects. When the anaesthetist greets the patient, a subconscious response is elicited that frequently doesn't reach conscious awareness. However, this response can be very potent, and the ability to utilize this aspect of brain functioning represents a powerful tool in the anaesthetists' armamentarium. This effect may exacerbate any anxiety or pain already present (see Chapter 3) or be as anxiolytic as a midazolam premedication.[2]

Most of the time, recognizing human subconscious responses is not particularly important, as these responses just allow us to get the job done! Much day-to-day functioning as anaesthetists is subconscious. This is the concept of *'being on autopilot'*—that is, the performance of a task without conscious effort. Examples in anaesthesia include central venous catheter placement or intravenous (IV) access. These motor skills are initially performed with varying degrees of conscious effort depending on the experience and skill of the anaesthetist. When we first learn a procedure the initial learning and performance of the skill is conscious, 'clunky', and takes time, as the procedure tends to be learned in chunks, as a sequence of steps. With experience the steps become more fluent until they become one smooth action skilfully performed with increasing accuracy and proficiency. This subconscious learning can be used by the anaesthetist clinically—for instance, by visualizing a vein prior to its cannulation.

The conscious mind responds to logic and direct command and is under volitional control. Subconscious processes are not usually considered to be under volitional control but can be accessed by using subconscious communication. The language of the subconscious is contained in metaphor, imagery, symbolism (see Chapter 5), and suggestion. Subconscious communication is 'below the radar' and awareness of it requires a shift in thinking—once recognized, subconscious communication can be utilized therapeutically.

When patients are extremely anxious they are sometimes unable to obey a conscious command such as, *'Lie still'.* In this situation, the use of suggestion is frequently more effective. For example,

> *'In a moment, you will find that you will be able to lie still.'*

Subconscious non-verbal cues include the anaesthetist's own calmness, posture, vocal tone, and confidence being conveyed to patients while managing their distress or pain effectively. An example of an inadvertent negative subconscious cue would be handing a patient a sick bowl *'in case you feel nauseated'.*

There are times when it is useful for anaesthetists to recognize their own subconscious responses, as these can both enhance and detract from optimal performance. Once recognized, the subconscious behaviour can be temporarily controlled if necessary. There can then be consideration given to whether to use a strategy that may be more helpful or even therapeutic. Subconscious responses that are frequently helpful include intuition, anxiety in moderation, and the ability to compartmentalize or dissociate from external stimuli, and focus on a single task—for example, difficult intubation.

Subconscious responses that can be unhelpful include excessive anxiety, and dissociation from external stimuli resulting in focusing on a single task, such as repeated attempts to intubate during a difficult intubation when, in fact, the patient is hypoxic and needs mask ventilation with 100% O_2—a 'fixation error'. These responses occur spontaneously and frequently.

Dissociation

Most people appreciate that there are times during consciousness when they switch off the 'logical brain' and enter 'daydream-type' thinking or they 'tune out'. In fact, we tend to function subconsciously most of the time—for example, during routine activities such as driving home on 'autopilot' and arriving home without realizing it consciously. The ability we all have to function automatically—that is, subconsciously—frees up the conscious part of the mind to focus on other things such as planning tomorrow's 'neuro' case. The teleological basis for this ability lies in being able to filter the massive amount of information continuously presented to the individual.

This allows the conscious mind to focus on what it perceives to be important—facilitating learning, logical thinking, and problem-solving. During activities where logical thinking is not a requirement, the subconscious comes to the fore. This is characterized by dissociation from the external environment—being 'in your own world'. Paradoxically, at times of extreme stress, the subconscious tends to take over when the conscious part of the mind becomes so overwhelmed by external inputs that it ceases to function logically. An example of this is going into an exam and not being able to recall or vocalize the dose of morphine.

Time—distortion and progression

When dissociated, time is experienced differently. This phenomenon can be explored by comparing experiential time with clock time. When this occurs, we experience time as much shorter or longer than clock time. This is referred to as time distortion. During periods of boredom, time appears to pass much more slowly. Likewise, in dreams it is common to experience a large number of events in a very short time span. Hence the expressions, '*Time flies by when you're having fun*' or, alternatively, '*A watched kettle never boils*'.

Our perception of time, like other perceptions, is open to alteration by suggestion. In circumstances where the anaesthetist may wish to emphasize benefit and de-emphasize negative aspects of an experience for a patient, suggestions can be made to associate and affect time in a positive and helpful way. For example, as stated in Chapter 10 the woman in labour can be asked to focus on the 'rest' that follows each contraction and it can be suggested that, '*In this way the rests can start seeming to last longer than they really are and the contractions to seem to last for a much shorter time …*'.

Our sense of the passage of time combined with memory and imagination can allow us to think into the future, and this expectance can generate useful perceptual and behavioural experiences. For example, suggesting to patients that they can,

> '*look forward to a rapid recovery where they can look on the experience and feel it all went a little easier than they had thought*'.

Imagery and imagination

Imagery and imagination is one way of communicating with the subconscious and can be used to elicit responses that allow people to do things that they had thought to be out of their control. For example, if one consciously asks the salivary glands to secrete, nothing happens, as the autonomic nervous system is not under conscious voluntary control. However, communicating subconsciously by imagining a favourite meal or sucking on a lemon soon causes the salivary glands to secrete. This example can be used as a metaphor that encourages patients to appreciate that they frequently can do more than they think they can. Some people, especially children, find it very easy to enter an imaginary world where to all intents and purposes this becomes their reality or real world. This is the basis for distraction techniques that allow the patient to dissociate from their immediate environment.

For example, an anxious patient waiting to go into the operating room said,

> **Patient:** '*I wish I could run away but I can't.*'
> **Anaesthetist:** '*If you could run away. Where would you run to?*'
> **Patient:** '*I'd run up the stairs.*'
> **Anaesthetist:** '*What would be at the top?*'
> **Patient:** '*A beautiful view.*'
> **Anaesthetist:** '*Tell me about the view … is it night-time or day-time?*'
> **Patient:** '*It is night-time I can see the lights … it's beautiful!*'

The anaesthetist has listened reflectively, accepted the patient's reality, and utilized the patient's desire to run away, in order to facilitate an imaginary 'escape'. By entering the patient's world, the anaesthetist has helped the patient distance herself from the stress of the immediate environment and allowed her to relax and cooperate with her care.

The question then arises—are there other ways that anaesthetists can use the subconscious with patients in a therapeutic way? A powerful example of the use of imagery is the use of the switch-wire technique.[4,5]

Trance logic

Many stressed patients interacting with the anaesthetist are in a dissociated trance-like state. Their capacity to think logically and rationally is reduced and in this state, patients can respond with a wider range of abilities that although illogical, can be therapeutic. Such responses allow patients to frequently find they can do more than they think they can and more than the anaesthetist thinks they can. Patients are both vulnerable and receptive to suggestion. This can be utilized therapeutically by the anaesthetist.

For example, a patient being preoxygenated can be asked to breathe in the oxygen and, knowing how it is helping their safety, each time they breathe in they can also breathe in some strength and control. Each time they breathe out they can breathe out anything unhelpful into the room. Of course, it is completely illogical to think we can breathe feelings in and out but trance logic allows this to happen in a very matter-of-fact way when communicated as a suggestion.

Formulating suggestions

Suggestions are verbal or non-verbal cues that lead to subconscious changes in perception, mood, or behaviour which can be therapeutic or inadvertently harmful. For example, when injecting local anaesthetic if patients are warned '*This will sting!*' they are more likely to perceive the injection as a '*sting*' when compared to patients told '*The local anaesthetic numbs the skin*'.[6] The latter communication provides the meaning behind the procedure, rather than predicting the perceptual experience of an injection in a negative way that is likely to increase pain and suffering. There are numerous opportunities to avoid inadvertent negative suggestions ubiquitous in anaesthesia practice and replace them with a more therapeutic approach when interacting with patients.[7] Suggesting that patients will find that they can lie perfectly still during an anaesthetic procedure can be far more effective than reasoning with them.

Anaesthetists frequently use suggestions without realizing they are doing so. An example where communications with patients are likely to focus attention in a negative way is when, patients are repeatedly asked for their '*pain scores*' or whether they are '*in pain*' or '*feel sick*' (see Chapter 3). Repeating an image or experience over and over again usually results in it spontaneously being realized as a suggestion. For example, if the anaesthetist says, '*Every time you breathe out, you can blow a bit of tension into the atmosphere and find yourself relaxing*'. The patient subconsciously focuses on 'breathing' when the anaesthetist says, '*breathe out*'. Chest wall relaxation is a physiological truism that facilitates a relaxation response by the patient as every time the patient breathes out to functional residual capacity, the chest wall is maximally relaxed, and a subconscious '*Yes*' is generated in the brain. After 5–6 such *Yes's*, patients usually subconsciously relax.

Direct suggestions

These tend to take the form '*You will find that . . .*', '*You will be able to . . .*' or '*You may be surprised that . . .*' At induction of anaesthesia, the anaesthetist could suggest to the patient,

'*You may be surprised how much better you feel when you wake up.*'

Indirect suggestions

Such as, '*Most (Some) people find that …*' or '*A patient I saw last week found that …*' The implication here is that the patient too will experience the same thing.

At induction of anaesthesia, the anaesthetist could suggest to the patient,

> '*Patients having this surgery, frequently tell us how much better they feel when they wake up.*'

Linked suggestions

Suggestions may involve linking two perceptions or behaviours with one another. This means that when you do one thing that is conscious, something else will happen that is subconscious. For example,

> '*When **you** focus on your breathing* [conscious], *each time **you** breathe out you will find yourself relaxing automatically* [subconscious].'

A direct suggestion tends to capture the attention of the conscious mind, gets logically processed, and can then be rejected. However, patients are more likely to respond to a direct suggestion under extreme stress when the conscious mind is focused elsewhere.

Indirect suggestions are more permissive. For example,

> '*When **people** focus on breathing, each time they breathe out they find themselves relaxing automatically.*'

This indirectly implies that if the patient focuses on breathing, then relaxation will also occur.

Communication interventions

Seeding an idea

Seeding an idea prepares the patient in a way that enhances the probability of a response occurring with a suggestion. Examples of seeding are expressions of confidence in the anaesthetist made by nursing staff and others, prior to the pre-anaesthetic visit.

> **Nurse:** '*Dr S is really good at putting drips in—you won't feel a thing …*'

This generates an expectation that the cannulation will be comfortable and straightforward. Another example of seeding is when the patient with nausea is asked to '***settle***' into the chair or '*allow yourself to **settle** into a more comfortable position*'. This seeds the **stomach settling down** indirectly.

Truisms and the development of a 'Yes set'

A truism is a statement that is difficult to refute—for example, '*Oxygen is good for you!*' This statement can then be utilized to encourage the patient to start feeling more in control. '*Knowing how good oxygen is for you, each time you breathe in, you will find yourself breathing in some strength and control you didn't even know you had*'. Physiological truisms can be utilized to elicit a subconscious '*Yes*' in the brain. As each '*yes*' is acknowledged subconsciously by the patient, a therapeutic change in perception or mood can be elicited. For example, during preoxygenation, patients can be asked to focus on their breathing … '*and each time you breathe out you can find yourself relaxing as you blow away anything unhelpful into the mask … every time you breathe out your will find yourself relaxing even more …*', re-enforcing statements encouraging the therapeutic response of relaxation can be achieved by pacing the suggestion in line with exhalation. '*That's right … that's good … well done … That's okay …*'

A '**Yes set**' can be elicited by communicating a series of truisms which generate subconscious '*Yes*' responses. These can be utilized to elicit therapeutic perceptions and behaviours that would otherwise be difficult to achieve. For example, prior to IV cannula insertion, rather than suggest that the patient's arm can go numb, the anaesthetist can suggest a series of small changes in perception that culminate in numbness. For example, the anaesthetist can say,

'*As the tourniquet is placed on* **the** *arm* [use of **the arm** rather than **your** arm helps dissociate the arm from the patient's body and suggest implicitly arm anaesthesia] *a change in sensation may occur* [subconscious *yes*].

Then, as the tourniquet tightens the arm starts to tingle [subconscious *yes*].

Then, it feels a little more different [subconscious *yes*],

a change of sensation … perhaps a little sleepy [subconscious response leading to a perceptual change],

perhaps heavy … and numb or even anaesthetic [perceptual response to the suggestion]. *This allows the drip to be positioned more comfortably than otherwise*'. (See Chapter 15.)

Repetition

Repetition in a variety of forms is one of the most useful ways that people retain important information, both consciously and subconsciously. This learning response can be facilitated by using a variety of phrases that mean the same thing. For example, during preoxygenation, if the anaesthetist's suggestion for relaxation with breathing appears to be effective, this can then be reinforced by saying; '*That's good!*', '*Well done!*', or '*That's right!*' coinciding with the patient's exhalation (Pacing).

Reversed effect

When patients find themselves unable to cooperate with anaesthetic care, asking them to do the opposite of what is required frequently allows them to respond in a useful way. For example, a patient who says, '*I can't relax*' can be asked '*Not to relax*', as a way of facilitating a subconscious 'relax' response. Similarly, during an inhalational induction of anaesthesia, children can be asked '**not** *to blow up the balloon too hard*'. This will usually result in the child taking deeper breaths and therefore speeding up the induction (see also Chapter 11). This is especially the case with anxious patients who try not to feel anxious.

The word '*not*' isn't processed by the subconscious. This means that when the anaesthetist asks the child, '*not to blow up the balloon too hard*', this is a subconscious suggestion for the child to blow harder!

Double binds

Double binds are statements of comparable alternatives that can facilitate a sense of control by allowing stressed patients the perception of choice when there isn't any. This is a technique most successfully used with children.

For example, when leading a child into theatre the anaesthetist can ask the child,

'*Would you like to climb up onto the bed all on your own or would you like Daddy to help you?*'

Either choice usually results in the child on the bed. Another example would be,

'*When you are lying still on the bed, would you like to hold Mummy's left hand or her right hand?*'

If a hand is chosen, the child is subconsciously communicating that they will (probably) lie still on the bed!

Failure words

The harder one tries to do something, the less chance there is of succeeding. '**Try**' is a failure word and should be used with caution. It implies an attempt, with the probability of failure.

As Yoda says, '*Do or do not ... There is no TRY*'.

However, the two words '**Try**' and '**Not**' can be used therapeutically. For example, when the anxious patient is asked to, '*Try not to relax*' the patient consciously will fail '*not to relax*' but subconsciously the patient **will relax** as the '*not*' isn't processed by the subconscious. The confusion this statement generates tends to facilitate the non-logical processing of the subconscious. Another example is if an anxious patient states that he cannot keep his arm still during arterial line placement, the anaesthetist can ask him, '*Try not to **stay relaxed and still** and it will just seem to happen*'.

'Starting' versus 'Finishing'

Choice of words is important. Warning patients that you are about to start a procedure such as IV cannulation tends to generate anticipatory anxiety. An alternative approach that allows patients to be goal focused to the end of the procedure is to suggest, '*Would it be okay to **finish** positioning the drip?*' This can be said before touching the patient. This principle can be applied to any potentially painful procedure such as epidural insertion.

Key points

1. A shift in thinking is required to become aware of subconscious communication and then to utilize it therapeutically.

2. Suggestions make up many of the communications commonly encountered in anaesthetic practice and acute care.

3. Language structures that act therapeutically can be readily learned and include: double binds; developing 'Yes sets'; seeding and suggestion.

References

1. Hansen E, Zech N, Benson S (2020). [Nocebo, informed consent and doctor-patient communication]. *Nervenarzt*, **91**(8), 691–9.

2. Cyna AM, Andrew MI, Tan SG (2009). Communication skills for the anaesthetist. *Anaesthesia*, **64**(6), 658–65.

3. Nowak H, Zech N, Asmussen S, et al. (2020). Effect of therapeutic suggestions during general anaesthesia on postoperative pain and opioid use: multicentre randomised controlled trial. *BMJ*, **371**, m4284.

4. Cyna AM (2003). Induction of labour using switchbox imagery during hypnosis. *Aus J Clin Exp Hypn*, **31**(1), 74–87.

5. Cyna AM, Tomkins D, Maddock T, Barker D (2007). Brief hypnosis for severe needle phobia using switch-wire imagery in a 5-year old. *Paediatr Anaesth*, **17**(8), 800–4.

6. Varelmann D, Pancaro C, Cappiello E, Camann W (2010). Nocebo-induced hyperalgesia during local anesthetic injection. *Anesth Analg*, **110**(3), 868–70.

7. Allen JG, Cervi E (2014). Evidence-based language. *Brit J Anaesth*, **112**(1), 175.

Chapter 5

Narrative and metaphor in anaesthesia

Audrey Shafer

'If I can ease one Life the Aching
Or cool one Pain . . .
I shall not live in Vain.'
Emily Dickinson, Complete Poems[1]

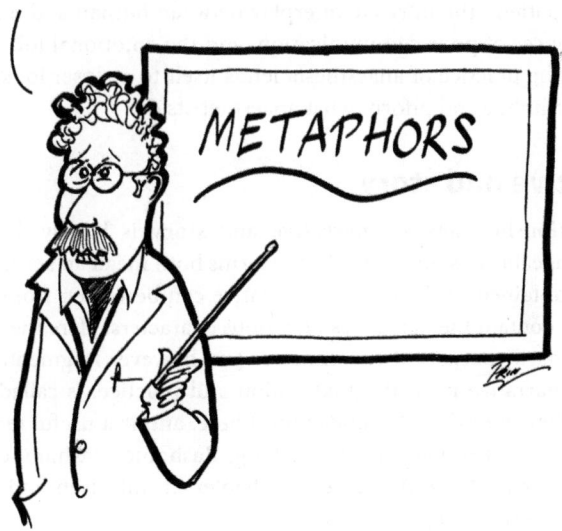

What this chapter is about

Health humanities is an interdisciplinary field of study which uses the tools of the arts, humanities, and social sciences to understand, interpret, and analyse the experience of health, illness, healthcare, and caregiving.[2] By placing such experiences in broad, complex, and dynamic contexts, health humanities seeks to explore more deeply the many ramifications of the human condition, including embodiment and mortality. Anaesthetists appreciate both these aspects of the human condition, yet it can be difficult to communicate about such meaning-laden, intense topics when one is engaged in keeping the patient alive.

Narrative and metaphor are core not only to the study of health humanities, but also to the study of medicine and how we communicate. Narrative and metaphor are integral to how we think, how we analyse and process information and how, in fact, we perceive and thus act.[3,4] With its compression and crystallization of communication with the patient, the intricate interplay between human and machine, the draconian consequences of poor communication, and the emotional toll of a high-stress environment, the practice of anaesthesia lends itself to a closer look at how narrative and metaphor imbue and inform what anaesthetists do.

Narrative and story

The relationship between **narrative** and **story** is largely determined by context. Interchangeable in some respects, the terms both mean an account of events, and each can be contained in the other. A narrative can be woven from various stories and a story can contain the narratives of various characters. Here the term narrative is most used primarily because it encompasses text however fragmentary. Dialogue, and the study of narrative in medical education and practice, is called '*narrative medicine*'.[5] Nonetheless, '**story**' is also understood here, and is a useful term, particularly in relation to a point of view or the retelling, Rashomon fashion, of an experience from differing perspectives. As noted in Chapter 2, inflection and emphasis change the meaning of even a single sentence.

The idea of differing perspectives deserves special attention in the anaesthetist–patient relationship. The 'narrative incommensurability'[6] between doctor and patient is one of the prime driving forces behind the need for good communication pre- and postoperatively. That is, the unknowableness of another person, indeed a stranger, for whom we anaesthetists assume vital and personhood responsibilities during the operation, makes clear and comprehensive communication that much more important.[7]

People develop not only as individuals but also as social beings. Just as we try to understand another's actions through, among other ways, the mirror neuron system, we try to understand another's perspective, recognizing that we are, by definition, distinct.[8]

During the course of the anaesthetist's relationship with patients, the patient's perspective is essentially and dramatically changed by what we do. We cloud the patient's sensorium to a degree not achieved, legally or routinely, by other physicians. The dynamics of the change in the patient's perspective and his or her ability to convey desire and choice, are what make us, in part, guardians of what we knew of the patient prior to induction.

The idea of story, of a beginning, an ending—and a middle—is also particularly germane to the practice of anaesthesia, and may well be part of the attractiveness of the profession to its practitioners. There is something tidy and satisfying about induction and emergence as beginning and ending, with maintenance of general anaesthesia as the middle, and perhaps the pre- and postoperative periods as preface and epilogue.

The patient also experiences these time points, but may place them in the larger history of his or her medical journey. One of the telling differences in narratives written by surgical patients, and by anaesthesia residents asked to imagine they were the patient just cared for, is the framing, in the patient narratives, of the operative and perioperative experience in the context of prior surgeries and recovery processes.[9] Furthermore, patients are far more likely to rank highly their concerns about their families as a cause for preoperative anxiety, compared with what surgery or anaesthesia residents imagine are their patients' top concerns.[10] A patient is apt to place the surgical experience not only in the continuum of his life, but also in the middle of his life experience – family, work, and other aspects of life which hold meaning and significance. A surgeon, however, begins the progress note as, for example, POD #4 (Post-Operative Day 4) no matter how long the patient had been hospitalized prior to the day of surgery, or when the diagnosis was made, or any number of other time points which may mark the start of the patient's story of illness.

It is human nature to seek meaning in life. A recitation of a series of events is enlivened by the connections, perceived or imagined, behind the series. This is plot. This is meaning-making. From the moment we start thinking about a case through to closure, we feel at the end of the day when all has gone well, we try to tie all the pieces of anaesthesia care together into a coherent whole. We notice something odd—for instance, the patient lying in the holding room has the blanket pulled over his mouth, and we think, perhaps he is embarrassed because his false teeth are out. Our approach to that patient is altered. And this is just the beginning of the complex dynamic that characterizes the series of interconnected events as we interact with the patient, the operating theatre team, other staff, and the 'props' (i.e. various devices and machines).

Life is messy and demarcations blurred, which is why telling the story of a trip is easier than recounting what you did during a week some months prior to the trip. The boundaries of typical anaesthesia care make it journey-like. If all goes well, drama and conflict are prevented. A smooth, seemingly easy anaesthetic makes even the remarkable nature of what we do appear routine. We do not seek to make bestseller adventure tales of our anaesthetics. Nonetheless, the natural boundaries of anaesthesia care make even an 'uneventful' anaesthetic story-like, punched out of the rest of our lives and of our patients' lives.

Narrative as a way of knowing

When compared to 'logico-scientific knowledge', knowledge gained from an appreciation of narrative has been touted to honour the individual—to illuminate the universally true by *'revealing the particular'* rather than by *'transcending the particular'.*[11] Narrative knowledge, therefore, is similar to case-based ethics, or casuistry, in that the particular archetypal situations on which the reasoning is based, are given prominence.

However, medical knowledge, even evidence-based medicine, is more narrative based than may be suspected.[3] The power of anecdotal experience cannot be overestimated, whether it is one's own, or 'told' to one via informal story, or via formal presentation at a morbidity and mortality conference, or by reading a case report. These narrative-based experiences underlie anaesthesia skill building such as interpretive reasoning, clinical judgement, as well as storing and retrieving information and knowledge.

Furthermore, medicine is a practice. We *'**know**'* to decrease sedative doses in the elderly because of observing the effect of titration. We also *'**know**'* to decrease such doses from reading the anaesthesia literature, which is filled with studies of individuals coalesced into groups. For instance, pharmaco-kinetic and -dynamic studies are performed using individual patients and volunteers. Any translation of those results needs to be applied back to the particulars of the patient before us—their age, habitus, debility, organ function, and so on.

Knowledge is iterative, reinforceable, malleable, and imperfect. If knowledge were not, then the delivery of anaesthesia care would be formulaic and robotic. We would gain nothing from the phenomenon of *'eyeballing'* a patient, that is comparing the patient as described in the electronic record with the person before us, and we could do push-button anaesthesia. By acknowledging that much of science is based on probabilities (the so-called p-value), one acknowledges that determining where a particular patient is on the continuum of anaesthesia—stimulation, consciousness, paralysis, pain perception, and so on, is an acceptance of the importance of the particulars of that patient at that moment. This is narrative knowledge.

The anaesthesia record is a valuable form of communication which is largely non-narrative in form; electronic anaesthesia records pull data from monitors integrating with other hospital data systems.[12] It can be reassuring to view a checkmark, or clicked notation by the previous anaesthetist, indicating no difficulties with laryngoscopy and intubation for a particular patient with a potentially difficult airway. However, a brief narrative as adjunct to the formulaic record is an effective form of communication across time for those circumstances where unexpected difficulties have arisen and the patient now requires another anaesthetic. Similarly, the narrative given to the recovery room nurse or intensive care team is formulaic in nature, but the specifics of the pre-operative status of the patient and intraoperative events make the narrative unique to the patient.[13]

Narrative in education, well-being, and reflection

Just as one cannot fully understand mathematics by reading a chapter in a textbook, one cannot understand the impact of narrative in anaesthesia without doing the prob-lems. In this case that means, telling stories, playing with language, and possibly even facing the terror of the blank page. Writing has been touted as a way of improving reflective practice, sharpening critical thinking skills, and preventing professional burn-out.[14,15] Anaesthesia trainees, asked to write narratives of challenging informed consent situations they had encountered, can use those narratives as the basis for improving preoperative communication with patients.[16] Acknowledging challenges via narrative tools can enhance our ability to recognize and respond to similar situ-ations in future anaesthetics.[17]

A growing literature on possible health benefits of writing about emotionally troub-ling experiences has led to initial investigations of the effects on patients of writing about their cancer pain.[18] Conceivably, therapeutic writing or themed reading can provide adjuvant means of communication for patients under the care of pain special-ists.[19] Even professional writers lament the difficulty of verbalizing the experience of pain.[20] A fascinating study of the use of a personal diary for patients in the intensive care unit invited entries by staff and relatives of the patient. In this study, designed to address problems of long-term psychological trauma of survivors of critical care, and their family members, intensivists found that both the writing and the document itself were therapeutic.[21]

Other uses of narrative include the inculcation of professional values, such as a com-mitment to optimal patient care, via reading or relating historical tales of remark-able anaesthetists.[22] These tend to be complete narrative texts. At the other end of the spectrum are the so-called unruly or post-modern texts—those which use electronic media in the form of blogs, postings, mixed media, and multiple authors whose only connection is via cyberspace.[23] These websites or other electronic media all rely to some extent on narrative which is used for intradepartmental communication, patient information, community building, social and professional networking, and a host of other purposes (see Chapter 22).

Narrative comments are also used for performance evaluation, largely in training programmes. Of note is the correlation between the presence or absence of negative comments on professionalism—including communication skills—and overall per-formance. During training, no anaesthesia resident whose overall performance was evaluated as excellent (top 30%) had received negative comments regarding profes-sionalism as opposed to 21% of residents.[24] Attention to implicit bias, for example the lower use of descriptors associated with leadership, such as *'confident'* or *'decisive'* when evaluating female versus male anaesthesia residents is indicative of a gender gap not only in evaluations, but also in potentially fewer opportunities for advancement by women in later leadership roles.[25,26] Indeed, throughout medicine, competency and communication skills are inseparable.[27]

Metaphor: ubiquity and importance

From business structure to computer science to courtroom evidence regarding criminal motivation, neuroscience is increasingly informing many branches of knowledge. Hence, it is not surprising that neuroscientific tools are being used to investigate language, and more specifically, metaphor processing.[28] In a fractal-like spiral, metaphor, which is essentially connection-making between two or multiple concepts, is being studied by imaging which neural centres and interconnections activate on functional scans as people 'process' metaphors.[29,30] Depending on how figurative or literal the metaphor, how novel or hackneyed, how open-ended or closed the context, and how reinforced or negated by gestural or non-verbal cues, different brain loci are recruited.[31-33]

There are a number of classification systems for metaphor depending on the historical, philosophical, or linguistic bent of the academic. Therefore, the range of metaphor presented in now classic texts such as Lakoff and Johnson's *Metaphors We Live By* constitutes a probable range of neuro-excitory responses. Neuro-linguists study brain activation patterns for different types of metaphor, for instance whether a metaphor is nominal-noun based, such as '*the recertification exam was a breeze*', or predicate—verb or motion based, such as '*the patient sailed (or flew) through the anaesthetic*'.[34] A metaphor embedded in our language, such as '*under anaesthesia*', makes **anaesthesia** into a '*something*' one can be within and below, that is, an ontological and orientational metaphor.[35] This form of metaphor would most likely be processed quite differently from a metaphor which is novel, innovative, or surprising and which more directly conjures up a host of associations. For instance, if the anaesthetist describes the anaesthetic plan in an uncommon way, saying for example, '*I'll be your bartender for the next hour, here's your first drink*'. The anaesthetist should be aware that multiple brain loci are stimulated to process the metaphor due to the less common metaphor employed, let alone possible negative connotations associated with alcohol by some patients.

This is not to say that humour has no place in anaesthetist–patient communication. On the contrary, humour can be extremely useful not only as a distraction or to lessen the stress of the moment, but also as a way to connect, person-to-person. Humour can instil confidence if used appropriately and can imply that the anaesthetist is so comfortable with his or her own abilities that multiple tasks can be handled such as starting the intravenous line and joking about something else.

Much humour relies on metaphor and forming new, off-beat connections between ideas, words, and situations. Just as one would not tell off-colour jokes to a patient in the holding area and risk alienating and angering that patient, the anaesthetist should think about what one says to, and how one speaks with, the patient in terms of metaphoric implications, including any possible negative effects.

Metaphor: dehumanizing, patronizing, yet persistent

Common classifications of medical metaphors include war and machine (Box 5.1) or engineering metaphors.[36] Because of the physical nature of anaesthesia practice and the alterations in patient sensorium thus caused, anaesthetists can readily view the patient as object: something to be controlled. This overlaps with aggression or war metaphors, something that resembles a container, and/or something mechanical.[35]

The direct connections between the patient and the anaesthesia and other machines, including infusion pumps and computerized record-keeping machines, make the anaesthetised patient particularly prone to mechanical descriptors and human/computer metaphoric transformations. These have increasingly been reviewed in cultural studies of embodiment.[37]

The projection of people-related terms onto their environments, including machines, for example, '*the sigh or wheeze of the ventilator bellows*', is a natural outgrowth of human conceptions of their world. But the obverse, machine onto person, viz. a productive academic '*churns out papers*', an efficient surgeon can be called '*a machine*', a short procedures room likened to '*a factory*' with patients '*on an assembly line*', all contribute to the linguistic blending of humans and machines. The translation of the patient into physiologic data represented on the anaesthesia monitors can mean a temporary metaphoric transformation of patient into machine. When the surgeon asks how the patient is doing, the anaesthetist glances at the vital signs and says, '*Fine!*' Further, when we present a case at conference, the patient '*becomes*' the projected anaesthesia record.

Patients also use metaphors to organize their thoughts and desires regarding healthcare. If they have a medical problem they expect the doctor to '*fix it*'. They might have something wrong with their '*ticker*' or '*plumbing system*'. They may ask for the '*knock-out*' drugs, or feel '*like a pincushion*' after multiple intravenous line attempts. Terrain metaphors are common as well. After all, sick patients enter not only the hospital but also the land of the ill, leaving '*A country as far away as health*'[38] where '*the*

Box 5.1 Metaphors in anaesthesia

War

'*Arterial stick or stab*'
'*Patient is resistant to the drugs*'
'*Knock out the patient*'

Machine

'*Tube the patient*'
'*Hook the patient up to the monitors*'
'*Patient is on cruise control*'

memory of your health is like an island, going out of sight behind you'.[39] Patients may ask to go to 'La La land'.

No matter the classification system, metaphors which turn the patient into an object can be particularly dehumanizing. Jargon shortcuts used to communicate with other professionals frequently employ metonymy (e.g. part for the whole—'He's a Mallampati 3').

It is not always wise to assume the patient is oblivious to the shop talk around him or her. For instance, as the anaesthetist enters the room with the patient, a nurse asks, for later charting purposes, 'What's his ASA?' and the anaesthetist responds, 'He's a 2'. This exchange may not be interpreted by the awake patient in a positive way. Even if the patient is fully anaesthetized or not present, it is wise to think about the language used to describe patients and cases as we communicate with colleagues. 'She's a full stomach!' 'Tank her up!', 'It was a peek and shriek', or 'Open and shut case'—a metaphor for an exploratory laparotomy/oscopy aborted due to tumour load.

A prime reason to consider the objectifying language that we use is to sort out emotions when something goes awry. If one is used to describing patients as if they were body parts, then when one encounters airway difficulty, it is easier to slide into blaming the patient for the oxygen desaturation or other problems—'**He is** a difficult airway' rather than '**He has** a difficult airway', or '**His airway** is difficult'.

It is unrealistic to believe or even desire an end to jargon, short-cut language, or metonymic references. But it **is** realistic to examine one's own practices. What language choices are made? In what context? To whom? Who else is in earshot?

We constantly make and try to interpret language choices. Not only figurative but literal language also requires interpretation. What does it mean that the radiologist wrote 'not enlarged' for the aorta, rather than 'normal'?[27]

The point is not to avoid metaphor—metaphor is too integral to how we think and talk, and enables communication. When we begin relating a case to a colleague by stating 'What a train wreck!' we have set the stage for the narrative of the difficult case that ensues. Our colleague instantly knows what we mean, sympathy is generated, and the specifics of the arduous anaesthetic are better appreciated. Yet we should also realize that by comparing the patient to a '**disaster zone**' and the image of massive railway carriages 'jackknifed', we have instinctively protected ourselves from some of the blame, stress, second-guessing, and other negative effects of being a provider of anaesthesia care, even when we feel we've provided the best possible service.

Using metaphor to understand difficult communication situations

Rather than shy away from communication in difficult situations, such as dealing with a demanding patient, a patient with 'do-not-resuscitate' (DNR) orders who is scheduled for an operation, or a patient nearing end of life, it behoves us to take the time and emotional energy to deal with them.[40,41]

Understanding the anaesthetist–patient relationship in a metaphoric way can help explain why difficult situations are so complex. Discussions about patients who are near the end of life are fraught with emotion. Patients may fear abandonment—a charged and associative word, or there may be a lack of clarity about '*informed*' consent where the gambling metaphors of '*odds*' and '*risks*' can be understood differently by different individuals with various spiritual and moral beliefs.[42]

Because metaphor can help clarify an unfamiliar situation by inviting comparison with one that is more familiar, judicious use of metaphor can open discussion in a non-threatening way.[43] For example, the '*anaesthetised state*' can be contrasted to the '*sleep state*' to explain why resuscitating drugs and intubation may be necessary for a patient with a DNR request where the need for a general anaesthetic is contemplated as a back-up plan: '*Unlike sleep, sedation and anaesthesia can make your blood pressure go down and your breathing slow down—we will need to be able to treat that.*'

The statement, '*No one dies on my watch*', spoken in response to whether or not DNR orders will be suspended in the perioperative period, is both a military and paternalistic metaphor.

Such a statement closes discussion because it assumes:

1) the anaesthetist knows best;

2) the anaesthetist is at all times in command and control;

3) the anaesthetist, just like a general, is not to be questioned.

Death is seen as the enemy, to be defeated at all costs. However, difficult decisions need to open the discussion, not close it, thus promoting interaction, not absolutism.

'*We're all on the same team*'.[44] Team metaphors acknowledge the complexities of interpersonal dynamics, goals, procedures, and practice. There are loyalty and leadership issues. Metaphors need scrutiny, but not necessarily flat-out rejection, at points of murkiness or failure.[45] In fact, rigidly adhering to metaphor connections as if they were one-for-one analogies limits the imaginative force and meaning-making inherent in metaphor. For instance, if one continues with the sports team metaphor, one wonders where the patient fits in—as another team member? As the playing field?

Metaphor: embedded in practice, perception, and research

Examples of deeply embedded metaphor in anaesthetic practice occur, for example, in the presentation of data by anaesthesia machines, and our interpretation of that data. In essence, communication between machine and anaesthetist. The metaphor, proximal is similar, (and the opposite—dissimilar is far apart) is found in language such as '*even though she's a first-year resident, her skills are close to a third year's*'. Our natural and manmade environments generate and reflect this concept—think of a flock of birds or the organization of syringes in one drawer of the cart. This metaphor, along with '*up is more*' guides much of the visual displays of the monitors, for instance the grouping of ventilatory data in one part of the screen. We find controls or displays which do not follow such basic metaphors to be counterintuitive or illogical. Attempts to improve performance by adding visual metaphors to monitors, such as representing normal values by sized rectangles, may not improve the anaesthetist's ability to diagnose the problem.[46]

Because, however, we bring objects close to each other in order to search out differences, purely visual comparisons can accentuate our perception of difference when objects are physically close.[47] The benefits of arranging similar-looking vials into proximate bins in an anaesthesia cart drawer because we will be more likely to scrutinize the label and avoid a drug swap may, however, be outweighed by the lack of muscle memory of reaching for lookalikes in disparate parts of the drawer.

The '*up is better*' metaphor underlies the synaesthetic translation of the colour of oxygenated blood to pitch.[35] Other auditory stimuli in the operating room, such as loud music, can reduce the effectiveness of this beat-by-beat communication of patient well-being. Red, meaning ***stop***, is used for colouring visual alarm status and as an aid to how much to pump up the pressure bag. Internationally, the lack of colour coding standardization of gas cylinders, and even across manufacturers in a single country, demonstrates a failure to use a consistent colour metaphor.[48] For example, in the USA, oxygen is green, and has led to faulty communication and catastrophic error.

Tidiness in the anaesthesia workspace is used as a metaphor for competence of anaesthetic care. In legal proceedings, the anaesthesia record can be regarded as a metaphor for the care provided; '*an illegible or scantily completed chart infers care that was likely substandard and inattentive*'. [49]

Lastly, embedded metaphors influence how well research results are communicated and how accurately they are interpreted. Theories of visualization emphasize the importance of underlying metaphors on data presentation for user comprehension. For example, treemap (nested rectangles) as opposed to node-link charts.[50] Algorithms, such as the difficult airway or preoperative cardiac testing for non-cardiac surgery, rely on branching metaphors, or decision tree visualization. Anaesthesia researchers can affect practice by understanding what visual metaphors are assumed when communicating research results via graphs and charts. Consideration of metaphors used, for example, to explain pain, such as pain pathways, with nerves like connecting wires, can help us to comprehend how understanding can be limited and channelled by the choice of metaphor.[51]

Summary

From the moment the anaesthetist is consulted, or looks at the operating room schedule, the care of that patient is placed in the context of experience and knowledge. The story is built by reading the patient records, reviewing prior anaesthesia records, and talking with and examining the patient. We set the scene in the operating room, preparing our equipment and pharmacopoeia for whatever twists we envision the plot of the anaesthetic care may take. We relay the story, using a wide variety of narrative constructs, to a relief anaesthetist, a recovery room nurse, the patient and family, or, potentially, to colleagues at a morbidity and mortality conference. Metaphor is embedded in the language used, how we think about mechanisms underlying anaesthesia and how we translate data into patient care. Examining the narrative and metaphoric structures which underpin our thought processes can clarify such processes and improve communication.

Key points

1. Language is integral not only to how we express our thoughts, but also how we think.

2. Narrative structure and the elements of story, such as character, tone, plot, and context, are fundamental to medical knowledge, recall, and clinical reasoning.

3. The essentials of anaesthesia care make such care both story- and journey-like.

4. Metaphors are ubiquitous in language and gesture.

5. Attention should be paid to the metaphoric basis of what is said and how sensory input is interpreted.

6. We need to be aware of the potential positive and negative effects of such metaphors on influencing patient perceptions, mood, and behaviour.

References

1. Dickinson E (1890, 1960). 'If I can stop one Heart from breaking' poem 919. In: Dickinson E. (ed.) *The complete poems of Emily Dickinson*. Boston, MA: Little, Brown & Co.

2. Jones T, Wear D, Friedman LD, eds (2014). *Health humanities reader*. New Brunswick, NJ: Rutgers U Press.

3. Montgomery K (2006). *How doctors think: clinical judgment and the practice of medicine*. New York, NY: Oxford University Press.

4. Lakoff G, Johnson M (1980). *Metaphors we live by*. Chicago, IL: The University of Chicago Press.

5. Charon R (2006). *Narrative medicine: honoring the stories of illness*. New York, NY: Oxford University Press.

6. Hunter KM (1991). *Doctors' stories: the narrative structure of medical knowledge*, p. 123. Princeton, NJ: Princeton University Press.

7. Stanford SER, Bogod DG (2016). Failure of communication: a patient's story. *Int J Obstet Anesth*, **28**, 70–5.

8. Iacoboni M, Mazziotta JC (2007). Mirror neuron system: basic findings and clinical applications. *Ann Neurol*, **62**(3), 213–18.

9. Shafer A, Fish MP (1994). A call for narrative: the patient's story and anesthesia training. *Lit Med*, **13**(1), 124–42.

10. Shafer A, Fish MP, Gregg KM, Seavello J, Kosek P (1996). Preoperative anxiety and fear: A comparison of assessments by patients and anesthesia and surgery residents. *Anesth Analg*, **83**(6), 1285–91.

11. Charon R (2001). Narrative medicine: a model for empathy, reflection, profession, and trust. *JAMA*, **286**(15), 1897–1902.

12. Rozental O, White RS (2019). Anesthesia information management systems: evolution of the paper anesthetic record to a multisystem electronic medical record network that streamlines perioperative care. *J Anesth Hist*, **5**(3), 93–8.

13. Kopp VJ, Shafer A (2000). Anesthesiologists and perioperative communication. *Anesthesiology*, **93**(2), 548–55.

14. Bolton G (2007). Narrative and poetry writing for professional development. *Aust Fam Physician*, **36**(12), 1055–6.

15. Liu EY, Batten J, Merrell SB, Shafer A (2018). The long-term impact of a comprehensive scholarly concentration program in biomedical ethics and medical humanities. *BMC Med Educ*, **18**(1), 204–13.

16. Waisel DB, Lamiani G, Sandrock NJ, Pascucci R, Truog RD, Meyer EC (2009). Anesthesiology trainees face ethical, practical, and relational challenges in obtaining informed consent. *Anesthesiology*, **110**(3), 480–6.

17. Shafer A (2009). "It blew my mind": exploring the difficulties of anesthesia informed consent through narrative. *Anesthesiology*, **110**(3), 445–6.

18. Cepeda MS, Chapman CR, Miranda N, et al. (2008). Emotional disclosure through patient narrative may improve pain and well-being: results of a randomized controlled trial in patients with cancer pain. *J Pain Symptom Manage*, **35**(6), 623–31.

19. Hovey RB, Khayat VC, Feig E (2018). Cathartic poetry: healing through narrative. *Permanente J*, **22**, 100–6.

20. Woolf V (2002). *On being Ill* (original pub. 1926). Ashfield, MA: Paris Press.

21. Bäckman CG, Walther SM (2001). Use of a personal diary written on the ICU during critical illness. *Intensive Care Med*, **27**(2), 426–9.

22. Bacon DR (2008). The historical narrative: tales of professionalism? *Anesthesiology Clin*, **26**(1), 67–74.

23. McLellan F (1997). 'A whole other story': the electronic narrative of illness. *Lit Med*, **16**(1), 88–107.

24. Rhoton MF (1994). Professionalism and clinical excellence among anesthesiology residents. *Acad Med*, **69**(4), 313–15.

25. Arkin N, Lai C, Kiwakyou LM, et al. (2019). What's in a word? Qualitative and quantitative analysis of leadership language in anesthesiology resident feedback. *J Grad Med Educ*, **11**(1), 44–52.

26. Matot I, De Hert S, Cohen B, Koch T (2020). Women anaesthesiologists' attitudes and reported barriers to career advancement in anaesthesia: a survey of the European Society of Anaesthesiology. *Br J Anaesth*, **124**(3), e171–e177.

27. Groopman J (2007). *How doctors think*. New York, NY: Houghton Mifflin Company.

28. Giora R (2007). Is metaphor special? *Brain Lang*, **100**(2), 111–14.

29. Shibata M, Abe J, Terao A, Myamoto T (2007). Neural mechanisms involved in the comprehension of metaphoric and literal sentences: an fMRI study. *Brain Res*, **1166**, 92–102.

30. Mashal N, Faust M, Hendler T, Jung-Beeman M (2009). An fMRI study of processing novel metaphoric sentences. *Laterality*, **14**(1), 30–54.

31. Cornejo C, Simonetti F, Ibáñez A, et al. (2009). Gesture and metaphor comprehension: electrophysiological evidence of cross-modal coordination by audiovisual stimulation. *Brain Cogn*, **70**(1), 42–52.

32. Schmidt GL, Seger CA (2009). Neural correlates of metaphor processing: the roles of figurativeness, familiarity and difficulty. *Brain Cogn*, **71**(3), 375–86.

33. Cardillo ER, McQuire M, Chatterjee A (2018). Selective metaphor impairments after left, not right, hemisphere injury. *Front Psychol*, **3**(9), 2308–17.

34. Chen E, Widick P, Chatterjee A (2008). Functional-anatomical organization of predicate metaphor processing. *Brain Lang*, **107**(3), 194–202.

35. Shafer A (1995). Metaphor and anesthesia. *Anesthesiology*, **83**(6), 1331–42.

36. Coulehan J (2003). Metaphor and medicine: narrative in clinical practice. *Yale J Biol Med*, **76**(2), 87–95.

37. Skara D (2004). Body metaphors – reading the body in contemporary culture. *Coll Antropol*, **28**(Suppl 1), 183–9.

38. Plath S (1960). Tulips. In: Hughes T (ed.) *Collected poems*, pp. 160–2. New York, NY: Harper & Row.

39. Hoagland T (1992). Emigration. In: *Sweet ruin*, pp. 69–70. Madison, WI: University of Wisconsin Press.

40. Kirklin D (2007). Truth telling, autonomy and the role of metaphor. *J Med Ethics*, **33**(1), 11–4.

41. Burns JP, Truog RD (2016). The DNR order after 40 years. *NEJM*, **375**(6), 504–506.

42. Hug CC Jr (2001). End-of-life issues and the anesthesiologist. *Int Anesthesiol Clin*, **39**(3), 39–52.

43. Periyakoil VS (2008). Using metaphors in medicine. *J Palliat Med*, **11**(6), 842–4.

44. Hilligoss B (2014). Selling patients and other metaphors: a discourse analysis of the interpretive frames that shape emergency department admission handoffs. *Soc Sci Med*, **102**, 119–28.

45. Evans HM (2007). Medicine and music: three relations considered. *J Med Humanit*, **28**(3), 138–48.

46. van Amsterdam K, Cnossen F, Ballast A, Struys MMRF (2013). Visual metaphors on anaesthesia monitors do not improve anaesthetists' performance in the operating theatre. *Br J Anaesthesia*, **110**(5), 816–22.

47. Casanto D (2008). Similarity and proximity: when does close in space mean close in mind? *Mem Cognit*, **36**(6), 1047–56.

48. Pauling M, Ball CM (2017). Delivery of anoxic gas mixtures in anaesthesia: case report and review of the struggle towards safer standards of care. *Anaesth Intensive Care*, **45**(1), 21–8.

49. Crosby E (2007). Medical malpractice and anesthesiology: literature review and the role of the expert witness. *Can J Anesth*, **54**(3), 227–41.

50. Ziemkiewicz C, Kosara R (2008). The shaping of information by visual metaphors. *IEEE Trans Vis Comput Graph*, **14**(6), 1269–76.

51. Neilson S (2016). Pain as metaphor: metaphor and medicine. *Med Humanit*, **42**(1), 3–10.

Section 2

Routine clinical applications

Chapter 6

The preoperative visit

Andrew Watson

'Chance favours the prepared mind.'
Louis Pasteur

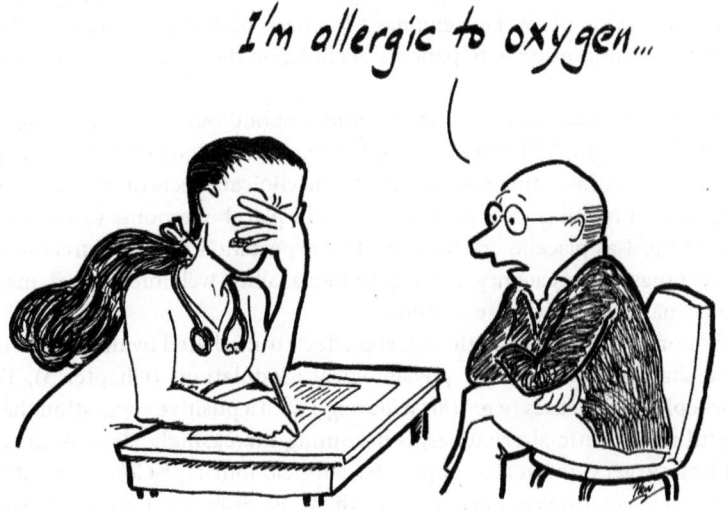

What this chapter is about

Preoperative communication and its influence on patient expectations and outcomes

The importance of preoperative assessment and preparation for surgery is reflected in the rapid growth of perioperative medicine as an anaesthetic subspecialty.[1] As the population ages and care for sicker patients increases, anaesthetists have emerged as champions of quality and safety in preoperative assessment. Traditionally the emphasis in the literature has been on gathering information, optimizing physiology, and obtaining informed consent. Less emphasis has been placed on the gains to be made in the way we communicate with patients in clinic, on the ward, or in the anaesthetic room.

Consciously or subconsciously, expectations about outcome are being shaped during every interaction (Chapter 4). A rapidly expanding body of literature exploring how placebos work, show that around 30% of the clinical effects of even our most potent analgesics for treating acute pain are due to the placebo response to a simple direct suggestion.[2-4] Just as placebo creates a positive expectation of a 'real' treatment, procedural warnings that create negative expectations, albeit well intentioned, may result in non-pharmacological adverse outcomes.[5]

This phenomenon, known as the nocebo effect, is mediated by discrete neurobiological mechanisms and specific physiological modulations (Chapter 3). The evidence for replacing phrases (e.g. *'This will sting'*) with a positive suggestion that offers meaningful therapeutic alternatives, is becoming increasingly clear. Acute anxiety surrounding surgery predicts a rough post-surgical journey.[6] Communication that sets positive expectations appears to have the most dramatic impact on pain, fear, and anxiety. Preoperative anxieties about pain respond to positive suggestions of comfort.[2,3] Conversely communications creating negative expectations in clinical medicine are common. These have been shown to have a powerful effect on reducing the therapeutic benefits of standard treatments, and exacerbate their side effects.[2-4]

Even with limited time, anaesthetists can still communicate effectively with patients with the aim of setting the scene for a more positive experience. It is an ideal time to address prior negative anaesthetic experiences, anxiety, pain, awareness, and fears of intraoperative death (see also Chapters 14, 15, and 16).

This chapter focuses on simple, practical tools to enhance communication in the preoperative setting. Having workable templates in the form of 'GREAT' and 'LAURS' during consultation is useful for ensuring that routine visits flow in an efficient manner and to maximize the value we can add to the perioperative journey. When employed they guide and direct interactions without limiting the ability to improvise. The words and context can be adapted to fit the individual patient, the doctor's own style, and the unique circumstances of every consultation whether in the clinic, day surgery unit, or at the bedside.

'GREAT' and 'LAURS' templates communicating comfort, anxiolysis, and control

Using 'GREAT' as the main framework, the principles of 'LAURS' can be applied throughout.

'LAURS' comes into its own with challenging interactions whether due to patient factors, a personality clash, or stress. Opportunities to use 'GREAT' and 'LAURS' occur through each stage of an anaesthetist's structured interaction and are explored next.

Greeting

The anaesthetist is about to see Mrs Margaret Collins, an 80-year-old former nurse booked for elective repeat excision of a basal cell carcinoma of the scalp. She is an active and generally well woman.

> **Anaesthetist:** '*Mrs Margaret Edith Collins* (ushers her into the room) *Good morning, my name is Doctor Andrew Vernon and I am an anaesthetic doctor. Would you like me to call you Mrs Collins, Margaret, or something different?*'
> **Patient:** '*Oh—I only get called Margaret when I'm in trouble; my friends call me Edith.*'

Opening a consultation using a patient's first name may be perceived as conveying warmth and caring to some patients who might prefer this to the more formal or 'distant' use of the last name. To another, the use of the first name may appear overly familiar and even indicate less competence. By asking how someone likes to be addressed we are showing respect for individual choice. Clarifying the patient's preferred name is a simple way to establish rapport.

Health services may have in place administrative systems for documenting the patient's preferred name and recording it on the case file. If not already in place, it could be a thoughtful addition for the anaesthetist to have the name documented.

Rapport

Rapport is a primary goal in successful communication between patient and clinician.[7] No one size fits all and, despite the common time limitations prior to anaesthesia, it is essential to connect, build trust, and a sense of safety.

> **Anaesthetist:** '*Is it okay if I call you Edith then?*'
> **Patient:** (Nods)
> **Anaesthetist:** '*Are you okay if we ask a few questions about your health and explain how we might provide you with the safest anaesthetic care possible.*'

An individualized approach can usually be established in the greeting and followed by expressing appreciation for the difficulties that have been overcome in making it to hospital on time.

Edith's demeanour may indicate that it has not been a good morning.

> **Patient:** '*I had to get up at 6:30am and the long wait here is killing my back.*'
> **Anaesthetist:** '*Our apologies for the long wait, it sounds like a really tough morning.*'
> **Patient:** '*It really has been.*'
> **Anaesthetist:** '*Are you happy for us to continue or would you like a pillow for your back first?*'
> **Patient:** '*It's okay, just keep going doctor.*'
> **Anaesthetist:** '*I'm really glad you are here now so we can make a plan to keep you safe and comfortable on the day of surgery and address any concerns you may have.*'

The anaesthetist has accepted the patient's reality and offers a solution, reframing the experience to focus on safety and comfort as the immediate goals.

Expectations

The core of a pre-anaesthetic visit is to gather information in the form of medical history, examination, and review of the medical record and investigations. The end result is to identify any key risk factors and make a safe anaesthetic plan.

Before proceeding with our own anaesthetic questioning, it is worthwhile to find out if the patient has any issues that are pre-occupying their mind regarding their anaesthetic. It can also save time in a busy environment by focusing at the very beginning on the patient's view of the world which may even completely change the course of the conversation (e.g. an opera singer whose greatest concern is the potential for vocal cord injury from intubation rather than her diabetes management). This places the patient at the centre of the conversation, acknowledging that the patient has experiences and skills that the anaesthetist respects and values.

> **Anaesthetist:** '*Before we go further, is there anything that needs clarifying? Do you have anything that's uppermost in your mind that you'd like to address before I ask my questions?*'
> **Patient:** '*Will I have to lay flat during the surgery—my back is going to bother me, you see?*'

Often our enquiry does not necessarily elicit a question about anaesthesia, but staying curious and using the listening and acceptance of 'LAURS' serves two purposes. Firstly, we learn about the patient's expectations, whether negative or positive, and secondly it frees up attention to listen and take on board any information that we need to convey later. Immediately voiced expectations of concerns can be dealt with upfront, paving the way for the anaesthetist to be able to focus on the medical history, examination, review of the charts, and investigations. In this way the discussions can move seamlessly into a mutual agreement about an anaesthetic plan.

It may be that the patient is disgruntled.

> **Patient**: *'No I don't have anything to ask. I've already talked to the surgeon (thinking he's taller and better looking than you) and you have all my records. I've been waiting two hours as it is.'*
>
> **Anaesthetist**: *'Sorry for the long wait, thank you for waiting to see me. It's good you've had a helpful discussion with the surgeon. Is it okay if I ask you a few questions specifically regarding your anaesthetic?'*
>
> **Patient**: Nods (subconscious '*Yes*')
>
> **Anaesthetist**: *'The questions are important for making a plan to keep you safe and comfortable.'*

The anaesthetist moves on promptly to pertinent questions (see Chapter 7).

Running late is a common problem in pre-anaesthetic clinics and patients are often stressed by the experience. Listening, acceptance, and thanking them for waiting demonstrates respect and usually diffuses the situation, facilitating a more therapeutic consultation. Gently highlighting the difference between surgery and anaesthesia shifts the dialogue towards safety, comfort, and the goal of facilitating recovery. The anaesthetist notes from the medical record that the patient has had several prior operations.

> **Anaesthetist**: *'I see you have had a number of surgeries—how were your anaesthetics? Were there any issues?'*
>
> **Patient**: *'After surgery, I get nauseous for about two days.'*

This open-ended inquiry offers an opportunity to establish what is uppermost in the patient's mind when considering previous anaesthetics. It provides a window to discuss nausea, pain, and previous poor rapport or unmet expectations, without steering the patient through a generic list of problems where inadvertent negative suggestions may be communicated. Rather it opens the door to a more individual risk-benefit discussion (see Chapters 9 and 15). 'GREAT' and 'LAURS' approaches can be used in different situations and contexts including, considering ways to communicate when establishing informed consent (Chapter 7).

The symptom of nausea provides an example of how '**LAURS**' can be used as a tool to reduce adverse perceptions and symptoms. Phrases like '*We have strong medicines to help you **stop feeling sick**'* or '*You won't feel sick*' are an invitation to think of nausea—bringing it to the forefront of consciousness, and can actually make it more likely to occur.

> **Anaesthetist**: *'Have there been any times where your stomach has been settled after the operation without this bothering you?'*
>
> **Patient**: *'Yes when I had my wrist done two years ago.'*
>
> **Anaesthetist**: *'Can you tell me what happened on that occasion? How soon after were you able to drink? When did you first have some food?'*

Focusing on a good experience and breaking it down associates the patient with this anaesthetic rather than creating negative expectancy from a previous postoperative nausea and vomiting (PONV) experience. One effective approach is to invite people to become absorbed in experiences that are incompatible with nausea, such as using guided imagery of their favourite food. The patient at this stage can be asked what they normally like eating. If they give an example, say, 'Chocolate ice cream', it can be suggested that, 'When patients eat an ice cream, in their mind prior to anaesthesia they often wake up hungry and feel like eating and drinking much sooner than otherwise' (indirect suggestion).

> **Anaesthetist**: 'We will give you some medication to allow your stomach to feel more settled this time round so that you can eat and drink as soon as you feel ready after the surgery—is that okay?'
> **Patient**: 'Yes that would be good.'

Generating a further 'Yes' makes a settled stomach more likely as the patient is implicitly buying into an expectancy of this happening—albeit subconsciously.

What if the patient states that they have never had a positive experience?

> **Patient**: 'I have nausea after every operation.'
> **Anaesthetist**: 'Okay, I see from your anaesthesia record there are things we can modify to help you feel more settled this time. Most people who have had similar difficult experiences find that with newer medications they can wake up surprised that their tummy feels much calmer than they thought it would be and even feel hungry.'
> **Patient**: 'Okay, thank you.'

These responses focus on a solution, not the problem. The inclusion of the words, 'most people' is part of an indirect suggestion that the patient too can experience 'being ready to eat'. Such suggestions are especially useful when reinforced on the day of surgery with a simple discussion about their favourite foods and actively visualizing this experience: the food's taste and appearance, the company, the pleasurable experiences with eating and so on, which further magnify this response.

Another voiced issue may be concern about the ability to mobilize post-surgery.

> **Patient**: 'Last time I couldn't move much for a day or two.'
> **Anaesthetist**: 'That, of course, can happen on occasion. However, the anaesthesia techniques we use these days allow most people to recover sooner than they think. The sensations after surgery can give you useful information. Firstly, they signal to you that the operation is over, the problem dealt with, and healing is underway. Your job is to let us know if you need any medications to help you move more comfortably to a speedy recovery.'

This approach encourages the patient to focus on postoperative sensations as indicative of healing and recovery rather than injury and disability. '**Pain**' is generally not a helpful word to use when describing postoperative sensations. However, if the patient uses the word '*Pain*' it is important to acknowledge it. Framing nociceptive input post-surgery as a normal part of tissue healing rather than associating it with tissue injury and disability, reinforces the expectation of some sensations as acceptable and encourages the patient to become an active participant in recovery. Offering patient-focused positive suggestions for being able to breathe deeply, eat and drink normally, and gradually mobilize may facilitate an earlier return to function. Adoption of the healing mindset gives new meaning to analgesic medication as a tool to facilitate a return to normal independent activity, rather than to numb all sensations.[5]

Addressing concerns

Patient concerns may be voiced and addressed at any stage. An immediate response prevents the patient from forgetting something important or failing to listen to vital information when they are pre-occupied by their fears. It is not uncommon for patients to be plagued by negative perceptions often shaped by friends, media, or even surgeons' comments. Listening and accepting current beliefs and perceptions offers an opportunity to reframe expectations.

Edith's initial basal cell carcinoma (BCC) resection had been done four weeks prior and subsequent to the histology report a wider resection is now required.

> **Anaesthetist:** '*Is there anything else you're concerned about?*'
> **Patient:** '*Yes, I needed to be put to sleep halfway through last time. I had local initially, but I felt some pain and I don't want to go through that again. I'm really worried though. I'm a nurse and I've seen many friends' brains deteriorate after general anaesthetics, I don't want to take any risk to my mind and I know local is safer.*'
> **Anaesthetist:** '*If I understand it correctly, you would prefer to avoid a general anaesthetic if you could be comfortable with a local anaesthetic.*'
> **Patient:** (Nods) '*Yes, you heard me well, Doctor.*'
> **Anaesthetist:** '*It sounds like the most important thing to you is that you feel comfortable throughout the surgery so that you can recover quickly and walk out of the hospital independently. Is that correct?*'

The anaesthetist has acknowledged the patients' concerns but reframed the consultation from what Edith **does not** want (cognitive decline), to outcomes she **does** want (being safe, comfortable, and independent). Note also how the anaesthetist observes how the patient expresses her response using the words '*You **heard** me well*' and matches her words using the auditory perceptual language in his answer (i.e. '*It **sounds** like*' . . .).

The patient's key concern has been identified, rapport deepened, and frame shifted from fear and catastrophizing to exploring options and how anaesthesia can be adapted to meet her needs.

Alternatively, Edith might say something like: '*What do you think I should do*' or '*You're the doctor, you know all about these things. Whatever you think best?*' This can be an opportunity to provide basic information and options, reassure and reframe unhelpful misperceptions, while still involving them in their care.

> **Anaesthetist:** *'Between us we should be able to come up with a pretty good plan to make this a different experience for you. We could start with a local anaesthetic and see how you go. There is the option to add some sedation and only convert to a general anaesthetic if required. You will be the one in control and we will ensure we don't do anything without your permission and only proceed when you are comfortable.'*

The use of the word *'we'*, and emphasis on the patient granting permission conveys that while they have sought our advice on decision-making at this point, patients still have some control on the day.

Alternatively, the anaesthetist could use a simple technique described as follows, to identify and reinforce the patient's strengths.

> **Anaesthetist:** *'Would it be ok if I asked something a little unusual and a little different?'*
> Edith nods.
> **Anaesthetist:** *'I would like to invite you to recall an episode where you did something you were particularly proud of, something you are comfortable to share.'*
> Pauses and waits.
> **Patient:** *'The birth of my children, I can remember them like it was yesterday.'*
> **Anaesthetist:** *'A significant memory . . .'*
> **Patient:** *'It wasn't easy, but I did it.'*
> **Anaesthetist:** *'Yes, many people describe labour as a very challenging experience. You dealt well with that.'*

By facilitating immersion in these past experiences, the anaesthetist has triggered memories of the strengths the patient has and brought these to the forefront of the mind. The anaesthetist's goal here was not to guide the patient to a particular anaesthetic but to connect them with the past experiences and tools they have to make a confident decision. Subconsciously appreciating these strengths, the patient can gain a sense of control realizing they have more skills and resources to call upon in this situation than they might have appreciated. The conversation can at this stage explore the options available and summarizes the pre-anaesthesia evaluation and plan.

Tacit agreement

Agreement that is understood without being stated is the core of a discussion where trust has been established. This may be informal or formalized by signing a consent form. Either way, at the end of every clinician–patient interaction a tacit agreement is forged. The patient can be thanked at this stage reconfirming that we are all on the same page and no other issues need dealing with at this time.

> **Anaesthetist:** *'Are you okay with our plan to use local anaesthesia and add in sedation if required to keep you safe and comfortable?'*
> **Patient:** *'Yes, that sounds okay.'*

Where rapport, trust, and tacit agreement have been reached during the pre-anaesthetic visit, patients often express the hope that the person they are talking to will be their anaesthetist on the day of surgery. However, it may not be clear who the treating anaesthetist will be on the day.

Communicating this to the patient in a way that inspires confidence rather than creating anxiety, requires reassurance that the relevant and important details of the conversation in the medical record have been recorded.

> **Anaesthetist**: '*I may not be your anaesthetist on the day so I have made a detailed note of our conversation and the plan we discussed today. The anaesthetist on the day of your surgery will review the notes I've made on our conversation and assessment and you'll be able to ask any further questions.*'

In cases where the anaesthetist of the day may have different approaches it is useful to facilitate communication by alerting that anaesthetist to any strong preferences the patient may have and avoid expectations of an anaesthetic that may not be offered on the day.

Opportunities to actively assist and enhance the perioperative patient experience and recovery

As Shafer notes, 'anesthesiology, in so many ways, is *crystallized medicine*. We rarely, if ever, have the luxury of multiple visits to connect with patients and family'.[8] Patients engage as part of the healthcare team when they feel cared about as a unique individual. The importance of giving patients as much choice as possible, even if this is in the form of a double bind, cannot be overemphasized. Choices, no matter how small, offer patients some perception of control over their care. There is a range of techniques that can be applied to utilizing patients' strengths, reframing unhelpful thoughts, and making suggestions to create a positive expectancy that can lead to an improved experience (Table 6.1, Chapter 2).

Table 6.1 A summary of the conversation

Greeting	Asking patients their preferred name establishes rapport. This also provides an element of control at the start of the interaction.
Rapport	Enhanced by using the 'LAURS' of communication—particularly listening and acceptance. Utilizing perceptions and strengths. Reframing and suggestion facilitate increased choice, safety, and comfort.
Expectation	Clarifying expectations of doctor and patient facilitates mutual decision making and goal setting.
Addressing concerns	Enhances rapport and promotes a therapeutic outcome.
Tacit agreement	Thanking the patient is a powerful way of completing the interaction as the shared understanding and agreed plan for the day of surgery and early recovery is confirmed.

Note the 'LAURS' concept weaving in and out of the 'GREAT' structure

> ## Key points
>
> 1. Good communication helps the patient to prepare as an active participant in their perioperative care and makes a tangible difference to comfort and recovery.
> 2. Patients interact best with the anaesthetist when they feel respected, listened to, and understood.
> 3. The pre-anaesthetic visit is a good time to reframe fears or negative expectations and utilize strengths to create positive expectations that will allow the patient to feel they will be actively participating in their recovery.
> 4. 'GREAT' and 'LAURS' provide a structure that can be adapted to a range of patients to facilitate a sense of safety, respect, and control.

Incorporating the 'GREAT' and 'LAURS' templates in the preoperative visit allows a structured approach that increases trust and rapport in a limited time, while enhancing the traditional focus on safety and patient comfort.

References

1. Oprea A (2021). Editorial: perioperative medicine: a bridge (not) too far! *Curr Opin Anaesthesiol*, **34**(3), 306–8.
2. Schedlowski M, Enck P, Rief W, Bingel U (2015). Neuro-bio-behavioral mechanisms of placebo and nocebo responses: implications for clinical trials and clinical practice. *Pharmacol Rev*, **67**(3), 697–730.
3. Benedetti F, Mayberg H, Wager T, Stohler C, Zubieta J (2005). Neurobiological mechanisms of the placebo effect. *J Neurosci*, **25**(45),10, 390–402.
4. Moerman DE (2002). Explanatory mechanisms for placebo effects: cultural influences and the meaning response. In: de Craen AJM (ed.) *The science of placebo. Towards an interdisciplinary research agenda*, pp. 77–107. London: BMJ Books.
5. Bingel U, Wanigasekera V, Wiech K, et al. (2011). The effect of treatment expectation on drug efficacy: imaging the analgesic benefit of the opioid remifentanil. *Sci Transl Med*, **3**(70), 70ra14.
6. Giusti EM, Lacerenza M, Manzoni GM, Castelnuovo G (2021). Psychological and psychosocial predictors of chronic postsurgical pain: a systematic review and meta-analysis. *Pain*, **162**(1), 10–30.
7. Howe L, Leibowitz K, Crum A (2019). When your doctor 'gets it' and 'gets you': the critical role of competence and warmth in the patient-provider interaction. *Front Psychiatry*, **10**, 475.
8. Schafer A (2009). 'It blew my mind'—exploring the difficulties of anesthesia informed consent through narrative. *Anesthesiology*, **110**(3), 445–6.

Chapter 7

Consent

Scott W. Simmons and Allan M. Cyna

'If it is not right do not do it; if it is not true do not say it.'
Marcus Aurelius

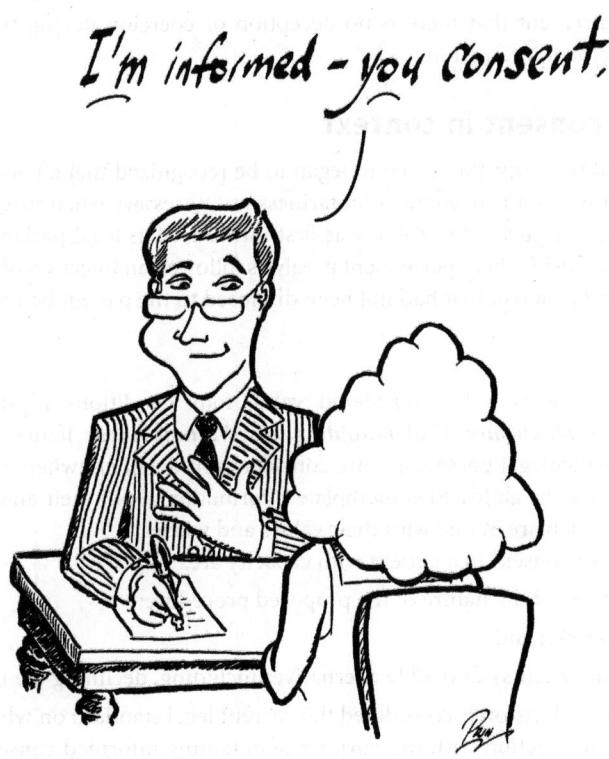

What this chapter is about

Patient consent for anaesthesia is the foundation of the therapeutic relationship and the ultimate expression of trust in their doctor. The patient is literally placing their life in the anaesthetist's hands. '*Informed consent*' has developed primarily as a medicolegal construct over the last 50 years and applies to two related, but nevertheless different, settings: medical practice and biomedical research. Ethically and legally, it is a fundamental requirement that there is no deception or coercion during the patient or research participant interaction.[1]

Informed consent in context

It was not until the early 1900s that it began to be recognized that a patient's right to bodily autonomy, and the need for voluntariness was necessary when surgery was proposed.[2] The term '*informed consent*' was first introduced as legal parlance following the Salgo case of 1957 where permanent paralysis followed an injection of radiological dye into the aorta—a risk that had not been disclosed to the patient beforehand.[2]

The legal

In brief, for consent to be considered valid, four conditions need to be fulfilled: **Capacity**, **Disclosure**, **Understanding**, and **Voluntariness**. Issues around consent from a medicolegal perspective are considered in detail elsewhere.[3] Patients are presumed to have the ability to contemplate information about their anaesthesia and make choices which are in line with their values and wishes.

Key features of consent in a patient with capacity are:

◆ comprehension of the nature of the proposed procedure;

◆ its *material* risks; and

◆ the risks and benefits of possible alternatives including, declining the procedure.

The Montgomery decision is considered the current legal standard on which to base a doctor-patient interaction with the purpose of obtaining informed consent.[4] The key requirement in this decision is for the doctor to ensure that the patient is aware of any material risks involved in any recommended treatment, and of any reasonable alternative or variant treatments.

The test of *materiality* is *whether, in the circumstances of the particular case, a reasonable person in the patient's position would be likely to attach significance to the risk, or the doctor is or should reasonably be aware that the particular patient would be likely to attach significance to it.*[4]

In essence, relevant information needs to be communicated to the patient in a way that has regard to the patient's capacity to **understand** it. Withholding such information because of concerns for the patient's welfare, '*Therapeutic Privilege*', is likely to be restricted by the courts, to circumstances where there is a likely severe detriment to the patient.

The clinical

'*The manner and context in which information is conveyed is as important as the information itself*.[2] This statement applies irrespective of whether informed consent is in the context of clinical practice or research.

The ethical

Contrast the goals and risk-benefit assessment of a social media influencer seeking facial surgery as a means of increasing their followership versus a similar person with a congenital or acquired facial injury who aspires to eat, drink, and smile like their friends. In their decision-making, both will have their individual and unique beliefs and values to weigh up. Clinicians need to take this into account when communicating in a way that is underpinned by trust, respect for the patient's autonomy and their individual circumstances—a fundamental concept of the ethical practice of medicine.[5] Sir William Osler advocated four principles to guide the physician.[5] These equate to a recognition of the importance of:

◆ science;

◆ a doctor's professional behaviour;

◆ the bedside manner or patient-centred approach to the therapeutic relationship; and

◆ *primum non nocere*—do no harm.[6]

Neurobiological advances and clinical research investigating how communication of risk might adversely affect patient outcomes, are emerging.[6-8] It is becoming increasingly clear that an imprudent choice of words can adversely affect patient care.[8-10] This has clinical, ethical, and potential legal implications for how we communicate, and may present a paradox when attempting to meet the needs of patients while fulfilling perceived medicolegal requirements by the hospital and governing medical bodies.[11]

The practical

Although, modern clinical practice has become dominated by medicolegal concerns related to **material risk** disclosure, it would be wise to temper the discussion if patients are to avoid being overwhelmed by excessive and/or incomprehensible generic information. Pre-emptively listing a vast number of possible complications that may beset a patient is unlikely to assist a legal defence if patients feel bombarded with excessive information they don't understand. This serves only to confuse and impair clinical communication in the unlikely event of a complication occurring. Paradoxically, the risk of being sued may increase as the patient remembers feeling overwhelmed. Attempting to explain every possible option of medical management does not automatically result in a patient being informed.

Balancing medicolegal requirements and communication in practice

Common themes that emerge when researching why patients might sue their doctors include:

- the patient's desire to prevent similar incidents from happening to others;
- not being informed how and why an injury occurred;
- financial compensation for pain, suffering or to provide future care for injuries; and
- to hold someone responsible.[12]

Patients who like and trust their doctor may be less likely to sue them. Doctors therefore need to be cognisant when communicating information and ensure that it is meaningful and understood by the patient. Anaesthetists frequently overestimate patients' understanding of information provided when obtaining informed consent.[13] The focus of clinical care requires doctors to listen to patients and keep their wishes and values at the centre of every interaction. Implications for follow-up and things to think about when communicating should a complication occur are discussed in Chapter 13. Ideally, information regarding anaesthesia should be provided well ahead of the day of surgery[3] and all patients given the opportunity to be seen in a pre-assessment clinic. Unfortunately, constraints of a busy system mean that it is not uncommon for the patient to meet an anaesthetist for the first time on the day of surgery. Although most patients want to know some basic information around what to expect, the need and desire for detailed information particularly about risks, is highly variable and many patients are happy to trust their treating clinicians to do the right thing by them.[14]

Surprisingly, little attention has been paid to how to communicate with patients in a therapeutic way that fulfils both clinical and legal obligations. The literature and anaesthesia information sheets focus almost exclusively on disclosure of the risks of harm.[3,15] A 'LAURS' approach can go a long way towards optimizing communication in this context, irrespective of patient circumstances, values, proposed procedure, or timing.

'LAURS' provides a basis for moving from paternalistic practices, where doctor or lawyer knows best, to one where doctors and patients share in the decision-making by establishing agreed, shared objectives. This shifts the *informed consent* discussion from a problem-based discussion, the purpose of which is to defend the doctor and organization against litigation, to one where the patient–doctor communication is *solution-focused* and *therapeutic*. Utilizing this perspective to guide how much, and in what form, information should be provided, consent is achieved by creating a sense of common purpose and a therapeutic alliance that encompasses both outcome and process.

The current medicolegal paradigm assumes that patients come as a blank canvas to a traditional face-to-face consult. This reflects a degree of paternalism and denies the reality that for most patients *informed consent* is happening in the context of their own preconceived perceptions and beliefs. Handing patients an information sheet with a list of incomprehensible complications, together with only fragments of useful knowledge, from an individual patient's perspective is likely to be wholly inadequate, especially in the context of the patient already being exposed to a variable amount of misinformation.[16]

The risk discussion

In the context of providing anaesthesia, there is usually only one choice on the menu. Whether or not to have an anaesthetic cannot be considered in isolation of the procedure and it is rarely appropriate to ask, '*Would you like the operation with or without an anaesthetic?*'[17,18] (see Chapter 23). Declining a laparotomy for an acute abdomen has very different implications to declining an arthroscopy for a painful knee. The potential benefits of a minor, and entirely elective procedure may not be worth the risk of an anaesthetic, whereas considerable anaesthetic risk may be acceptable for a potentially life-saving operation. Many anaesthetists have a list of material risks of anaesthesia that they give or discuss with all patients including mentioning the possibility of death. Others argue that this approach fails to take into account the patient's needs or desire for this type of information,[19] its context, or the possibility of nocebo effects.[20]

If a patient is at increased risk of a particular complication or clearly wants more information, it becomes more important to be explicit—especially if surgery is elective and the discussion is taking place prior to the day of surgery. There are as many possible approaches to this vexed question as there are anaesthetists.

> '*Have you been told any risks of anaesthesia?*'
> '*What can you recall?*'
> '*Do you have any particular concerns?*'
> '*We can discuss relevant risks in your particular circumstances and address any other concerns you may have ... Is that okay?*'
> '*My expectation with this common procedure in someone fit and healthy is for everything to proceed in a very straightforward, safe and comfortable way for you ... Yes, anaesthesia does carry risk.*'
> '*Are there any risks you are concerned about?*'
> '*Is there anything I can say about risks that would stop you going ahead?*'
> '*I am expecting that given the precautions we are taking, everything will go smoothly for you*'.

It is usually unhelpful for patients on the day of surgery to be informed of generic information about the risks of anaesthesia such as *Death, Paralysis, Nausea*, and *Pain*, for the first time without individualizing these risks in the context of how they are being mitigated by the anaesthetic care being proposed.

For example,

> '*From my perspective, the only relevant risk or concern in your case is your asthma. For that, we will be giving you a nebulizer prior to your surgery to help ensure your*

airways are dilated and relaxed so that you can breathe more easily throughout the procedure and for when you wake up in recovery. Is that okay with you?'

Not

'You are at risk of having an asthma attack!'

Risk disclosure can be communicated in the context of explaining what the anaesthetic options are.

'Okay, so you need to have this hip done.'

'Have you heard of a spinal anaesthetic? What this involves is . . . we find with most people, this is the safest and most comfortable approach, and if required we can give a little sedation.'

'Do you have any questions or concerns?'

Even after a full explanation of the risks and benefits, the patient may make an autonomous decision to decline the procedure and even if this is not in their best interests, the patient's decision needs to be respected.

Evaluating risk

Many factors influence our assessment of risk and few of them are rational. Self-inflicted risk is generally tolerated better than externally inflicted risk and rare but serious risks tend to be overemphasized. Strategies to improve comprehension include:

♦ Plain language and avoidance of jargon in both verbal and written communication.

♦ Data presented as frequencies rather than percentages. '*1 in 10 patients will suffer a particular side effect*' is more easily understood than '*10% of patients will suffer the side effect*'.

♦ Presenting information from both positive and negative perspectives (e.g. '*a 90% chance of eating and drinking*') is likely to be better received than a '*10% chance of nausea and vomiting*'. However, if nausea and vomiting is a concern, this must be communicated directly:

'I note nausea and vomiting have been a problem for you previously. Can I ask if you recall any time you recovered from the anaesthetic with a settled stomach and were able to eat and drink more easily afterwards?'

Patients frequently recall a time when nausea did not occur, and going through this positive experience in detail allows them to focus on the same therapeutic outcome happening this time.

♦ Visual aids such as graphs and pie charts may be helpful. Pictograms have been shown to be the best-understood and most effective way of communicating absolute numbers.

♦ The order in which risks are presented can skew their perceived significance. The recency effect means that information presented last will be retained more reliably. Hence, presenting benefits first and risks last may affect the patient's perception of the magnitude of risk and vice versa.

A 'GREAT' 'LAURS' approach

Dr James Rorshach is a consultant anaesthetist of 20 years standing. He is currently working in a busy district general hospital and enjoys the diversity of practice that brings, including a small amount of obstetrics. As he approaches the day admission area, he notices that the first patient is a woman—Sarah Jones, with metal work in her lumbar spine, is scheduled to have a caesarean. Perusing her anaesthesia form, Dr Rorshach notes that she has been to the high-risk clinic and been seen by a registrar who had indicated that a general anaesthetic was most likely, but that ultimately the final decision would be with the anaesthetist on the day. Following his review of the notes, James briefly introduces himself to the patient and her partner, Bill.

Greeting

'Good morning, I'm Dr Rorshach, I am the anaesthetic consultant looking after you during your caesarean today. Can I confirm your name please and what operation you are having? ... I do know, but just need to confirm we are all on the same page'.

Confirming with the patient their name and procedure may bring up other procedures planned such as tubal ligation, so this is always a good question to ask.

Rapport

James: 'So, are you okay if I call you Sarah?'

This starts the consent process and confirms the preferred name to address the patient and generates a first 'Yes' as part of a 'yes set' (see Chapter 4). It promotes a sense of control and initiates the building of rapport between patient and doctor. Finally, using the name with which the patient is most familiar will likely improve responsiveness perioperatively including when waking up from a general anaesthetic if required.

Expectations

Sarah Jones was 38 years old and having her first baby. The pregnancy had been complicated by gestational diabetes and near term, the baby was large. Her obstetrician had advised on a caesarean birth as the safest option. This was, after all, a very special baby, following almost 10 years of assisted reproduction therapy and multiple failed attempts at becoming pregnant. She had also overcome other adversity, having experienced a major back injury following a fall as a teenager. She had been left with metal screws and a small plate in her lower back which was often painful, and she frequently had pain going down her left leg.

Sarah: 'When we saw the other doctor in the clinic, I said I would like to be awake so I could be involved with the birth of my baby, and my partner, Bill could also be there. The doctor did say something about needles in the back not working particularly well, but we both stressed to him that this will be the most important day of our lives and we are prepared to do whatever it takes.'

James recalled a medicolegal case of a woman who had been too timid to speak up during a caesarean with an obviously inadequate regional block,[21]. This had been followed by his medical indemnity organization emphasizing that, based on claims history, awareness with perhaps more than anything else, pain under regional anaesthesia was something that all anaesthetists should be on their guard against.[22] There was also neurological injury,[1] postdural puncture headache[23] ... the list seemed endless.[24] James recognized that this couple were very adamant in their wish to both be present for the birth. He focused on the pertinent risks of complications in Sarah's specific case, responding to questions in a truthful way while still offering a solution-based approach.

After identifying Sarah and Bill's goals, James goes on to summarize his thoughts and expectations so that there can be a respectful, mutually agreed plan on how best to move forward. This requires taking into account information regarding pros, cons, risks, and benefits. The goal here is to ensure that if a particular type of anaesthetic is a safe and available option, then the information conveyed allows for an informed decision by the patient and preferably, her partner. It appeared clear that from both James's and Sarah's perspective that neuro-axial anaesthesia rather than a general anaesthetic would still be their first-line choice despite the risk of a less than perfect block.

Addressing concerns

Questions and concerns may be voiced early on in the consultation and, while some anaesthetists ask the patient to hold off until they've provided risk information, it is nearly always preferable to allow the patient to get initial questions and concerns addressed and out of the way. This avoids patients trying to remember important questions which may stop them listening to information about the procedure or worse, forget a vital concern they wished to have addressed. Unvoiced fears such as awareness, pain, and death can be addressed indirectly. For example, in the introduction to the patient when explaining the anaesthetist's role in their care, the anaesthetist might say,

> **James:** '*The anaesthetist's role is to maximize safety and comfort by careful monitoring and administration of medications throughout the operation through to you arriving safely in the recovery room.*'

The implication here is that patient safety and comfort are primary goals during and after the procedure and that the patient will reach the recovery room with these goals achieved.

> **James:** '*Do you have any other questions?*'

> **Sarah:** '*Will the spinal hurt?*'

> **James:** '*Some women tell me it does! However most find it a lot more comfortable than they thought it might be-especially once we have finished popping in some local anaesthetic to numb the skin before we place the spinal anaesthetic. Also, given your previous surgery, it may take a little longer to find the right spot in your back, so we will allow more time for that.*'

'Given you are at increased risk of needing a sleeping general anaesthetic we may need to supplement the spinal with an epidural top-up called a CSE or give medication into the drip or if required get you off to sleep at some point during the operation—this is the main concern from my perspective as an anaesthetist.'

'Do you know of any other risks of a spinal?'

'Would it be okay to talk about some other risks and what we might do to minimize their occurrence?'

'I usually talk to patients about the risk of a headache which is uncommon with a spinal and some patients raise concerns about nerve damage or becoming paralysed, which is extremely rare. We can discuss these further if you wish.'

The point here is a tailored conversation for this specific individual.

'The most important thing to know from my perspective is that if a sleeping anaesthetic is required Bill will need to leave the operating room so we can have room to look after you and the baby as safely as possible.'

Tacit agreement

Having established that the patient is comfortable with the proposed anaesthetic and understands the risks and benefits, agreement is made. Many healthcare systems do not require a separate signed consent form for anaesthesia. For those that do, one way of doing this is to sum up while adding notes to the form. For example, the anaesthetist might say:

'Are you okay to sign the consent form?'

'I am just jotting down our discussion about the spinal anaesthetic' ... writing it down on the form ... *'and the risks we have discussed'*.

Integrating 'LAURS' into consent

Listening

In order to support a meaningful consent, the doctor needs to be able to absorb and process the information being offered by the patient (i.e. listen specifically for the patient's values, goals, and concerns). It was very apparent in this case that Sarah placed immense value on having a birth experience that involved her partner. A general anaesthetic, even perfectly administered, was therefore totally contrary to this goal (see 'Expectations', earlier).

Acceptance (NOT acquiescence)

Patients frequently have realities, beliefs, and concerns that are not appreciated by the anaesthetist. This makes it essential to focus on listening to patients in a way that optimizes the chances that patient priorities and concerns are identified, and misperceptions discussed in a respectful way. By accepting the patient's current mindset, the clinician can move respectfully towards achieving a common understanding.

Recommendations that support patient values usually allow safe and informed decision-making.[21] Involving Sarah and Bill in decision-making about aspects of their anaesthesia care facilitates patient choices that may be radically different from other 'reasonable patients' seemingly in the same circumstances. Accepting that being awake for the birth was the single most important thing for Sarah and Bill, enabled James to positively engage with a range of possible alternatives and discuss what these might look like within the bounds of safe anaesthesia care.

Utilization

Using Sarah and Bill's language and responses allows James to tailor information in a relevant and meaningful way. Building on Sarah's profound desire to participate in the birth of her baby created the opportunity for James to undertake problem-solving specific to what has become a shared goal. Options could include conversion to general anaesthesia as a planned event immediately after her baby's birth, or the addition of multiple modes of analgesia supplementation in addition to the regional block if this proved necessary and was acceptable. Both courses might be considered a form of anaesthetic failure. If patients have understood and consented for such an eventuality, should it occur, it is not a failure!

Reframing

Ideas of risk to the patient can be presented in a variety of ways—some therapeutic and some potentially harmful.

Negative framing: '*There's a very high chance that the block will fail and you will need a general anaesthetic and miss out on seeing the baby*'.

Positive framing: '*If we put a range of options in place we can work very closely together, to help give you the best chance possible of seeing your baby being born safely and comfortably with general anaesthesia being immediately available to you if required – How does that sound to you?*' This usually generates another, '*Yes*' and builds on the rapport between Sarah, her partner, and the anaesthetist.

Suggestion

Supporting patient decision-making at a conscious and subconscious level that is consistent with Sarah and Bill's core values and goals, will be markedly enhanced with both direct and indirect suggestion (see Chapters 2–4, 23) directed at a therapeutic outcome. For example,

> **Anaesthetist:** '*We will do everything we can to keep you as comfortable as possible during the procedure so that you can look forward to seeing and holding your baby. There are lots of strategies that can help you stay awake comfortably and safely. For example, there is medication we can place in the drip . . . gas and oxygen that you can breathe in by mask. It is helpful to know that any sensations you feel are usually telling you that you are getting closer to seeing your baby for the very first time. If anything is bothering you, let us know by just saying '*Stop!*' and we will stop what we are doing and help you get more comfortable prior to proceeding and finishing the operation. We will be checking in*

with you regularly and if at any time you feel the need for a sleeping anaesthetic, then it will be immediately available to you.'

'So, just to summarize, the plan is ... that we won't be doing anything without your permission and during the caesarean you will let us know if there is anything you need or any way we can help if something bothers you during the pro- cedure ... Remember ... we will be with you at all times ... Is there anything else we need to address? Do you Sarah or you Bill have any other concerns or ques- tions? Is this all okay with you?'

Consent as an ongoing process

Obtaining ongoing consent from the patient needs to continue well beyond the signing of the consent form. In many ways the initial tacit agreement and signing of a consent form, where required, is only the beginning of the consent process. Although not a legal requirement, many patients benefit from being asked permission before each time they are touched, or a procedure is about to start.

Examples of what the anaesthetist might say as part of an ongoing consent during anaesthesia care are given next. The degree of patient anxiety and their responses to the various communications will determine what to say and how frequently. Anxious patients tend to feel out of control, and gaining permission at each stage allows them to be actively involved in their care and provides space and time to gather thoughts be- fore moving to the next stage. The anaesthetist might say when performing the spinal anaesthetic procedure,

'Is it okay to clean the skin with antiseptic?'
'Position the drapes?'
'Is it okay to touch your back?'
'Finish placing some local anaesthetic under the skin?'
'Can we numb the area I am touching so that we can finish the spinal as safely and comfortably as possible?'
NOT *'Sting coming!'*

Patient: *'Can you stop for a moment ... '*

Anaesthetist: *'No problem. Just take a couple of deep, slow breaths so you can* **feel** *a bit more* **in control** *(suggestion) ... blow a little tension into the room and as you breathe out, just* **feel yourself relax** *(suggestion) without trying to do anything else ... when you are ready for me to* **finish** *(Goal directed commu- nication allows the patient to focus on the end of the injection of local anaes- thesia) ... just let me know with a Yes.'*

Other examples of communications that are likely to increase patient rapport are:

'Are you okay if we start taking you into theatre?'
'Is it okay for you to sit up on the bed and rest your feet on the stool?'
'Are you okay if I examine your back?'

'Is it okay to paint your back with antiseptic to keep things clean and sterile so we can finish the spinal as comfortably and safely as possible?'
NOT *'This will be freezing and make you jump!'*
'Are you okay for us to position the ECG stickers here?'
'Can we place the blood pressure cuff on your right arm?'

In the context of a GA:

'Is it okay to place the oxygen mask on now?'

Confirming consent in this way allows for further *'Yes'* set generation that invariably increases a patient's sense of control and also allows subconscious therapeutic changes in perception to be realized.

Consent and the nocebo effect

There is increasing evidence for potential harm in the mere disclosing of risk. This underscores the significant moral liability of the caregiver when creating a nocebo effect in the patient together with the gravity of responsibility to prevent it.[25] While patients must be given every opportunity to have concerns addressed, and questions responded to in a frank and honest way, the necessity of repeating negative risk information in both written form[15] and verbally, on the day of surgery should be limited.[11] This is particularly relevant when suggesting symptoms such as *Pain, Nausea,* and *Itch,* when anaesthesia induction approaches and patient anxiety escalates.[9] It is usually possible to provide risk information in a way that is reassuring rather than anxiety provoking.

Rather than tell a parent that their child will need pain killers during and after their surgery, one could say,

'As pain is a concern, we will give some medicine before and during surgery to ensure Jonny wakes up from the anaesthetic as comfortably as possible and further medication will be available in recovery should this be required.'

Likewise, rather than tell patients that they might have nausea and vomiting, they could just as truthfully be informed that, *'Most patients find that they can eat and drink as soon as they feel like it'* (indirect positive suggestion—see Chapters 2 and 4) or that,

'We will give medication during anaesthesia to help the tummy settle' and allow the patient to *'feel like eating and drinking a bit sooner than otherwise'.*

Overwhelming patients with a generic list of anaesthesia risks is not only potentially harmful but is confusing and, paradoxically, may be decreasing patient autonomy, and even increase litigation. Krauss calls for *'calibrated and nuanced language for procedural disclosure to communicate truthful* (therapeutic) *information that positively influences the patient's affective state while minimizing nocebo responses*.[9] In this way, informed consent can be primarily focused on optimizing anaesthesia care rather than the more common approach of viewing consent primarily, or only, through a legal lens.[26]

Documentation

Consider documenting key medical issues, specific relevant risks discussed from both the anaesthetist's and patient's perspective and treatment choices offered. Some colleges and medical regulatory bodies may require specific documentation.

Emergencies

The principles of 'GREAT' and 'LAURS', albeit in condensed form, still apply in an emergency. The key issue here is to check-in with the patient after the overall picture of what is planned has been explained in general terms as well as its risks and benefits and those of possible alternatives. Maintaining effective communication in time critical situations can be challenging, but nonetheless requires keeping the patient apprised of what is happening and why. For example, when placing IV access, it can be explained that *'the drip is to replace some of the blood and rehydrate you and give medications to keep you safe and comfortable for when you arrive in the recovery room'*.

Where to from here?

Adhering to the science, behaving professionally, and truly listening to what patients are telling us, will likely meet our ethical, clinical, and medicolegal obligations, and reduce litigation.[27]

Key points

1. Establishing patient consent is all about effective communication.
2. Communicating consent is a continuous process that allows patients to feel more in control and respected throughout their care.
3. Unless proven otherwise, it should be assumed that all adult patients, and in some cases children, have the capacity to make decisions about their treatment and care. A lack of capacity determination is decision specific at a particular time-point.
4. Informed consent is part of the ongoing relationship between the patient and anaesthetist.
5. At its core a patient-centred approach that respects the individual patient's values and wishes is a fundamental premise of communicating consent.

References

1. McCombe K, Bogod D (2021). Regional anaesthesia: risk, consent and complications. *Anaesthesia*, **76 Suppl** 1, 18–26.
2. Bazzano LA, Durant J, Brantley PR (2021). A Modern History of Informed Consent and the Role of Key Information. *Ochsner J*, **21**(1), 81–5.
3. Yentis SM, Hartle AJ, Barker IR, et al. (2017). AAGBI: Consent for anaesthesia 2017: Association of Anaesthetists of Great Britain and Ireland. *Anaesthesia*, **72**(1), 93–105.
4. Orr T, Baruah R (2018). Consent in anaesthesia, critical care and pain medicine. *Brit J Anaesth Educ*, **18**(5), 135–9.
5. Silverman BD (2012). Physician behavior and bedside manners: the influence of William Osler and The Johns Hopkins School of Medicine. *Proc (Bayl Univ Med Cent)*, **25**(1), 58–61.
6. Arrow K, Burgoyne LL, Cyna AM (2022). Implications of nocebo in anaesthesia care. *Anaesthesia*, **77** Suppl 1, 11–20.
7. Chooi CS, White AM, Tan SG, Dowling K, Cyna AM (2013). Pain vs comfort scores after Caesarean section: a randomized trial. *Brit J Anaesth*, **110**(5), 780–7.
8. Amanzio M, Corazzini LL, Vase L, Benedetti F (2009). A systematic review of adverse events in placebo groups of anti-migraine clinical trials. *Pain*, **146**(3), 261–9.
9. Krauss BS (2015).'This may hurt': predictions in procedural disclosure may do harm. *Brit Med J (Clinical research ed)*, **350**, h649.
10. Lang EV, Hatsiopoulou O, Koch T, et al. (2005). Can words hurt? Patient-provider interactions during invasive procedures. *Pain*, **114**(1–2), 303–9.
11. Simmons S, Cyna AM (2017). 'Medicolegal' or 'patient-centred' consent? *Anaesthesia*, **72**(7), 917–8.
12. Huntington B, Kuhn N (2003). Communication gaffes: a root cause of malpractice claims. *Proc (Bayl Univ Med Cent)*, **16**(2), 157–61; discussion 61.
13. Babitu UQ, Cyna AM (2010). Patients' understanding of technical terms used during the pre-anaesthetic consultation. *Anaesth Int Care*, **38**(2), 349–53.
14. Morrison C, Munk R, Lo JJS, Przybylko T, Hughes R, Cyna AM (2019). Parental understanding of their child's risk of anaesthesia. *Brit J Anaesth*, **123**(1), e5–e6.
15. Guscoth LB, Cyna AM (2022). Nocebo language in anaesthetic patient written information. *Anaesthesia*, **77**(10), 1113–9.
16. Cheng WY, Cyna AM, Osborn KD (2007). Risks of regional anaesthesia for caesarean section: women's recall and information sources. *Anaesth Int Care*, **35**(1), 68–73.
17. Meurisse M, Hamoir E, Defechereux T, et al. (1999). Bilateral neck exploration under hypnosedation: a new standard of care in primary hyperparathyroidism? *Ann Surg*, **229**(3), 401–8.
18. Wong L, Cyna AM, Matthews G (2011). Rapid hypnosis as an anaesthesia adjunct for evacuation of postpartum vulval haematoma. *Aust N Z J Obstet Gynaecol*, **51**(3), 265–7.
19. Cyna AM, Simmons SW (2017). Guidelines on informed consent in anaesthesia: unrealistic, unethical, untenable … *Brit J Anaesth*, **119**(6), 1086–9.
20. Arrow K, Burgoyne LL, Cyna AM (2022). Implications of nocebo in anaesthesia care: a reply. *Anaesthesia*, **77**(8), 946.
21. Stanford SE, Bogod DG (2016). Failure of communication: a patient's story. *Int J Obstet Anesth*, **28**, 70–5.

22. McCombe K, Bogod DG (2018). Learning from the law. A review of 21 years of litigation for pain during caesarean section. *Anaesthesia*, **73**(2), 223–30.

23. Kwak KH (2017). Postdural puncture headache. *Korean J Anesthesiol*, **70**(2), 136–43.

24. McCombe K, Bogod DG (2020). Learning from the law. A review of 21 years of litigation for nerve injury following central neuraxial blockade in obstetrics. *Anaesthesia*, **75**(4), 541–8.

25. Cohen S (2014). The nocebo effect of informed consent. *Bioethics*, **28**(3), 147–54.

26. Yentis SM (2017). AAGBI Consent for Anaesthesia 2017 guidelines - a reply. *Anaesthesia*, **72**(5), 657–8.

27. GMC (2020). Shared decision making and consent are fundamental to good medical practice. Available at: https://www.gmc-uk.org/ethical-guidance/ethical-guidance-for-doctors/decision-making-and-consent/the-seven-principles-of-decision-making-and-consent. (Accessed 22 March 2023).

Chapter 8

Perioperative care

Suyin G.M. Tan, Andrew F. Smith,
and Allan M. Cyna

'Every breath you take, every move you make,
I'll be watching you.'
Sting

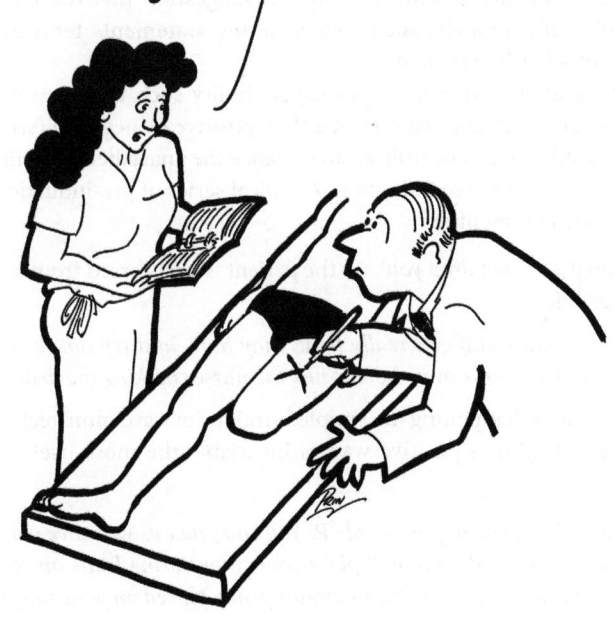

Hang on, Prof – the left foot can't be the right foot because the right foot's the only one left...

What this chapter is about

The perioperative period can be a life-changing event for many patients, the effects, for better or worse can be lifelong. The anaesthetist's communication at this time can have a profound impact on the care of patients in the matter of both short-term cooperation and long-term perceptions of their hospital experience.

Induction

Induction of anaesthesia is a stressful time for many patients. There is an inevitable loss of control when the patient hands this over temporarily to the anaesthetist. In order to enhance cooperation, anaesthetists will reap unexpected benefits by avoiding the use of negative language (see Chapter 3).[1] Well-meaning staff may, however, sabotage an otherwise smooth induction by telling patients, '*There is nothing to worry about*' with the implicit suggestion that there is '*something to worry about*'. Unfortunately, such well-meaning statements tend to yield the opposite effect of what is intended.

Patient stress at this time increases suggestibility such that comments frequently function as inadvertent suggestions—be they positive or negative (see Chapters 3, 4, and 23). Suggestibility can be utilized to enhance the anaesthetist's ability to provide a smooth, safe, and stress-free induction. A typical series of pre-induction communications may go something like,

> '*Don't worry we won't drop you*'. As the patient is transferred from a trolley to the operating table.

> '*The blood pressure cuff gets really tight, may hurt, and try not to move while it's pumping up. That noise over there is just the nurse checking the drill!*'

Explaining what is happening in simple, straightforward non-technical language, and communicating in a positive way, is invariably the more useful approach. For example:

> '*Welcome to the operating room, Mr P. You can relax as we move you to this other bed—you are quite safe. We will place some monitoring leads on so we can keep you safe and comfortable. A pulse monitor gently placed on your finger, an ECG on your chest and a blood pressure cuff on your arm. As the blood pressure cuff tightens and we take its reading this often allows patients to relax knowing how closely we are looking after them.*'

This is an indirect suggestion that the patient can relax as the blood pressure cuff tightens.

> *'Although operating rooms aren't the quietest places, all this activity is just everybody getting ready to ensure that things go smoothly, safely and, as comfortably as possible for you.'*

Cannulation

Although having an IV cannula inserted is usually straightforward for many patients, negative suggestions are frequently encountered in this context, and theatre staff may require training in how to avoid them. It is useful to ask the anxious patient to focus on a spot with the eyes directed away from the arm that is to be cannulated. Suggestions for subconscious *'arm anaesthesia'* (see Chapters 4 and 15) can be elicited in many patients to facilitate comfortable insertion.

Preoxygenation or inhalational induction

There are several strategies to consider when using a mask. Many patients feel more comfortable if they are allowed to hold the mask themselves. In any event, the anaesthetist should be wary of placing the mask on the patient's face without permission. It is helpful to avoid touching the face initially while the patient becomes familiar with the mask. This is an excellent time not only to inform patients of the benefits of oxygenation but also to link deep breathing with relaxation, and an element of control.

Preoxygenation presents the anaesthetist with an opportunity for some therapeutic suggestions. For example, the anaesthetist could say,

> *'The oxygen is full of goodness. Each time you take a deep breath in you can feel stronger, more in control. Each time you breathe out, feel yourself relax and become a little more comfortable as the mind drifts into a bit of a daydream.'*

As the patient breathes in, the anaesthetist can reinforce the effect by saying, *'That's right!'* *'Well done!'* *'Good! It's healthy to fill your lungs with oxygen'.*

Inhalational induction is commonly used with young children (see Chapter 11). Patients can be asked to take slow gentle breaths or, if they prefer, they can blow the gas away.

Propofol induction

Intravenous injection of propofol is frequently accompanied by a negative suggestion, *'This is going to sting!'* (see Chapter 3). An indirect positive suggestion might include something like, *'People sometimes feel a cool feeling, sometimes a warm feeling'.* A more neutral suggestion might be simply, *'You may feel something in a moment as you drift off to sleep',* or *'You will feel what you feel'.*

Communications at induction to enhance recovery

Asking patients about hobbies, work, sport, and other activities that they enjoy can be utilized. It can be suggested to patients that if they imagine doing their favourite activity as they drift off to sleep, they can wake up in recovery surprised that things went a little easier than they might have anticipated.[2]

> *'It's okay for you to go off to the beach or somewhere else you would rather be. When people take themselves to a favourite place or do a favourite activity they usually relax more easily and find themselves recovering more quickly.'*

Similarly, imagining enjoying a favourite food or drink during the induction can be suggested as facilitating eating and drinking as soon as the patient feels like it, postoperatively—an anti-emesis suggestion (see also Chapters 3 and 23). The anaesthetist can suggest, *'As people wake up from surgery, knowing that the problem has been dealt with allows them to appreciate that, as the wound heals, any sensations are telling them they are on the road to recovery'.*

If a urinary catheter or vaginal examination is required prior to induction in an anxious patient, it could be suggested that, *'As you breathe out you will find the legs flop apart without even thinking about it. There is nothing you need to try and do and nothing you need think about—as it will just seem to happen all on its own!'*

This suggestion frequently facilitates relaxation of the lower part of the body which the anaesthetist can re-enforce as soon as any positive responses become evident by saying something like *'Good!'*, *'Well done!'*, or *'That's right!'*

Eyes open or closed

During induction, some anaesthetists insist on asking patients to keep their eyes open for as long as they can. This can be uncomfortable for some patients and fails to give them an opportunity to develop an internal focus away from the external environment of the operating theatre with its bright lights, multiple personnel, and visible instruments of 'torture'.

A helpful communication might be, *'You can close your eyes if you wish and just take yourself somewhere you would rather be—perhaps a favourite holiday place or just somewhere comfortable at home if you prefer'.* Unconsciousness can be confirmed by asking the patient to take a deep breath and waiting for a response.

Communicating with patients during potentially painful procedures and during procedures under regional block is discussed in Chapters 10 and 23.

Using 'GREAT' in an emergency

One of the biggest problems in an emergency is that communication tends to break down and frequently is omitted altogether (see also Chapters 7, 10, and 17). It is at this time that clear communication and the use of a structured approach are at their most useful. The emergency version of '**GREAT**' (see Chapter 2) can be used to communicate effectively within the short time available.

Greeting

> **Dr G:** *'Hi, I am the anaesthetist, Dr S. Gonzales. I just wish to confirm, you are Mr Ian Extremis?'*
> **Dr G:** *'Do you know what operation you are having?'*
> **Mr E:** *'Yes, they are going to cut my belly to repair that big blood vessel.'*

Rapport

Dr G: '*We are doing everything we can to get you through this as safely and comfortably as possible.*'

Expectations

Dr G: '*I need to ask you some questions while I examine you so that the anaesthetic is as safe for you as it can be* ... Dr Gonzales performs a focused history and examination. *I understand that you have been told that this is a life-threatening illness and that we need to act quickly. We are very shortly going into the operating room and will be placing some monitoring, giving oxygen, blood, etc. ... As with any anaesthetic there are risks, but the biggest risk is that without treatment it is likely you will die.*'

Addressing concerns

Dr G: '*Do you want me to go into more detail about the anaesthetic risks?*'
Mr E: '*No, I know I've got to get this done.*'
Dr G: '*Are there any questions you wish to ask?*'
Mr E: '*Does my family know I am here?*'
Dr G: '*Yes, I've been told your wife is outside waiting to see you.*'

Tacit agreement

Mr E: '*I know you will do your best for me.*'
Dr G: '*We will. Thanks.*'

Inevitably in a crisis, there are a lot of communications occurring literally and metaphorically, over the patient's head. The important thing here is to remain aware that everything and anything said may be negatively misinterpreted or inadvertently suggested to the patient (see also Chapters 3, 12, 16, and 23).

Anaesthetist (referring to suction tubing): '*This one's buggered we may have to chuck it!*' **Patient** hears: '*I'm buggered and am going to die!*'

The same principles of communication apply whether for emergency or elective surgery. Explaining what is happening and reassuring patients that everything is being done to ensure their comfort and safety, will increase rapport and cooperation.

There is now good evidence that communicating with patients using therapeutic suggestions intraoperatively may be of value in improving recovery.[3]

Recovery

The recovery room, where patients can recover from anaesthesia and surgery and be cared for by specialist staff, has been developed as a dedicated area within the operating theatre complex. This section draws on the author's (AFS) own research and aims to raise awareness of the importance of communication in the recovery room or post-anaesthetic care unit (PACU).

The recovery room environment

The recovery room is seldom quiet and calm. Observations in the recovery room have revealed many activities, both clinical and non-clinical take place simultaneously.[4,5] Two main communication tasks are identified. Communicating with the patient emerging from anaesthesia and communication between staff.

Communication with patients

Effective communication must start with setting the right tone. Ideally, patients should return to consciousness in a quiet, softly lit environment, spoken to quietly, and with privacy and dignity maintained. It must be a cause for concern that awakening takes place with bright fluorescent lights directly in the supine patient's line of sight and is often accompanied by a tug-of-war with the patient's airway device sound-tracked by shouts of *'Open your mouth so I can take this tube out!'* Fortunately, awareness is still clouded by the residual effects of general anaesthesia. Although there are standards for staffing and equipment, published guidance is limited on how to talk to the patient emerging from anaesthesia.[5]

Recovery routines have been classified into *'functional'*, where the anaesthetist or nurse use talk to assess the patient's clinical state, or *'descriptive'*, where an attempt is made to describe to patients what they might expect to feel.

This might include helpful information such as, *'I'm just giving you some oxygen to breathe until you're properly awake'*. Patients should be allowed to wake up naturally with constant gentle reorientation. It is essential that patients are not repeatedly asked for *'pain scores'*.[6] Similarly, providing a vomit bag or sick bowl *'just in case'* may be a non-verbal cue to experience nausea or to vomit.

Communication between anaesthetists and recovery staff

Handing over has a number of functions. Within nursing, four have been identified.[7]

Informational—catching up on patients' progress, maintaining continuity of care.
Social—social or emotional support, stress relief.
Organizational—immediate plans for shift, controlled drugs, and prescriptions.
Educational—both explicit learning and enculturation.

Two further functions have been identified, *transfer of responsibility* and *checking or audit*.[4]

Nurses and anaesthetists may have differing expectations and sometimes conflicting agendas for handover. The anaesthetist may be more concerned with the next patient on the list and may simply trust the recovery nurse to 'pick up' what needs to be known. The nurse, on the other hand, is coming to the patient fresh and with no prior knowledge and wants to be satisfied that all the information necessary to do a good job has been communicated.

This transfer of responsibility does not always coincide with the transfer of information. Anwari surveyed 276 patients admitted to the PACU.[8] Professional behaviour had four elements:

- whether the anaesthetist stayed to see the first set of monitor readings;
- whether the patient was left in a satisfactory and stable condition;
- whether the anaesthetist returned to review the patient; and
- whether clear instructions for the recovery room care were given.

Anaesthetists perform well on the professional behaviour element but are less likely to hand over all information sought.[8] The Australian and New Zealand College of Anaesthetists (ANZCA) have provided recommendations for good handover practice (see also Chapter 17). Despite evidence of the increased morbidity and mortality associated with handover,[9] neither the ANZCA[10] nor the Association of Anaesthetists in the UK guidelines refer specifically to how to optimize communication during handover.

Using 'GREAT' to structure the acute pain round

In terms of communication skills, the pain round is the clinical context which requires the most of an anaesthetist. Although the doctor–patient interaction is the focus, it is equally important to remember that communication occurs between members of the pain team and the patient's 'home team'. This particularly applies to written documentation of management plans and drug regimes. The aim of the interactions with patients on the pain round is to ensure adequate analgesia, recognize and treat side effects, promote patient recovery, reassure, and comfort patients, and respond to queries or concerns they may have.

Greeting

The first step is to orientate oneself to the patients—know their names, the procedure they have undergone, and what their analgesic regimens are. Ask patients what they like being called. Secondly, the environment should be optimized. It is never ideal to conduct a pain round assessment through the shower door! Distractions such as the TV should be eliminated where possible. Having confirmed a patient's identity and introduced oneself, the next step is to explain the purpose of the consultation.

> 'Hello Mrs Brown, I'm Dr James from the Anaesthetic Department. Our team visits people after their operations to make sure that they are **comfortable** ...'

Careful choice of words helps to avoid negative suggestions which can increase the patient's awareness and expectation of pain.

> 'Hello Mrs Brown, I'm Dr James from the **Pain** Service, I've come to see how much **pain** you are in ...'

This generates a totally different expectation. It is not uncommon to see patients who have been happily watching TV, or chatting on the phone, suddenly begin to wince and grimace once you introduce yourself as the 'Pain Doctor' and start asking for 'Pain scores!' Subconsciously they are responding to the expectation that they should have pain and this is likely to augment rather than diminish symptoms.[11,12]

Rapport

Rather than asking, '*How much pain have you got?*' or '*Where does it hurt?*' Other statements that can be far more helpful in increasing rapport, utilize open-ended questions such as,

> '*How are you feeling this morning?*'

This gives patients the opportunity to talk about issues that concern them rather than the doctor setting the agenda. Often patients will utilize this opportunity to air concerns regarding procedures or other aspects of their illness, rather than pain.

Expectations

The efficacy of the analgesia regimen, the presence or absence of side effects and relevant physical examination such as checking the epidural site, make up this part of the interaction. An assessment of patients' physical capacity to mobilize and cough or breathe deeply adds a further indication of their degree of comfort. Patients are often uncertain as to what to expect, and offering a brief, positive description of the postoperative course is useful to many patients.

> **Anaesthetist:** '*It's now the third day since your operation Mr Smith and I can see you are doing well. You've been up to the shower and you have had your drain removed. I think that by tomorrow you will be drinking and eating and we will be able to replace the PCA with some tablets.*'

Generating positive, realistic expectations of a patient's progress is a powerful way to assist recovery.

Addressing concerns

Enquiring of patients, '*What can we do to make you more comfortable?*' often elicits complaints about urinary catheters and nasogastric tubes rather than a request for more analgesia. Obviously, if patients have inadequate analgesia this should be addressed immediately and any changes in the analgesic regimen explained to them. The ability to reframe a patient's experience in a positive way is very helpful in eliciting a therapeutic effect.

> **Patient:** '*Doctor, I feel terrible—really nauseated—I don't think I can keep anything down ...*'
> **Anaesthetist:** '*That's okay, Mrs Brown, I note the surgeons have reviewed you this morning and are pleased with your progress. Lots of people feel like this after surgery. Just remember you haven't eaten for more than 24 hours. A body needs fuel to keep it going and to heal wounds. Perhaps you might feel better if you have a little something to settle your stomach.*'

It is important to ensure that a surgical complication is unlikely. In this therapeutic communication the doctor is reframing the patient's nausea as a need for the body to have food.

There is an acknowledgement of the complaint, '*That's okay*' followed by a general statement, '*lots of people*'. This is then followed by a more specific and yet generally true statement regarding the patient's need for food. Having engaged the patient's subconscious responses of '*Yes*' to the preceding statements, the suggestion that eating may be beneficial is more easily accepted by both the conscious and subconscious mind. This also allows the patient to take a more active role in controlling their nausea rather than being a passive recipient of ondansetron.

Some anaesthetists may throw up their hands in horror and think, '*Why not just give some anti-emetic?*'

Yes, anti-emetics do work, but may cause side effects and often are no more effective than a placebo. The generation of positive expectation of the treatment, usually by suggestion, is the key to eliciting a therapeutic effect.[12] So, whether the patient has some food or some ondansetron, or even both, the suggestion that '*Something will settle the stomach*' is likely to help.

Symptoms such as pain and nausea, the two problems most commonly encountered on the pain round, are inherently subjective, have a strong emotional subconscious component and are therefore usually most amenable to therapeutic suggestion (see Chapters 3, 4, and 23).

Tacit agreement

The interaction ends with a tacit understanding that the patient's needs have been met and that follow-up will ensure that this is maintained.

> **Anaesthetist:** '*Okay, Mrs Brown, it seems we are both comfortable with that! Dr Smith will be reviewing you tomorrow and we are happy to call by anytime you feel we can help.*'

Some dos and don'ts

- Don't ignore or belittle patients' concerns or complaints.
- Do listen to what they have to say, even if it appears irrelevant or minor, acknowledge the problem and check that you have understood. '*So the way I understand it is—you've been having difficulties getting the nurses on night duty to give you the oxycodone.*'
- Do be careful when 'normalizing' a patient's experience. While informing a patient what to expect postoperatively, and thereby taking the opportunity to generate positive expectations, it is important that pain and nausea are ***not*** presented as inevitable, and therefore 'normal'.

'*Well of course the chest drain is excruciatingly painful for the first couple of days, but once it's out, you will feel much better!*'

This is seeding the idea that the pain won't go until the drain is removed. The subconscious often latches onto these seemingly innocuous comments, so be aware that words can hurt but words can also heal (see Chapter 3).

Or preferably,

'After your operation, the chest drain is usually left in for a couple of days. Everyone feels differently—some people take a while to get up and about, but most people are comfortable enough to get up and shower the next day'.

◆ Do allow the patient autonomy in controlling symptoms. A blood pressure of 230/120 mmHg requires treatment even if the patient is asymptomatic. A pain score of 6/10 or even 8/10 isn't quite the same thing.[11] Often the process of acknowledging symptoms, excluding underlying pathology (e.g. wound haematoma), reassuring the patient and discussing treatment options helps to allay patient anxiety and relieves distress.

While analgesic pharmacotherapy should be given where indicated, the use of therapeutic communication and the generation of positive expectations is likely to help enhance analgesic efficacy as well as diminish side effects.[13]

Key points

1. Communications with patients at induction can have a profound impact on anaesthetic care in both short-term cooperation and long-term perceptions of their hospital experience.

2. Anaesthetists and patients will reap unexpected benefits by avoiding negative language at induction.

3. Patients emerging from anaesthesia should expect a calm, quiet environment with reassurance and reorientation.

4. A good handover to recovery staff is essential if patient risk is to be minimized.

5. A structured communication on the pain round enhances the quality of anaesthetist–patient interactions.

6. Communication generating positive expectancy is likely to augment analgesia and recovery.

References

1. Arrow K, Burgoyne LL, Cyna AM (2022). Implications of nocebo in anaesthesia care. *Anaesthesia*, **77 Suppl 1**, 11–20.

2. Evans C, Richardson PH (1988). Improved recovery and reduced postoperative stay after therapeutic suggestions during general anaesthesia. *Lancet*, 2(8609), 491–3.

3. Nowak H, Zech N, Asmussen S, et al. (2020). Effect of therapeutic suggestions during general anaesthesia on postoperative pain and opioid use: multicentre randomised controlled trial. *Brit Med J*, **371**, m4284.

4. Smith AF, Pope C, Goodwin D, Mort M (2008). Interprofessional handover and patient safety in anaesthesia: observational study of handovers in the recovery room. *Br J Anaesth*, **101**(3), 332–7.

5. Smith AF, Pope C, Goodwin D, Mort M (2005). Communication between anesthesiologists, patients and the anesthesia team: a descriptive study of induction and emergence. *Can J Anaesth*, **52**(9), 915–20.

6. Chooi CS, White AM, Tan SG, Dowling K, Cyna AM (2013). Pain vs comfort scores after Caesarean section: a randomized trial. *Brit J Anaesth*, **110**(5), 780–7.

7. Kerr MP (2002). A qualitative study of shift handover practice and function from a socio-technical perspective. *J Adv Nurs*, **37**(2), 125–34.

8. Anwari JS (2002). Quality of handover to the postanaesthesia care unit nurse. *Anaesthesia*, **57**(5), 488–93.

9. Jones PM, Cherry RA, Allen BN, et al. (2018). Association between handover of anesthesia care and adverse postoperative outcomes among patients undergoing major surgery. *JAMA*, **319**(2), 143–53.

10. Baker AB (2008). Patient responsibility and the anaesthetist. *ANZCA Bulletin*, **17**(2), 12–13.

11. Nguyen T, Slater P, Cyna AM (2009). Open vs specific questioning during anaesthetic follow-up after Caesarean section. *Anaesthesia*, **64**(2), 156–60.

12. Schweiger A, Parducci A (1981). Nocebo: the psychologic induction of pain. *Pavlov J Biol Sci*, **16**(3), 140–3.

13. Pollo A, Benedetti F (2009). The placebo response: neurobiological and clinical issues of neurological relevance. *Prog Brain Res*, **175**, 283–94.

Chapter 9

Pain

Meredith J. Craigie and Mark P. Jensen

'If you are distressed by anything external, the pain is not due to the thing itself, but to your estimate of it; and this you have the power to revoke at any moment.'
Marcus Aurelius

What this chapter is about

The conundrum of talking about pain

Pain is essential for survival. It is one of many protective outputs of the brain enabling us to exist and even thrive in the highly complex environments in which we live.[1] Yet despite pain's life-saving role, it is almost always perceived as unpleasant and undesirable. Pain is hard to ignore, and accommodating chronic pain can be extremely challenging.

Almost everyone experiences pain, yet no two people ever have the same pain experience. A range of factors, including genetics, biological sex, gender, thoughts and emotions, attentional biases, learning history, values, and beliefs, can all influence the experience of pain, with or without a noxious stimulus. Pain occurs within a social context and has social implications; yet it remains a personal, subjective, and multidimensional experience (Box 9.1). Communicating our experience of pain can be difficult; it sometimes requires complex strategies to alert others and obtain the desired assistance. We all know about pain. But in reality, this knowledge is limited to our own experiences.

Box 9.1 International Association for the Study of Pain's definition of pain

The International Association for the Study of Pain states that pain is:

An unpleasant sensory and emotional experience associated with, or resembling that associated with, actual or potential tissue damage and is expanded upon by the addition of six key notes:

◆ Pain is always a personal experience that is influenced to varying degrees by biological, psychological, and social factors.

◆ Pain and nociception are different phenomena. Pain cannot be inferred solely from activity in sensory neurons.

◆ Through their life experiences, individuals learn the concept of pain.

◆ A person's report of an experience as pain should be respected.

◆ Although pain usually serves an adaptive role, it may have adverse effects on function and social and psychological well-being.

◆ Verbal description is only one of several behaviours to express pain; inability to communicate does not negate the possibility that a human or a nonhuman animal experiences pain[3].

Adapted with permission from Raja SN, et al., 'The revised International Association for the Study of Pain definition of pain: concepts, challenges, and compromises', *Pain*, 161, 9, 1976–82, Copyright International Association for the Study of Pain, 2020. https://journals.lww.com/pain/abstract/2020/09000/the_revised_international_association_for_the.6.aspx

One's understanding of pain is embedded in one's mental representations. These evolve throughout life in a dynamic, iterative manner in response to interactions with our environment. We develop complex models of pain that include image schemas and linguistic concepts, embedded in cultural traditions and socially defined interactions.[2] These working models influence interactions between the person with pain and those from whom help is sought.

In healthcare, however, the care provider's conceptual models and language evolve in response to education and clinical experience with pain and are often shaped by the paradigms of a clinician's health discipline. Differences in paradigms can potentially create and exacerbate a communication gap, as many clinicians may use a language not shared by those outside their discipline.

It is therefore not surprising that it can be challenging to find common ground for communication between the person with pain and healthcare providers. The most recent definition of pain offered by the International Association for the Study of Pain[3] aims to define this common ground. Although it is perhaps the most comprehensive definition to date, not all find it acceptable. The presence of qualifiers and explanatory notes of the definition reflects the complexity of the experience of pain,[4] which makes it all the more important to seek to understand patients' pain from their perspective.

Contrary conversations about pain in healthcare settings

Many people experience interactions with healthcare systems as 'an adversarial struggle'.[5] In the past, providers had a limited understanding of the importance of communication in healthcare and the motivating forces underlying this communication.[6] Discrepancies leading to dissatisfaction exist between patients' and health practitioners' expectations that can impact treatment choices and outcomes.[7] Healthcare providers do not always understand why patients do not carry out instructions, especially in the management of chronic health conditions. However, if the desired outcome is not immediately obvious, patients may not follow instructions because they do not think they are essential at that point. In reality, people will only willingly do something consistent with their own goals and values.[7,8]

Problems can arise when the healthcare provider fails to explore and understand the values of the person with pain, especially when these differ from their own. Healthcare providers may place a premium on being seen as knowledgeable about medical matters and having good technical skills. They may value the biomedical model of pain and therefore focus more on diagnosing and treating 'finding and fixing' a medical problem, focusing less on the whole person. Thus, active management of pain may be a low priority, and the health care plan may not address the patient's most important needs. Preconceived ideas about how much pain should be experienced in a particular situation, often arising from personal experiences, family modelling, and other social and cultural constructs, can complicate the problem. Formal teaching during tertiary education in healthcare adds another layer of preconception, often depending on the paradigms of that discipline.

Communication can be thought of as a combination of behavioural and verbal strategies. Behaviours include body language, the extent and nature of eye contact, facial expressions, posture, and movement towards or away from the other person. Verbal strategies include the use of specific words, as well as vocalizations such as moaning, crying, or screaming.

Verbal language is critical in communication about pain. Words can promote a sense of control and enable healing, or they can frighten and disempower. Therefore, healthcare providers must recognize and understand the effects of the various language constructs used in communication about pain.

What patients tell us about pain and how do they do it?

Patients with pain rely primarily on verbal language to communicate their experiences and obtain emotional support and professional help.[8] However, both patients and their healthcare providers commonly report problematic communications resulting in patients feeling misunderstood and disbelieved.[5,7,8]

The language of pain is steeped in the use of metaphor and simile that attract the listener's attention. This can explain poorly understood concepts, and provide a basis for shared understanding.[9] It has been argued that pain is an embodied experience and that the use of metaphor facilitates empathy by eliciting a simulation of the speaker's pain experience.[10] The likelihood of producing the desired response may depend on the nature of the metaphor and its detail, creativity, and textual complexity. Many factors, including biological sex, gender, age, and time from the injury, or onset of the pain-provoking illness, also influence the metaphor[11] (see Chapter 5).

Metaphors and similes can be considered helpful, dependant on patient and context.[6] Descriptors based on concepts of tissue damage or the metaphor of 'pain as a personal attack'[11] are frequently used by patients. Some of the most common are presented in Box 9.2. They may start with a simple analogy that engages the listener and then layers of more complex or extreme imagery are built. Some similes and metaphors

---

Box 9.2 Examples of metaphors and similes used by patients with pain

Pain as reflecting tissue damage

A sharp stabbing, twisting pain

Pain is a red-hot poker

Burning, searing pain

A gnawing pain in the stomach

Pins and needles

Stomach tied in knots

Headache like head in a vice

Blinding headache

Pain as personal attack

My feet are killing me

Pain is the devil

Switches flicking on and off

Neuropathic pain is purgatory

Pain like a lightning strike

Something crawling inside

Like pouring hot water on the skin

Pain is a punishment

show that patients consider their pain separate from themselves, indicating an external locus of control.[11]

Although such metaphors allow patients to communicate the severity of their experiences, they can also contribute to greater pain severity, feelings of victimhood, and reinforced fears. One communication goal would be to help the patient reframe these metaphors and similes into descriptors that are less affect-laden. When possible, clinicians can offer alternative pain descriptors when speaking with patients such as, '*uncomfortable sensations*' or '*feelings you would like to change*'. Communication about pain qualities also provides the opportunity to suggest or seed the idea that these qualities can and do change.

For example, if a patient says, '*This stabbing pain is killing me!*', the clinician might say, '*Wow! That sounds really scary. It sounds like one of the goals of treatment would be to change the quality of these sensations to something softer—like a dull feeling or even more comfortable*'.

Painful communications

Experiencing pain can be frightening for many people, and fear is a powerful driver of behaviour. Healthcare providers may not be aware of their patients' fears or how easily a patient may become afraid just by hearing a single careless word or phrase. What may seem like an innocuous comment, not even remembered by the healthcare provider, can be so alarming that the patient is unable to remember anything else from the conversation. Even if one healthcare provider communicates well, thoughtless words from another may sabotage the message and undo earlier understandings (see Chapters 3 and 23).

During training, healthcare providers learn structured rituals for history-taking and physical examination. However, much less time is devoted to considering language and its structure. A typical example is the use of closed questions early in a consultation. Closed questions invite a single answer—often, '*Yes!*' or '*No!*' Such questions can interfere with meaningful communication, especially when dealing with complex or challenging topics.[12] Similarly, knowing a discipline's technical language is considered essential for healthcare providers. Over time this discipline-specific language becomes incorporated into the healthcare provider's daily language. However, using technical terms when talking to patients about pain, for example to describe '*nociceptive pathways*' or '*pain processing*', can be annoying and unhelpful, causing confusion rather than clarity.[13]

There are also many words and metaphors commonly used by healthcare providers that are demeaning, unhelpful, and disempowering, including '*sufferer*', '*victim*', '*attention-seeker*', and '*catastrophizer*'.[14] Metaphors can also paint graphic and frightening pictures, worst-case scenarios, or simply not help patients understand their pain experience. Some metaphors that the authors have heard colleagues say that are less than helpful are listed in Table 9.1 together with alternative comments.

Healthcare providers might assume that everyone understands what the term 'chronic pain' means. Patients, however, usually view pain as a symptom rather than a diagnosis[13] and may be perplexed by the absence of focus on diagnosis or specific

Table 9.1 Unhelpful metaphors commonly used in healthcare consultations

Words that clinicians use that could exaggerate or promote fear	Say instead ...
'The worst case I have ever seen'	'I have seen many cases like this. I think we can come up with **a plan** that **will help you be able to do more and hurt less.**'
'A slipped/crushed/blown out disc'	'The results of your scan are within normal range for someone of your age.'
'Collapsed ankle joint/arches/vertebra' 'The X-ray shows bone-on-bone' 'A pinched nerve in the back'	'The results of the scan suggest some ideas about what might be contributing to your pain. We have **treatments** that **can help strengthen the muscles, tendons, and structures that could help.**'
'Wear and tear'	'What you describe is common. We have treatments that can help strengthen the muscles tendons and structures that could help.'
'There's no choice; we have to operate'	Simply do not say this. There is **always** a choice!
'You'll have to learn to accept your pain'	'I think we can come up with a plan **that will help you do more and hurt less**.'
Words that deny a person's experience of pain	**Say instead ...**
'The surgery went well, so you shouldn't have that much pain'	'What you describe is common for someone who has had the surgery you had. Now is the time to come up with a pain management plan that **will help you be more comfortable**.'
'You should be used to it by now' 'It can't be that bad' 'I've seen worse cases' 'There's nothing to see on the scan' 'You're looking really well today' (said in the context of a patient reporting severe pain)	Do not make any of these comments. Instead communicate an understanding of the patient's experience, and provide a realistic hope for change. For example, 'I understand that the pain is bad now. I have seen this before—you are not alone. I have also seen patients in this situation get better. Shall we work towards that?'

curative treatment. Perhaps even more importantly, the idea that the pain will be present forever, which is implied by the term 'chronic pain', may not only be inaccurate but also provoke feelings of helplessness and despair.

Healthcare practitioners use metaphors to explain pain concepts and pain management plans, goals, and outcomes. The 'body as machine' is a prevalent metaphor.[6] It implies that, like a machine, every pain or ailment is an indication of damage, perhaps at the pain location, and like a machine, it can be fixed with the correct procedure or part replacement. This analogy becomes increasingly counterproductive when pain transitions from acute to chronic. For chronic pain, the source of any breakdown is often unclear, and purely biomedical treatments are unlikely to be curative. Yet the expectation for a cure remains, often leading to patient dissatisfaction with healthcare providers who may, in turn, feel frustrated, and blame the patient for not trying hard enough to 'get well'.[7]

Indeed, patients often view the persistence of pain as an indication that somebody did not fix the original problem correctly and that harm is ongoing. They may also believe that persistent pain means that the body will continue to break down, just like any machine that is not appropriately maintained. As a result, patients may seek multiple opinions and invasive treatments without resolution of the problem. Critically, healthcare providers who continue to use a 'body as machine' paradigm to manage persistent pain are likely to do more harm than good.

Metaphors involving negative or unpleasant descriptors are often used in conversations about pain. For example, the military metaphor of 'medicine is war' invokes concepts of struggle, weaponry, and battle; neurological metaphors of electrical circuits, keys and wires; and penetrating physical damage with sharp, hot objects dominate community and medical discourse (see Chapter 5). The simplification of pain into such mechanistic metaphors emphasizes the physiological to the detriment of pain's psychological and social aspects. It also ignores the role that contextual factors have on the experience and impact of pain. It does little to boost patients' self-efficacy, reduce anxiety, or quell worry and catastrophic thinking. On the other hand, some religious metaphors are positive and can promote acceptance and transcendence, helping to facilitate a pathway to recovery.

Healthcare providers' questions arising from the 'physician as expert' metaphor may have an accusatory tone and run the risk of eliciting defensive responses. For example: '*Why haven't you started an exercise programme?*'

Helpful communication to facilitate recovery from pain

Many commonly used paradigms come with significant limitations and risks, nicely summarized by the statement that '*health professionals who focus on fixing the damage/ disease but ignore the worried, help-seeking persons, do so at their peril*'.[6] However, developing an effective therapeutic relationship requires the healthcare provider to think and communicate beyond the biomedical framework.

Good foundations for communications about pain involve the healthcare provider being curious about the experiences of the patient, having feelings of compassion for them, and an awareness of the impact of their language. Having a clear structure to guide the conduct of consultations can be very useful, especially when they are likely to be challenging. However, the classical medical model of history-taking could be viewed as an inadequate framework for many consultations with persons experiencing pain.

The 'LAURS' model

Listening

Resisting the temptation to interrupt can be a particular challenge for healthcare providers.[15] Being present and actively listening without interrupting, provides the space for patients to share the narrative about their pain experience and feel like they have been heard, sometimes for the first time. In one study, the median time to the first interruption by the physician was 11 seconds (ranging from 3 to 234 seconds), with specialists interrupting more frequently than primary care physicians.[16]

Carefully crafted open questions may guide further exploration of that history and establish the patients' agenda, including their goals for the consultation. However, in the study by Singh Ospina et al., physicians elicited a patient's agenda in only 36% of primary care consultations and 20% of specialist consultations.[16] Perceived time pressures may drive this behaviour. When allowed to speak uninterrupted, most patients finish speaking within two minutes. Missing an opportunity to elicit patients' concerns about their pain may lead to assumptions, over-investigation, and unnecessary, ineffective, or even harmful treatments.

Healthcare providers often use **closed** questions in the misguided belief that this will ensure a more focused and efficient conversation. However, **open** questions invite the person with pain to tell their story, enabling much more to be learnt in a similar time. In short, the clinician who listens more during the interview learns much more than the clinician who speaks more. The words the patients choose, how they use them, and their tone of voice provides a wealth of information about how they perceive themselves, their emotional responses, resources, and their self-efficacy for implementing treatment plans.

For example, a question like, '*What do you think is causing your pain?*', especially when followed by, '*Tell me more about that ...*', will identify the patients' beliefs about the cause of their pain (e.g. '*a pinched nerve*', '*a bulging disc*', '*nerve damage*'). Firmly held beliefs may be consistent with what physicians have told the patient in the past. However, responding to such a key open question may identify concerns and fears that can interfere with progress. Open questions also provide important clues about the amount of reassurance the patient may need as treatment progresses.[17,18]

Most people use a variety of strategies, some of which may be useful, lead to less pain, and more function in the long term (e.g. regular exercise), while others are less helpful (e.g. pain-contingent rest or analgesic medication use), or possibly harmful in the long run.[19,20]

Helpful **open** questions could include, '*What would you like to get out of today's consultation?*' or, '*What concerns you most about your pain problem?*' A request to share experiences can be another way to indicate readiness to listen (e.g. '*Tell me about your pain*'). Other **open** questions like, '*How do you manage a pain flare-up?*' can be used to explore specific aspects of the person's day-to-day pain management choices. **Closed** questions early in the conversation are likely to shut down communication but can be helpful later when brief, specific answers are needed. For example, '*Are you still taking this medication?*'

Acceptance

Acceptance involves having a non-judgemental attitude while maintaining a calm acceptance of what the patient has to say, and being prepared to be corrected if there are misunderstandings expressed during the interaction. A reflective statement responding to a person complaining loudly about a lack of pain relief might be, '*It sounds like you're looking for an approach that could provide you with some pain relief*'. It is vital to follow such reflections as a 'best guess' of patients' experiences, with a pause giving them an opportunity to expand on this idea and clarify their needs.

Acceptance of what patients are saying can be very helpful, letting them know by reflecting back what you are hearing, you are attempting to understand. This is not the same as agreeing with the patient or encouraging harmful behaviour. Acceptance in this context acknowledges emotions, thoughts, and behaviours as they are. Patients can then be encouraged to focus on their more helpful responses and understand, and perhaps discourage, responses that are less helpful.

Compassion, a concept closely related to acceptance, involves seeking to promote and prioritize patient well-being, needs, and wishes[21,22] and to lessen feelings of rejection. By understanding the patient's perspective supporting their autonomy and affirming their strengths and efforts, the healthcare provider can assist patients experience therapeutic change (see section 'Motivational interviewing').

Utilization

Healthcare providers can utilize a person's descriptions or concerns about pain to identify a solution. This can be particularly helpful in the acute pain setting where pain can be used as a guide and motivator for increasing appropriate activity during recovery. Based on past experience, patients with chronic pain often express the fear that pain will worsen with increased activity. They may also believe that pain is a sign of physical damage. These fears can be acknowledged and utilized as reasons to gradually become more active. The healthcare provider could say, '*Your previous experiences make sense because muscles become weak and joints stiffen up after long periods of resting. So when you do even a small task, it can hurt. Any increased pain is actually a sign that a reactivation and strengthening programme is needed. Gentle activity programmes strengthen the muscles and lubricate the joints, reducing the risk of pain getting worse. The research is clear: maintaining an appropriate activity level reduces pain for most people in the long run*'.

The example above utilizes the pain experience as a strategy to identify appropriate activity goals. As an example of the utilization of a patient's metaphor about the pain, a patient might describe their pain as feeling like their '*stomach feels like a rope that is tied into knots*' (Box 9.2). The clinician could then say, '*A lot of patients tell me that they feel like the pain is a giant knot or their stomach is tied up in knots*'. This is very important to know, because patients can then be asked, '*What will loosen and relax the knots? And you know, we actually have many options. One is relaxation training, with which you can learn to get control over the feelings of tightness anywhere in the body. Another is the use of very focused stretching and strengthening exercises, because weak and tight muscles are more likely to get knotted up than stretched and strong ones. Some patients choose to both learn relaxation strategies and engage in a systematic strengthening and stretching programme ... What do you think?'*

Reframing

Escalating distress is common when pain does not resolve quickly or becomes more severe over time. Expressions of concern can be reframed to make the perception of pain more positive. For example, a person with persistent pain following knee replacement surgery may express concerns about an exercise programme. The response could be reframed as, *'Each time the pain increases a little when you do your exercises, your body is telling you that you are working hard towards recovery'.*

With reframing comes rephrasing. Healthcare practitioners can take on the role of coach, helping their patients rephrase a more realistic and reassuring inner monologue. Careful listening will enable the identification of unrealistic and alarming thoughts—thoughts that can reinforce a negative self-view and the accompanying negative emotions such as shame, fear, frustration, and resentment. Even simply changing a few words can effect significant change.

As an example, for the person stopping an activity early due to pain saying to themselves, *'It's ridiculous that I can't do this. I used to be able to do it before',* the clinician might say, *'It's ridiculous to think that I can do this right now without completing the exercise programme AND other recommended treatments. In the same way that it is ridiculous to expect an infection will be resolved after two doses of antibiotics without completing the course of treatment'.* Such rephrases can nurture a new inner dialogue, which can then facilitate the addition of a more supportive thought such as, *'I will be able to get stronger and stronger over time'.* Such thoughts are more likely to result in emotions that encourage resilience and persistence. (See also discussion of dealing with resistance in the section on motivational interviewing, later in this chapter.)

Suggestion

Patients bring their expectations and hopes, their memories of past consultations, and their emotions to the current consultation. By appealing to these thoughts and feelings, suggestion can be a strategy of gently inserting either directly or indirectly a new idea or observation that encourages the patient to consider an alternative view, therapeutic approach, or way of coping. Patients with pain and high levels of anxiety or distress are particularly responsive to suggestion. In response to the patient's stated goal of managing agitation or stress better, a direct suggestion might take the form of, *'You might be surprised how easy mindfulness mediation is to learn and how much calmer it will help you feel'.* Sharing information about other patients' experiences provides an indirect suggestion to a patient that they could expect a similar outcome.

For example, saying *'Patients who have stopped their opioids tell me that they can think more clearly, they are less sleepy, their mood is better, they don't need to take laxatives, and they generally feel a lot better. And their pain did not get worse; for some it was even less'.* This can encourage a patient to start an opioid tapering plan to counter concerns about medication withdrawal symptoms and increasing pain.

The 'GREAT' template

The 'Great' template (see Chapter 2) provides a simple yet comprehensive framework for conducting more effective conversations in any pain setting.

Greeting

Courteously greeting the patient along with any accompanying persons (e.g. family member or another support person), and politely acknowledging their relationships, sets the scene for a respectful encounter. Showing genuine curiosity and sensitivity towards the patient and whoever is with them at the start of the conversation, is more likely to facilitate a healthy therapeutic alliance and to identify goals.

Trust is essential for developing effective therapeutic relationships. As the healthcare provider approaches, the person seeking help looks for clues about the nature of the healthcare provider and whether they are trustworthy.[23] Likewise, healthcare providers are also observing patients to determine their trustworthiness. High levels of suspicion about the authenticity of complaints of pain are common, especially when pain has persisted for longer than expected.[24] Patient characteristics affecting pain and authenticity include sex, gender identity, age, ethnicity, facial features, likeability, and manner. Awareness of these contributors to unconscious, positive and negative, bias may enable healthcare providers to be more open-minded and to choose their words thoughtfully.

Rapport

Developing a harmonious working relationship is critical, especially in chronic pain settings. Establishing an achievable pain management plan is more likely when patients feel cared for and listened to. This is facilitated when the patient feels believed, their situation understood, and their health issues managed in ways that suit their needs. Utilizing the principles of 'LAURS', noted earlier, enables healthcare providers to develop rapport rapidly.

Expectations

A question like, 'What are you hoping to get out of today's visit?' can start the conversation.

A key element of communication with the patient is to evaluate the status of their experience and responses to current and previous pain management strategies. The detail required depends on the context, the goals of the interaction and the time available. Information gathering needs to be targeted and efficient, especially in the acute pain setting.

Communication continues into the next phase of the encounter, the examination. The healthcare provider should conduct a pain-orientated physical examination, including pain-orientated sensory testing.[25] It should be conducted with curiosity and open questions so that points from the history are clarified and reports of pain correlated with the physical findings. An **open** question like 'How does this feel?' compared with a **closed** one such as 'Does this hurt?' is more likely to elicit the patient's authentic experience. Areas of pain should not be tested repeatedly, as this may lead to pain exacerbations, which are likely to undermine the patient's confidence.

Patients will have a range of expectations influencing their satisfaction with the encounter.[26] An explanation for the pain consistent with contemporary pain science can lead to an improved understanding of the pain problem and validation that the **pain is real**—an essential outcome of a beneficial encounter.[26] Expectations of outcomes can be utilized therapeutically, employing the 'LAURS' framework.

As it can be challenging to explain pain in layman's language, healthcare providers frequently resort to metaphors to explain various aspects of the pain experience. In most clinical encounters, the person with pain may expect a diagnosis or at least an explanation of their pain experience.[7] Verbal metaphors such as, '*Pain is a complex multi-layered experience*' and '*Pain is a disease*' can be helpful in these encounters.[6]

Butler and Moseley's '*Pain is a protective mechanism*' is a newer metaphor replacing '*Pain is a danger signal*'.[1] This metaphor can be very helpful in acute pain settings to encourage engagement in rehabilitation and expanded in chronic pain settings to, '*Chronic pain is the result of an overprotective system*', encouraging a change of focus thus making the system less protective. These metaphors provide the basis for further understanding of the person's experience of pain by providing a framework for them to identify the actions, relationships, or therapies that increase or decrease their pain.

Addressing concerns

Offering an opportunity to ask questions allows the patient to express concerns not yet elicited or to clarify the treatment options before a draft management plan is made. It helps to avoid falling into the trap of assuming the person understood the plan, its reasons, and any technical language used. Acknowledging and directly addressing concerns can assure the person with pain that they have been heard and understood and that the healthcare provider is open to answering any questions. This makes it less likely that the patient will maintain the status quo through misunderstandings or fear.

Tacit agreement

Towards the end of the consultation, it is helpful to summarize what the patient has said and confirm the agreed plan with the patient. Summaries can be valuable for helping patients to understand their own '*Big picture*', a view that can provide them with the perspective they need to move forward.[17, 27] An accurate summary of, '*Where we go from here*' represents a tacit agreement that a therapeutic relationship has been formed. A balance of key ideas and options that support behaviour change while acknowledging ambivalence allows the patient to participate in ongoing decisions around their care.

Motivational interviewing

In contemporary pain management, the patient is often asked to change their behaviour to manage pain more effectively and become more functional. Engaging in the rehabilitation process takes a great deal of motivation and trust. Self-motivated lifestyle change is easily recommended but can be very challenging to put into action.

Motivational interviewing (MI) was developed specifically to seed and nurture motivation for positive behaviour change.[28] MI allows patients to voice ambivalence about a specific and challenging behaviour change while focusing on values and long-term goals.

It draws together many of the principles of 'LAURS'. These strategies include:

(1) asking open questions involving skilful **Listening**;

(2) affirming the patient with **Acceptance** of their behaviours and attitudes;

(3) skilfully reflecting back to the patient what the patient has communicated—**Utilizing** change talk that includes **Reframing**; and

(4) summarizing the key ideas expressed by the patient throughout and in particular at the end of the encounter. **Suggestions** for behaviour change can be inserted throughout the communication encounter as opportunities arise.

A fundamental principle underlying MI is to elicit from the patient their own reasons for change, for example, by asking open questions about the behaviour in question.[28] This is often called 'Change talk', defined as verbalizations for a desire to change, a belief that change is possible, reasons for change, a perceived need for change, and in particular, a commitment to change. Examples of 'Change talk' include stated reasons for making positive changes, 'I know I need to exercise to be able to get back to being able to carry my granddaughter', or 'Once I stop taking opioids, I will be able to think more clearly' as well as statements indicating a readiness to change, 'It's time that I do something about this', or 'Okay I'm ready to try something new', or even an intention to change, 'I am going to start going to the gym this week'.

Psychological theories provide a strong rationale for the importance of patients, rather than clinicians, arguing for change. For example, cognitive dissonance theory[8] asserts that when people are enticed to make public statements that differ from their previous statements, their beliefs and values shift in the direction of the new statements. Similarly, self-perception theory[29] argues that people learn about themselves through their actions. People know what they believe by what they hear themselves say, and see themselves do.

Once 'Change talk' is elicited, that is, once the clinician hears reasons for positive change that patients themselves state, the clinician can then nurture and reinforce those statements by reflecting them. The reflection can include a simple restatement of what the patient said, or the reflection can be more sophisticated and include ideas or emotions implied by the content of the patient's statements.

Here are some examples of a clinician asking **open** questions to elicit conversation that includes **change talk**, followed by reflections of **change talk**.

Clinician: 'What worries you most about your pain problem?'
Patient: 'It's taken over my life. I can't sleep any more, and I'm no longer working.'
Clinician: 'Which of these has been hardest on you?' (identifies the primary concern of the patient).
Patient: 'Missing sleep is really the worst. This makes it hard to do anything else, including getting back to work.'
Clinician: 'You really want to learn how to get a good night's sleep, so that you can get back to your life.'

The clinician reflects both an achievable goal for which there are interventions known to be effective while also reflecting a value to better understand what is important to the patient, as well as to enhance the patient's awareness of achievable goals.

Reflecting or paraphrasing **change talk** back to the patient, allows clinicians to reinforce statements that maintain a focus on the patient's desire, ability, reasons, perceived need, and commitment to change. This facilitates positive patient engagement and motivation for change and avoids confrontation and arguments that may arise from lecturing the patient.

It is not uncommon for a patient to state, '*I just want you to take the pain away*'. However, the patient may be expressing an unrealistic goal and communicating that treating pain should be the focus of the consultation.

There is a temptation to respond with a direct answer like, '*Well, removing your pain is not possible right now*', or even worse, '*I think you will have to learn to live with your pain!*'

However, reflecting and reframing the underlying sentiment with a statement like, '*It makes complete sense to me that you want to feel better*', perhaps followed by, '*I also want you to be able to do more and hurt less*'. Such a response helps defuse a situation where trust might easily be lost. Effective reflections decrease resistance to change and increase rapport and patient engagement.[17]

Clinicians commonly explore coping strategies in acute and chronic pain settings. Responses to open questions about how the patient copes can be used to explore problems and concerns about unhelpful coping strategies, and nurture and reinforce those that are more beneficial. The clinician can better understand the patient's beliefs by asking about both the benefits and costs of each coping response. A clinician voicing a strong argument against a particular strategy will likely backfire and reinforce the person's commitment to that strategy.

A typical example concerns exercise. Instead of arguing about the importance of exercise in response to a statement like '*I've done exercise programmes, they just make my pain worse*'. It would be more helpful to ask **open questions** which show curiosity about the outcomes of exercising versus not exercising, and then reflect back the change talk that is elicited.

> **Clinician:** '*I'm interested in hearing a little more about your experiences with exercise. What has been easy and what has been difficult about it?*'
> **Patient:** '*Right after the surgery, my doctor wanted me to walk every day. I was able to do it at first—for about 3 months. But then I fell and had to stay in bed for several weeks. After that, I couldn't walk without a lot of pain.*'
> **Clinician:** (reflecting on past success): '*So, you were able to maintain a walking programme for 3 months! During this time, how did your tolerance for walking change?*'

The clinician wants to know about the patient's perceptions of the effects of the walking programme. The clinician may reflect and/or ask for elaboration on perceived benefits and improvements. A lack of perceived benefit may be responded to with an affirmation that the patient's ability to maintain the exercise programme, despite no immediate benefits, suggests a lot of determination. Importantly, although the rule is to respond with a reflection statement, which statement is reflected depends on what words the patient says.

> **Patient:** '*Well, during the time I was walking regularly I was able to walk a little more each day. And I started to feel better. But then, once I fell, the whole pro-gramme went pear-shaped.*'
>
> **Clinician:** '*So, you felt better and were able to do more as you engaged in the walking programme. I wonder what it might take to start the walking programme again. Perhaps starting very easy and very slowly building up your strength, until you are strong again. Or perhaps have a programme that you know is safe, even if it results in some pain as you get stronger. Maybe there are other options. What are your thoughts about getting back into some kind of programme versus keeping things as they are?*'

Open questions are designed to elicit change talk and ideas for starting another pro-gramme, but one based on the patient's ideas and goals, not the clinician's.

Sometimes, when a patient seems dead set against engaging in an adaptive coping response such as regular exercise, it may be strategic to redirect the conversation to an area where adaptive change might be acceptable. This may only involve reframing an issue to keep the possibility of its future discussion.

For example, in response to a statement from the person with pain such as, '*I need all of my medications*', the healthcare provider could suggest reviewing the medica-tion list, '*You may be right. After we review all of your medications, you may decide to continue asking for prescriptions for these medications. That choice will be yours*'. The clinician is acknowledging the possibility of truth in the patient's statement and not pushing them into listing the reasons for not changing. This approach allows the clin-ician to emphasize patient choice while leaving open the possibility of more adaptive behaviour in the future.

Conclusions

The words we choose and how we use them can sometimes cause harm from thought-lessness, impacting patients in unknown ways long after conversations have ended. Misunderstanding the metaphors patients use to share their pain experiences and im-press on clinicians the distress they feel, perpetuates the stigma and victim-blaming that are common responses to reports of pain seemingly outside of clinicians' expect-ations of the '*correct*' amount of pain in a particular context. The 'LAURS' framework outlines useful communication skills that can significantly improve patient-clinician interactions, especially for those living with chronic pain. The steps in the 'GREAT' strategy enable a structured approach for conducting interviews, shows respect for the patient's autonomy, addresses their expectations and concerns, and ends with tacit agreement to work together. MI can enhance the 'LAURS' and 'GREAT' strategies, adding skills for eliciting and addressing patient-identified goals and barriers leading to improved function and recovery whether pain is acute or chronic.

> ## Key points
>
> 1. The words we choose and how we use them influence pain outcomes.
> 2. Patients frequently express their pain experiences through metaphor.
> 3. The 'GREAT' 'LAURS' framework can improve patient-clinician interactions and enable a structured approach that shows respect for the patient's autonomy.
> 4. Motivational interviewing skills can elicit and address patient-identified goals and barriers that can improve function and recovery in both an acute and chronic pain context.

Together this suite of communication strategies provides the clinician with a comprehensive range of communication skills for deeper and more satisfying conversations with patients and are more likely to result in positive therapeutic outcomes.

References

1. Butler DS, Moseley GL (2003). *Explain pain.* Adelaide: Noigroup Publications.
2. Prieto Velasco JA, Tercedor Sanchez M (2014). The embodied nature of medical concepts: image schemas and language for PAIN. *Cogn Process*, **15**(3), 283–96.
3. International Association for the Study of Pain (2020). IASP revises its definition of pain for the first time since 1979. Available at: https://www.iasp-pain.org/wp-content/uploads/2022/04/revised-definition-flysheet_R2-1-1-1.pdf
4. Raja SN, Carr DB, Cohen M, et al. (2020). The revised International Association for the Study of Pain definition of pain: concepts, challenges, and compromises. *Pain*, **161**(9), 1976–82.
5. Toye F, Seers K, Barker KL (2017). Meta-ethnography to understand healthcare professionals' experience of treating adults with chronic non-malignant pain. *BMJ Open*, 7, e018411.
6. Loftus S (2011). Pain and its metaphors: a dialogical approach. *J Med Humanit*, **32**(3), 213–30.
7. Calpin P, Imran A, Harmon D (2017). A comparison of expectations of physicians and patients with chronic pain for pain clinic visits. *Pain Practice*, **17**(3), 305–3011.
8. Festinger L (1957). *A theory of cognitive dissonance.* Stanford, CA: Stanford University Press.
9. Neilson S (2016). Pain as metaphor: metaphor and medicine. *Med Humanit*, **42**(1), 3–10.
10. Semino E (2010). Descriptions of pain, metaphor, and embodied simulation. *Metaphor and Symbol*, **25**(4), 205–26.
11. Hearn JH, Finlay KA, Fine PA (2016). The devil in the corner: a mixed-methods study of metaphor use by those with spinal cord injury-specific neuropathic pain. *Br J Health Psychol*, **21**(4), 973–88.
12. Lærum E, Indahl A, Skouen JS (2006). What is 'the good back-consultation'? A combined qualitative and quantitative study of chronic low back pain patients' interaction with and perceptions of consultations with specialists. *Rehabil Med*, **38**, 255–62.

13. Evers S, Hsu C, Sherman KJ, et al. (2017). Patient perspectives on communication with primary care physicians about chronic low back pain. *Perm J*, **21**, 16–177.

14. Painaustralia (2019). Talking about pain. Language guidelines for talking about chronic pain. Available at: https://www.painaustralia.org.au/static/uploads/files/talking-about-pain-lgfcp-16-07-2019-wfsumqrbtavy.pdf

15. Cyna AM (2018). A GREAT interaction and the LAURS of communication in anesthesia. *Acta Anaesth Belg*, **69**, 131–5.

16. Singh Ospina N, Phillips KA, Rodriguez-Gutierrez R, et al. (2019). Eliciting the patient's agenda- secondary analysis of recorded clinical encounters. *J Gen Intern Med*, **34**(1), 36–40.

17. Jensen MP (2018). Motivational Interviewing and pain management. In: Karoly P, Crombez G (ed.) *Motivational perspectives on chronic pain: theory, research, and practice*, pp. 407–44. New York, NY: Oxford University Press.

18. Jensen MP (2019). Using hypnotic reflective listening to identify effective suggestions for behavior change. In: Jensen MP (ed.) *Handbook of hypnotic techniques, Vol 1: Favorite methods of master clinicians*, pp. 140–70. Kirkland, WA: Denny Creek Press.

19. Riddle DL, Jensen MP, Ang D, Slover J, Perera R, Dumenci L (2018). Do pain coping and pain beliefs associate with outcome measures before knee arthroplasty in patients who catastrophize about pain? A cross-sectional analysis from a randomized clinical trial. *Clin Orthop Relat Res*, **476**, 778–86.

20. Tripp DA, Nickel JC, Wang Y, et al. (2006). Catastrophizing and pain-contingent rest predict patient adjustment in men with chronic prostatitis/chronic pelvic pain syndrome. *J Pain*, **7**(10), 697–708.

21. Singh P, King-Shier K, Sinclair S (2018). The colours and contours of compassion: A systematic review of the perspectives of compassion among ethnically diverse patients and healthcare providers. *PLoS One*, **13**(5), e0197261.

22. Sinclair S, Bouchal SR, Schulte F, et al. (2021). Compassion in pediatric oncology: A patient, parent and healthcare provider empirical model. *Psychooncology*, **30**(10), 1728–38.

23. Ashton-James CE, Nicholas MK (2016). Appearance of trustworthiness: an implicit source of bias in judgments of patients' pain. *Pain*, **157**, 1583–5.

24. Schäfer G, Prkachin KM, Kaseweter KA, Williams AC (2016). Health care providers' judgments in chronic pain: the influence of gender and trustworthiness. *Pain*, **157**(8), 1618–25.

25. Faculty of Pain Medicine, Australian and New Zealand College of Anaesthetists (2018). Pain-oriented sensory testing (POST) guidelines. Available at: https://www.anzca.edu.au/getattachment/554e8dd9-a45d-4f6d-8cdc-1b0793dba926/POST-Guidelines (Accessed 5 August 2022).

26. Guerts JW, Willems PC, Lockwood C, van Kleef M, Kleijnen J, Dirksen C (2017). Patient expectations for management of chronic non-cancer pain: A systematic review. *Health Expect*, **20**, 1201–17.

27. Jensen MP (2018). Enhancing motivation to change in pain treatment. In: Turk DC, Gatchel RJ (ed.) *Psychological approaches to pain management: a practitioner's handbook*, pp. 71–95. New York, NY: Guilford Press.

28. Miller WR, Rollnick S (2013). *Motivational interviewing: helping people change*. New York: Guilford Press.

29. Bem DJ (1967). Self-perception: An alternative interpretation of cognitive dissonance phenomena. *Psychol Rev*, **74**, 183–200.

Section 3

Specific clinical contexts

Chapter 10

Pregnancy and childbirth

Marion I. Andrew and Allan M. Cyna

'I have nothing to offer but blood, toil, tears and sweat.'
Winston Churchill, 13 May 1940

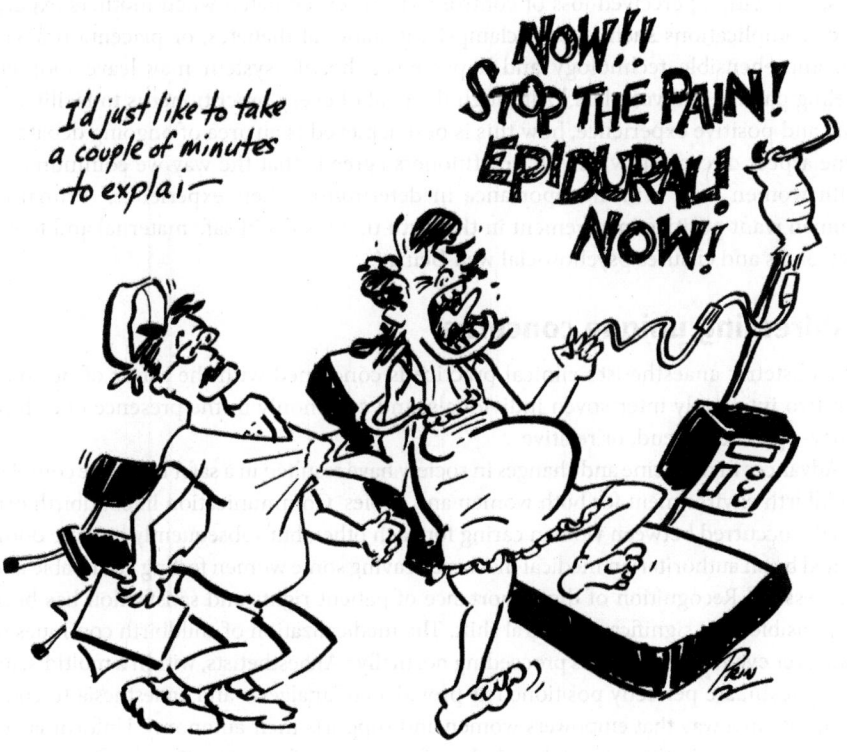

What this chapter is about

Setting the scene

Many women approach the birth of their baby with at least some apprehension. The increasing medicalization of childbirth[1] has left some women feeling dependent, helpless, and with a perceived loss of control.[2] This is exacerbated when mothers experience complications such as pre-eclampsia, gestational diabetes, or placenta praevia. Incomprehensible technology and a perceived hostile system may leave mothers feeling passive and voiceless.[3] Although the goal of every practitioner is to facilitate a safe and positive experience, how this is best achieved is an area of ongoing debate.[4–6] One aspect of care on which all practitioners agree is that the way we communicate with women is of critical importance in determining their experience.[7] Primarily, women want positive involvement in the birth that results in safe maternal and foetal outcomes and ensures psychosocial well-being.[6]

Addressing unique concerns

The obstetric anaesthetist's clinical practice is concerned with the safety of not one, but two intricately interwoven individuals, and commonly in the presence of a third party—partner, friend, or relative.

Advances in medicine and changes in society have resulted in a safer but more complex childbirth environment for both women and babies. Communication in childbirth originally occurred between women caring for each other, but subsequently became dominated by an authoritarian medical machine, leaving some women feeling vulnerable and 'processed'.[8] Recognition of the importance of patient rights and satisfaction has been responsible for a significant cultural shift. The medicalization of childbirth continues to take over even when labour is proceeding normally.[2] Anaesthetists, within a multidisciplinary team, are perfectly positioned as providers of analgesia and anaesthesia to communicate in a way that empowers women and supports their autonomy. Unfortunately, communication in the antenatal period is often presented in a negative way.[7,9]

Antenatal preparation

Women become highly focused on pregnancy and labour as the evidence looms ever larger in front of them. Pregnancy and childbirth represent a challenging psychological and physiological experience. This focus of attention on pregnancy makes women highly suggestible to subconscious communications and they show increased hypnotisability.[10] For this reason, positive and negative suggestions can function as powerful determinants of how women perceive pregnancy and childbirth.

There is a range of emotional responses to pregnancy—for some, joy and excitement, for others, fear and anxiety. Overlaying this, there may also be pre-existing generalized anxiety, social concerns, obstetric problems, and other complications. In addition, women often receive negative suggestions (see Chapter 3) from well-meaning relatives and friends regaling them with stories of their own experiences. '*I was in labour for 48 hours, it was torture!*'

While unable to change messages conveyed to mothers from friends and family, the anaesthetist can communicate in ways that encourage patient autonomy and control.

The first step when preparing women for childbirth is to encourage the woman's own abilities, resources, and potential. For very good reasons, athletes train to optimize physical performance and mental capabilities, allowing them to reframe experiences in a positive way despite the considerable effort, and sometimes pain, involved. After nine months of pregnancy the mother is, in essence, like a finely tuned 'athlete'. She does not know the day of the event or whether she is in for a 'sprint' or a 'marathon'. Either way, by the end of pregnancy, her body is optimized physiologically to cope with the demands of childbirth. Offering positive choices on how she might experience childbirth helps facilitate her control.

Written antenatal information is useful. Firstly because it gives women plenty of time to consider their options. Secondly, information provided early about anaesthesia risk encourages women to raise concerns and have them dealt with. The language used to provide information should avoid negative suggestions where possible (see Chapter 3).

The following clinical scenarios illustrate how '**GREAT**' and '**LAURS**' (see Chapter 2) can be applied to create a positive and more rewarding experience.

Sophie is pregnant with her first child and is very anxious about the approaching labour. She asks to see the anaesthetist in the antenatal clinic at 36 weeks' gestation. She expresses trepidation at the thought of experiencing any contractions, and wants to know if she can have an epidural the minute she comes into the hospital. She is '*extremely frightened of pain*' and says she has been called a '*wimp*' all her life.

> **Sophie:** '*I'm due in four weeks and I'll need an epidural as soon as I come in—can I book it now?*'

Possible standard replies might be:

> **Anaesthetist:** '*Of course, if you can't cope you can have an epidural as soon as you come in.*'
> or
> **Anaesthetist:** '*You can have an epidural, but you may not necessarily get it right away—and anyway, you would be best to wait till you are 3 cm dilated.*'

Neither of these responses addresses the real issue of fear of not coping. Both responses re-enforce Sophie's negative belief that she can't cope by the anaesthetist offering epidural as a panacea. Is there an alternative?

> **Anaesthetist:** '*Yes, this is a whole new experience … and you aren't sure that you can* **cope** *and feel that you will* **need** *an epidural straight away …*'

The anaesthetist has listened, reflected back, and then pauses to allow a response.

> **Sophie:** '*Yes, I was told by one of my friends that labour is the worst pain imaginable. I don't think I could* **cope**. *My friend was in labour for over 24 hours. I would never manage that. I don't want to be out of* **control**.'

> **Anaesthetist:** '*It is unusual to have a 24-hour labour … Everybody's labour is different and sometimes labour progresses more quickly than you think.*'

The anaesthetist accepts Sophie's reality and utilizes her language.

> **Anaesthetist:** '*Spontaneous labour begins gradually with rest periods between the contractions that can seem quite long—you may be surprised how "in* **control**" *you can be, using some very simple techniques.*'

The utilization of the **need for control** is recognized:

> **Anaesthetist:** '*Our job is to ensure you and your baby are comfortable and safe. One of the ways we can do this is to place an epidural. Some women find that if labour is progressing gradually and normally, they feel in control and may decide that an epidural may not be required.*'

This is an indirect suggestion that Sophie may not need one either. The anaesthetist has listened attentively and reflectively to Sophie, utilized the concern about prolonged labour and suggested an alternative experience is possible. The anaesthetist has also established that the issue here is one of confidence, the ability to **cope and control**.

> **Sophie:** '*I'm still* **not sure**.'
> **Anaesthetist:** '*It's okay to be "* **not sure**". *In that way you have left your options open, so that you can decide when the time is right.*'

By utilizing Sophie's uncertainty and reframing it into flexibility, choices, and autonomy, the anaesthetist provides suggestions that Sophie can be more confident in her own abilities and take time in making informed decisions regarding analgesia. Using language this way is designed not to dissuade women from having epidural analgesia, but rather to communicate, in a manner that engenders confidence, reinforces their resources, and offers more choice.

Labour

Anaesthetists' contact with women in labour is usually in the context of providing epidural analgesia. Communication with highly distressed women in labour is particularly challenging as they are frequently in a dissociated state and respond poorly to logical communication. Different forms of language are often necessary if useful responses are to be elicited.

Epidural analgesia

No opportunity to meet and begin establishing rapport with the labouring woman is ever wasted. To this end, it is often helpful for the anaesthetist to be visible as part of the team attending labour ward rounds and making anticipatory visits in situations where an intervention is likely. Open communication occurs when the anaesthetist engages with the patient and her partner in a way that shows respect for autonomy.

Women in labour are usually relieved and delighted to see the anaesthetist. Establishing rapport on this basis is straightforward, with introductions and acknowledgement that pain relief can be provided promptly. An unhurried, cool, professional anaesthetist talking confidently, calmly, and encouragingly is a source of great relief in itself.

Consent

In obstetric anaesthesia practice, verbal, and in some jurisdictions, written consent needs to be obtained prior to insertion of a labour epidural. Written patient information is increasingly the norm.[11] Written consent may have been obtained in the antenatal clinic, where explanations of the material risks pertaining to that particular woman can be given more fully (see also Chapter 7).

This solution provides factual information but does not address the woman's immediate concerns. The most pertinent aspect of consent is not so much facts and figures, but the human interaction based upon trust and confidence in a competent professional. Which risks are 'material'? What should be discussed? How should this information be presented? Although there are no easy answers to these questions for every patient there are some aspects that are worth considering.

Competence

It has been argued that it is impossible to obtain informed consent when women are in labour on the basis that they are not competent to give consent.[4] In the absence of a clear definition of 'competent', this remains controversial in this context. What is apparent is that the patient is vulnerable, is asking for help, her needs are relatively urgent, and she wants to feel confident that the doctor will perform the procedure safely and quickly. While labour is not an emergency, and insertion of an epidural is not a life-saving procedure, the issue of 'competence' arises because, in distress, the patient perceives the situation as an emergency. The labouring woman is often exhausted, medicated, and may behave as if she is irrational and unable to listen to explanations. Despite this and the distraction of contractions, she is usually capable of listening to a brief focused explanation of the procedure, its benefits, and risks. The anaesthetist can then confirm her wishes whether to proceed or not.

Sophie, now at term, has been admitted to the delivery suite with spontaneous rupture of membranes and in active labour.

> **Anaesthetist:** *'Hello Sophie, my name is Dr Love, I'm one of the anaesthetists. What can I do to help?'*

This allows the woman to state her wishes and respond rather than have the partner, relative, or midwife tell you what they believe the woman wants or needs.

> **Sophie:** *'I want a f***ing epidural! Quick, just do it!'*
> **Anaesthestist:** *'We will do this for you as quickly and as safely as possible. Do you have any particular concerns before we start? The good news is that epidurals usually allow women to become very comfortable and feel more in control ... have you read the information leaflet?'*
> **Sophie:** *'Yes, but I can't remember now!'*
> **Anaesthetist:** *'I'll just very briefly tell you about the risks or potential problems that can occasionally occur with an epidural ... Epidurals don't always work perfectly first time and may need adjusting or replacing ... Headache can happen occasionally in less than 1:100 women having an epidural. Very rarely nerve damage and paralysis can occur but I've never seen that complication in my 30 years of practice. My expectation is that the epidural will be straightforward and we can get you much more comfortable very soon." Do you have any questions about the epidural before we finish?'*
> **Sophie:** *'No—please just hurry!'*

While it is important to avoid negative language (see Chapter 3), this is nearly impossible when providing risk information (see Chapter 7). However, communication that focuses on the benefits of epidural analgesia immediately after the risk discussion, brings to the patient a helpful perspective. The consent process and how consent is obtained aims at supporting patient autonomy—not 'covering the anaesthetist's backside'. Unnecessary repeated emphasis of major risks can escalate anxiety in an already fraught situation. A 'jumpy' patient, focused on things going wrong rather than on things going right, is more likely to have a complication.

Enhancing patient cooperation during epidural insertion

Women often say that they are unable to cooperate and, while they may be begging for relief, they may insist that they are unable to keep still or sit up. In these circumstances, acceptance of the patient's perception is essential.

Some anaesthetists may become irritated and insistent, *'Well, you will have to sit up and keep still otherwise I can't do this. If you move, we could damage your spinal cord'.*

Although this strategy has the effect of terrifying women into sitting still, gentler communication allows the anaesthetist to more effectively support the patient in a way that enhances a therapeutic alliance and safety.

Sophie has agreed to proceed with an epidural.

> **Sophie:** '*Oh no! Here comes another one! No! Aaaaaargh—just put it in!*'
> **Anaesthetist:** '*Okay, let's get on and do this safely, comfortably, and as quickly as we can.*'

The anaesthetist communicates with the patient '**safety**', his concern, and '**speed**', her concern.

> **Sophie:** '*Yeah, yeah I can be paralysed! Please HELP ME—I can't* **listen** *to anything anymore!*'
> **Anaesthetist:** '*That's okay—you don't have to* **listen** *because you will still* **hear** *everything you need to allow yourself to relax and sit still.*'

The anaesthetist accepts that Sophie can't '**listen**', utilizes her language and reframes it so that even though she can't '**listen**' she can *still* '**hear**', suggesting she will be able to '**relax and sit still**'.

> **Anaesthetist:** '*Would you like to sit up now or after the next contraction?*' (A double bind—see Chapter 4). '*In a moment I will ask you to tell me when you are having a contraction—I can then* **finish** *positioning the epidural while you are sitting still. I will use local anaesthetic to numb the skin.*'

The anaesthetist puts research evidence[4] into practice by avoiding the use of negative language like, '*It will sting*', and encouraging the patient at each stage with the expectation that she will be able to achieve what is being asked even if she doesn't believe it herself. By talking about '**finishing**' the epidural the anaesthetist focuses on the end of the procedure which helps reduce anticipatory anxiety.

Communicating with women during a contraction

Communicating in a way that helps women to stay still while they are having strong contractions represents a pinnacle of achievement for the obstetric anaesthetist. Some practical dialogue follows to illustrate some techniques.

Women can be asked to focus on their breathing by counting their breaths silently during a contraction. This can be communicated with an indirect approach.

> **Anaesthetist:** '*As you know each contraction tells you that you are getting closer to seeing your baby. The other thing you know, is that each contraction is followed by a rest. Interestingly, women find that they can cope with each contraction one at a time and enjoy each rest as they build up their strength and confidence, counting breaths silently as you breathe in strength and control and blow away anything unhelpful into the room. This allows you to know when the rest is coming and as you focus on the rest, the contraction starts to seem much shorter and the rest that follows seem much longer than it really is.*'

For the woman who doesn't complete the counting of breaths before the contraction finishes, it is important for the anaesthetist to reframe this as a 'success'.

> **Anaesthetist:** '*How many breaths did you count in that last contraction?*'
> **Sophie:** '*Three, the contraction was too painful to concentrate.*'
> **Anaesthetist:** '*Good! Well done! Many women can't get past "one" the first time they attempt this. As each contraction passes you will find there comes a point when you will find yourself able to keep counting right through to the end of the contraction. The contractions then start to move into the distance and start to seem much shorter and the rests that follow each contraction start seeming much longer.*'

Encouragement to focus attention on the '*rest*' is a suggestion to dissociate from the contraction.

Time distortion

In their dissociated mental state, labouring women are often able to accept suggestions in a very concrete and unquestioning way. The suggestion of a much longer rest period is accepted concretely and experienced as a perceptual change distorting the passage of time aiding relaxation (see Chapters 4 and 22).

N.B. It is important to use the word '*seeming*' as some highly suggestible patients may reduce the frequency of their contractions with this suggestion.

Reframing contractions

The reframe involves a communication exchange providing an alternative meaning or interpretation of an experience (see Chapter 2). Table 10.1 shows how different meanings of the same perceptual experience can be interpreted. Metaphor can be particularly useful in this context, where the contractions can be described in a way that is positive. A contraction might be described as '*a powerful wave*' guiding the woman to focus on seeing the baby as the goal rather than enduring pain for pain's sake.

> **Anaesthetist:** (Using a confusional technique): '*As surely as day follows night these powerful waves of energy bring your baby closer and closer to you.*'

Caesarean section

The dynamic and acute nature of childbirth means that sudden changes may result in an emergent situation. A clear understanding of the procedure is achievable when communication is provided calmly, honestly, and with sensitivity to the effects of negative suggestions on the patient's distress, fatigue, and vulnerability.

Regional anaesthesia is nearly always the anaesthetic of choice. However, having an operation while awake is confronting for most people. Some women and their partners are extremely anxious, others are delighted to have escaped labour, while a few may feel cheated of a natural birth. Establishing the woman's perspective and acceptance of her reality builds rapport and gives her a degree of control. Appreciation that vast differences occur between women allows the anaesthetist to focus attention on the woman's major concerns and to tailor communication accordingly.

Knowing what to expect is an important part of preparation. The mind naturally rehearses all sorts of scenarios, often negatively, as a survival mechanism (see also Chapter 3). For this reason, explaining what the patient might feel, and attention to detail when testing the adequacy of the anaesthetic block, is essential. Particular care is required to avoid inadvertently leading the patient into perceiving a perception such as cold, that they would otherwise not have experienced. Irrespective of modality being tested, the choice of words and the use of **open** versus **closed** questions is critical to the proper assessment of the level of block.

Table 10.1 Different interpretations of the same experience

Experience	Positive interpretation	Negative interpretation
Labour onset	*'When contractions are regular and the cervix is dilating you are in established labour and well on the way to having your baby.'*	*'We can place an epidural before the contractions become too painful.'*
Labour contractions	*'One step closer to seeing the baby.'* *'The stronger the more effective.'*	*'An increasingly painful experience that is absolutely terrifying and almost unbearable.'* *'The stronger the more painful.'*
Rests between contractions	*'Focusing on the rests can allow them to seem longer than they really are and the contractions seem shorter than they really are.'*	*'The contractions seem continuous and ever more painful and excruciating as labour progresses.'*
Cx 3–4 cm	*'At this stage most women are entering the accelerated phase of their labour where the contractions become much more effective.'*	*'This stage of labour starts getting really painful and most women will need an epidural!'*
Full dilatation	*'This is the exciting part of labour where women are no longer passive observers but become active participants in the birth of the baby.'*	*'Most women find at this stage they are too tired to care as the pain becomes even more unbearable.'*
Pushing and crowning	*'All the rests that you have had during the first stage of labour has given you more than enough energy to push in the most effective way possible for you and your baby.'* *'As skin stretches it usually becomes numb and anaesthetic, allowing the birth to be as comfortable and safe as possible.'*	*'Most women at this stage are too tired to do anything let alone push.'* *'As skin stretches, it burns and the burning sensation is the worst experience of the entire birth.'*

Sophie has been in labour for 12 hours and has failed to progress. The obstetrician has decided that she requires a caesarean section. Her epidural is working well and it has been 'topped up' for the procedure.

> Anaesthetist: 'We have talked about what you might *feel* and I am now going to test the anaesthetic block so that we are both happy that it is working. We will only begin the caesarean when we are all confident that it is working well.'

If the level of block is tested using ice, asking the open question, 'What can you feel?' is more reliable, and is less like leading the witness than asking 'Is this cold?'.[12]

One way to test the block is outlined below and is aimed at preventing the anaesthetist suggesting a perception the woman otherwise wouldn't experience.

At the reference point (e.g. forehead), the woman can be informed, 'This is ice. What can you feel?' Then applying the stimulus to the lower abdomen, the anaesthetist asks, 'What can you feel?' If there is a 'No' response then say 'Can you feel touch?' and proceed to a level until the patient feels touch, and then ask, 'Can you feel cold?' 'Does it feel icy?' until the level is identified for 'Touch', 'Cold', 'Ice', and 'No change' from the reference point.

The drapes are placed, and Sophie is assessed as having a block to T3 with ice.

> Sophie: 'I don't think I **can do** this!'
>
> Anaesthetist: 'That's okay. I have tested the anaesthetic and I am confident that the block will ensure you are comfortable and safe during the procedure. There are things you **can do**. One of the things women **can do** is to imagine seeing their baby for the first time. How much hair, the palm of the baby's hand, the baby's eyes? You know you **can do** this!'.

'**You know**' is a suggestion that the woman subconsciously 'knows' she can manage getting through the caesarean and also knows there are things she **can do** to help herself.

> Anaesthetist: (As the baby is being born) 'Any sensations you might feel **can** remind you that you are getting closer and closer to seeing your baby.'

Communication with a borderline block

When the mother expresses a strong desire to avoid a general anaesthetic, many anaesthetists will not entertain allowing surgery to proceed in a situation where the block appears less than perfect. However, many mothers are highly motivated to be conscious for the birth of their baby and are able to cope with some degree of discomfort during the procedure. The importance of 'checking-in' with the patient is the key to managing the patient successfully with a less than perfect block.

> Anaesthetist: 'Although I think the anaesthetic is working reasonably well up to here (e.g. T6) it would be better if you were numb up to here as well (e.g. T4). I appreciate how important it is for you to see your baby being born. What do you think?'
>
> Woman: 'Does that mean I might feel pain?'

Anaesthetist: '*Yes, you might feel pain and if you are not coping, I can put you to sleep.*'

Alternatively—

'*Yes, you might feel some pain but if you do, we can help you with extra local anaesthetic and give medications into the drip to keep you comfortable once the baby is born. I am ready to give you a sleeping anaesthetic at any time you feel you want it. Is it okay with you for us to proceed? I am right here.*'

Understanding Sophie's motivation to stay awake the anaesthetist acknowledges honestly that the woman may feel pain but offers other solutions before letting her know that a general anaesthesia (GA) is possible. He avoids suggesting that she might not be able to cope, but instead informs the patient of a range of anaesthetic options supporting the patient's autonomy. Since Sophie asked about '*Pain*', the anaesthetist uses the word '*Pain*' in his response. Communicating with the partner is helpful, and a joint decision is preferred where possible. Similarly, the obstetrician needs to be informed of the borderline nature of the block (see Chapters 7 and 18). Infiltration with local anaesthetic by surgeons can supplement the block, and the anaesthetist can communicate to the obstetrician that this is not the time for teaching junior trainees. In all cases the primary consideration is maternal safety, the woman's wishes, and her autonomy— **not** the anaesthetist's fear of litigation! Once baby is born and in mother's arms it is unusual for a GA to be required or requested.

Communicating with partners

On occasion partners do not wish to be present for the birth. Far more commonly, partners are present, raising the emotional stakes. Some appear at home in this role while others are less comfortable and unsure how to support the woman. The anaesthetist's acceptance of a partner's chosen level of involvement may alleviate stress. Partners should be advised that they may be asked to leave the operating room if a GA is required, since '*more space and personnel are needed for mother and baby's safety*'.

Tips and tricks

It is not uncommon for women to have a variety of symptoms and concerns during the procedure. These can be helped with calm reassurance before resorting to pharmacotherapy.

Managing nausea

Woman: '*I'm feeling a bit sick*'.
Anaesthetist: '*Here's the vomit bowl.*'
Alternatively—
Anaesthetist: '*It's because your blood pressure is a bit low. I have just given you something to help you should feel more settled soon.*'

Difficulty breathing during caesarean section

Woman: '*I can't breathe!*' or '*It's hard to breathe*'.

Providing the patient is vocalizing and not whispering, and can take a deep breath when asked, there is likely no immediate concern.

> **Anaesthetist:** '*That's okay. Sometimes when the anaesthetic is working really well we lose the sensation in the chest that we are breathing even when we are. Can you place the palm of your hand on your chest and take a deep breath and feel the chest move up and down each time you breathe? The breathing soon will start to feel much easier.*'

While it is essential to assess whether a total spinal is developing, this is unlikely if the woman is vocalizing. If the patient is whispering, '*I can't breathe*', it's time to find the laryngoscope and the emergency drug tray!

> **Anaesthetist:** '*We are just giving you some oxygen and will get you off to sleep if this doesn't settle.*'

Pruritus with neuraxial opioids

Woman: '*I'm really itchy.*'
Anaesthetist: '*That's excellent. This usually means you can stay comfortable with the spinal medication as you recover from the caesarean. Knowing this, allows women to put it into the background . . . as the itching reaches a peak over the next little while and then settles . . . Is that okay for you?*'

It is unusual for women to ask for further treatment of itch after this explanation.

Using 'GREAT' in an emergency GA caesarean section

Because emergency GA for caesarean section is a stressful and technical challenge for the anaesthetist, good communication skills tend to be forgotten. Communication with patient, partner, obstetrician, and theatre team is a vital component of quality care.

Emergency theatre is alerted that there is a Category I call for prolapsed cord. Thirty seconds later the theatre doors swing open and amidst shouts of, '*Don't push!*' The woman on a trolley is wheeled hurriedly towards the operating table.

Greeting

> **Anaesthetist:** '*Hi, my name is Dr Gonzales. I'm the anaesthetist. We are here to keep you and your baby safe and I will be giving your anaesthetic. I'm just about to finish putting the drip in and the nurses are placing some monitors . . . Can you tell me what you like to be called?*'
> **Patient:** '*Susie . . . Is my baby going to be **okay**?*'

Rapport

> **Anaesthetist**: '*Susie, all these people here are doing everything possible to make sure you and your baby are **okay**.*'
> **Susie**: '*I'm **scared**.*'
> **Anaesthetist**: '*It's okay to be **scared**.*'

The anaesthetist utilizes '*scared*' letting her know she has been heard and understood.

Expectations

> **Anaesthetist**: '*I need to ask you some questions. Have you ever had a problem with anaesthetics? Teeth? Medication? Allergies? Can you open your mouth? In a few moments we will give you some oxygen and some medicine to get you off to sleep ...*'

Addressing concerns

> **Anaesthetist**: '*Have you anything to ask before we start your anaesthetic?*'
> **Susie**: '*Is the anaesthetic going to affect my baby?*'
> **Anaesthetist** (Pre-oxygenating): '*Sometimes anaesthetic does make the baby a little sleepy too. The "baby doctor" is here to look after your baby when he is born.*'

Tacit agreement

> **Anaesthetist** (Pre-oxygenating): '*Just let me know when you are ready ...*'

Almost any interaction can be structured to allow patients to feel a sense of control whether emergency, elective, or any other context, even that of bereavement and grief.

Bereavement and grief

Anaesthetists may be required to care for women where pregnancy or birth does not result in a good outcome. Such poor circumstances inevitably colour the experience of women in subsequent pregnancies.

History of previous stillbirth

A woman presenting antenatally with a past history of stillbirth can benefit immensely from attentive **listening. Acceptance** by the anaesthetist that her natural protective fear that the current pregnancy might also result in stillbirth is more reassuring than negating it . Negating fears does little to alleviate them. Identifying positive life experiences and skills developed since the stillbirth, can be **utilized** to **reframe** this pregnancy experience in a different way, and **suggest** a different perspective.

> **Anaesthetist**: '*I know I can't understand what you have been through, and I'm not going to tell you that the same thing can't happen again. But the risk is extremely*

low, given how closely you are being monitored in this pregnancy. What we do know is that once something like this happens, people develop skills and resources they may not have appreciated and are no longer the same person they were. I see you are well supported by family and friends and have overcome other challenges successfully. In the very unlikely event that the same thing happens again in this pregnancy, it cannot be experienced in the same way.'

It's important **NOT** to state explicitly that the experience will be better. The fact that it cannot be experienced in the same way implies it will be better as nothing could be worse.

Miscarriage, stillbirth, and genetic termination

There is little or no research or training on how best to communicate in this context and on how language impacts on grieving parents. Prevailing themes from interviews with parents after stillbirth, include the use of inappropriate language, a lack of sensitivity and privacy, and unhelpful diversionary techniques.[13] Poor communication in this area engenders mistrust, distress, and may even have a lasting effect on the grieving process.

Healthcare professionals often find it difficult to step back from their own discomfort to appropriately focus on what is most helpful to patients. Despite the workload pressure, finding a protected period of time (e.g. handing over the pager to a colleague) sets aside space for a gentle conversation.

With 'LAURS' as a foundation, 'GREAT' provides a structured approach.

The delivery suite senior midwife requests a consultation for pain relief with Sarah who has been diagnosed with an intrauterine foetal death at 38 weeks.

Greeting

Anaesthetist: *'Hello Ms Jordan, Mr Jordan. My name is Dr Martha Green and I'm one of the anaesthetic doctors.'*
Sarah: *'Oh hi! I'm Sarah and this is my husband Peter.'*
Anaesthetist: *'I am so sorry for your loss.'*
Sarah: (tearfully) *'Thank you, we just can't believe it. We're devastated!'*

Rapport (using Listening, Acceptance, and Utilization)

It is essential to **Listen** and allow time for parents to express their emotions while avoiding the urge to fix things, move on to practicalities, or convey that we understand how they feel. We can't.

Anaesthetist: *'Yes, I can't begin to imagine how hard this is for you.'*

In these cases, less is more. Listening reflectively is paramount, with just a few words of acknowledgement to let the patient know that their thoughts and feelings are important. Once the immediate emotion has dissipated, then proceed:

> **Anaesthetist:** '*We are here to help make her birth as comfortable for you as we can. Would this be the right time for me to ask a few questions and talk with you about options for doing that?*'

If parents use the baby's name or refer to '*Her*' or '*Him*' it shows acceptance and utilizes their relationship with this baby to provide a more personal approach. Asking for permission offers a degree of control to parents and slows the conversation to a pace that allows them time to think more clearly.

Expectations

> '*There are some pain relief options we can offer. Has anyone discussed these with you?*' '*Would it be okay to talk to you about these?*'

Standard phrases like, '*What we usually do in this situation is*', can sound insensitive. For these parents there is nothing usual or routine about this day. Avoiding repeatedly saying the word '***Pain***' minimizes nocebo effects (see Chapter 3). However, should the patient use the word '***Pain***' it is important to include it in the response confirming the woman has been heard. Responding with '***Pain relief***' allows us to honestly address a solution.

Addressing concerns

> **Anaesthetist:** '*Do you have any questions or concerns about these?*'
> **Patient:** '*I don't want to be in pain, this is hard enough.*'
> **Anaesthetist:** '*Yes, we can help you feel more comfortable. We have several ways to give pain relief* (Explain PCA, fentanyl, etc).
> **Patient:** '*Yes, I'd like an epidural.*'
> **Anaesthetist:** '*We can do that for you whenever you are ready*' (Anaesthetist explains the procedure and risks/benefit) '*Do either of you have any questions or concerns about the epidural or anything else that's bothering you?*'

Tacit agreement

> **Anaesthetist:** '*So the plan is an epidural to get you comfortable when needed. Is that okay?*'

The ability to maintain a calm and open demeanour while avoiding distractions takes time and a willingness to hand some control to the parents. Sensitive and unhurried communication can have beneficial effects on the grieving process.[13]

Key points

1. The anaesthetist can communicate in ways that encourage patient autonomy and control.

2. Women who may appear distracted by contractions are usually able to listen to brief focused explanations.

3. The anaesthetist should 'check in' with the patient at regular intervals to confirm her wishes.

4. Women in labour can usually do more than **they** think they can, and frequently respond to suggestion in ways that allow them to achieve more than **we** think they can.

5. Verbal and non-verbal communications delivered confidently and calmly can rapidly elicit subconscious responses that defuse an otherwise fraught situation.

6. Communicating in a way that helps women to feel in control, and cooperate with anaesthesia care, represents a pinnacle of achievement for the obstetric anaesthetist.

7. How we communicate with bereaved patients and families helps shape memories and can positively influence the grieving experience.

References

1. Miller S, Abalos E, Chamillard M, et al. (2016). Beyond too little, too late and too much, too soon: a pathway towards evidence-based, respectful maternity care worldwide. *Lancet*, **388**(10056), 2176–92.

2. Clesse C, Lighezzolo-Alnot J, de Lavergne S, Hamlin S, Scheffler M (2018). The evolution of birth medicalisation: a systematic review. *Midwifery*, **66**, 161–7.

3. Bejenke CJ (1996). Obstetrics. In: J B (ed.) *Hypnosis and suggestion in the treatment of pain: a clinical guide*, pp. 250–5. London: WW Norton.

4. Kannan S, Jamison RN, Datta S (2001). Maternal satisfaction and pain control in women electing natural childbirth. *Reg Anesth Pain Med*, **26**(5), 468–72.

5. National Institute of Health (2006). NIH state-of-the-science conference statement on cesarean delivery on maternal request. *NIH Consens Sci Statements*, **23**(1), 1–29.

6. Downe S, Finlayson K, Oladapo OT, Bonet M, Gülmezoglu AM (2018). What matters to women during childbirth: a systematic qualitative review. *PloS One*, **13**(4), e0194906.

7. Cutajar L, Miu M, Fleet JA, Cyna AM, Steen M (2020). Antenatal education for childbirth: labour and birth. *Eur J Midwifery*, **4**, 11.

8. Wennerström S, Dykes AK (2021). Parents who have received 'psycho-prophylaxis training' during pregnancy and their experience of childbirth—an interview study highlighting the experiences of both parents. *J Reprod Infant Psychol*, **39**(4), 408–21.

9. Cutajar L, Cyna AM (2018). Antenatal education for childbirth-epidural analgesia. *Midwifery*, **64**, 48–52.

10. Alexander B, Turnbull D, Cyna A (2009). The effect of pregnancy on hypnotizability. *Am J Clin Hypn*, **52**(1), 13–22.

11. Stewart A, Sodhi V, Harper N, Yentis SM (2003). Assessment of the effect upon maternal knowledge of an information leaflet about pain relief in labour. *Anaesthesia*, **58**(10), 1015–19.

12. Cyna AM, Simmons SW (2017). Enhancing communication in obstetric anaesthesia— listen, listen, listen. *Int J Obstet Anesth*, **32**, 87–8.

13. Nuzum D, Meaney S, O'Donohue K (2017). Communication skills in obstetrics: what can we learn from bereaved parents? *Ir Med J*, **110**(2), 512.

Chapter 11

Children

Catherine Olweny

'I had six theories about bringing up children; and now,
I have six children and no theories.'
John Wilmot

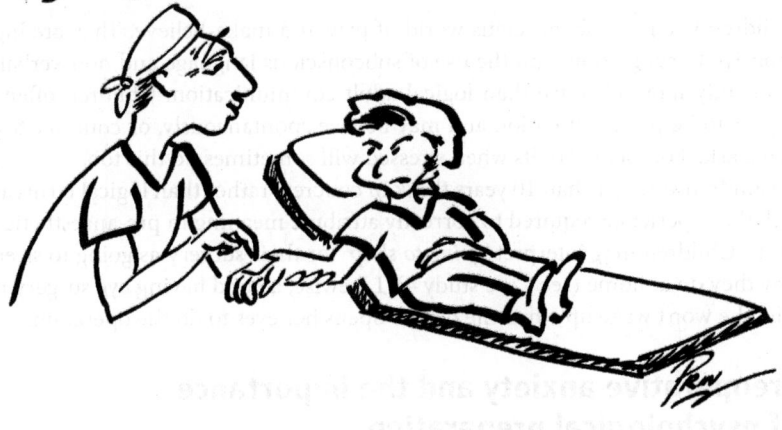

The challenge of working with children

When working with children the anaesthetist must establish rapport with the child, gain the confidence and trust of the parents, and convey important information without creating unnecessary anxiety or fear. Communication needs to occur at multiple levels to meet the different needs and concerns of patients and family members. Working with children necessarily involves a surrogate decision-maker, however, the emerging autonomy of the child needs to be recognized and respected. Communicating with children and involving them in decisions about their health respects their autonomy, builds resilience for future medical encounters and improves parental and child satisfaction.[1]

Children or adults: same but different!

Children live in a subconscious world of play and make-believe. They are highly responsive to suggestion, and the use of subconscious language and non-verbal cues is frequently more effective than logical adult communication. Children often do not appear to be paying attention and may behave spontaneously, or contrary to what is being asked of them. Adults when stressed will sometimes do this too.

Children younger than 10 years think in concrete rather than logical terms and may lack the experience required to correctly attribute meaning in pre-anaesthetic discussions. Children may interpret '*going to sleep*' for their surgery as going to sleep in the way they do at home (see Case study 4). Likewise, a child having eye surgery may ask why she won't wake up when the doctor opens her eyes to do the operation.

Preoperative anxiety and the importance of psychological preparation

Up to 80% of children experience anxiety preoperatively.[2,3] Risk factors for preoperative anxiety include age, with children between 1 and 5 years at greatest risk, high trait anxiety, temperament, parental anxiety, and previous negative encounters with healthcare providers.[2] Preoperative anxiety is associated with negative outcomes, including increased pain perception, analgesic requirement, nausea and vomiting, postoperative behavioural disturbance, and prolongation of recovery time. It has been estimated that 40–55% of children display new onset maladaptive behavioural changes following surgery.[2]

These behavioural changes include separation anxiety, sleep and eating disturbance, and aggression towards authority. In some children, behavioural changes persist at one year. Although we know that preoperative anxiety is associated with morbidity in both adults and children, little attention is usually given to psychological preparation largely because of cost and time restraints. Psychological preparation can reduce anxiety, facilitate a more positive experience for children and families, foster resilience, and decrease the use of sedation.

How to make communicating with kids, child's play!

Nearly all children will respond well to a warm and empathic doctor who shows a positive regard for the child, and listens to and accepts without criticism what the child has to say.[4]

The quality of paediatric healthcare improves when children are seen as intelligent, capable, and cooperative. Children often understand more about medical conditions and procedures than they are given credit for. Involving children in discussions about their health and in treatment planning, results in improved satisfaction, improved adherence to treatment plans and better health outcomes.[5,6]

Handing over their child to an anaesthetist can be emotionally distressing for a parent.[7] In addition, when a child attends the hospital for a procedure, families have frequently made complex arrangements for transportation, employment, and other children. Being mindful of the background stresses can help the anaesthetist communicate in a way that recognizes the experiences of families in their care.

Anaesthetists usually develop their communication skills over many years of trial and error. Much angst can be avoided by learning some simple techniques that can facilitate interactions even when only a short time is available. Flexibility in approach is paramount.

The preoperative visit

The preoperative visit is an opportunity to evaluate the medical and anaesthetic requirements of the planned surgical procedure and to assess the psychological and emotional needs of the child. The pre-anaesthesia interview has traditionally focused on information gathering, informed consent, and documentation. Rapport building is easily overlooked. The patient has a cognitive need to know and understand but they also have an emotional need to be known and understood.[6] To fulfil these needs, the physician must therefore communicate at a task-related level and an affective level, where the focus is on showing empathy and concern.[5]

Awareness of and a focus on the non-verbal aspects of communication helps build empathy and rapport.[1] Anaesthetists need to observe the non-verbal signals of both the child and the parents such as posture, eye contact, pace of speech, and response to questions and examinations. A systematic approach can help, similar to reading a chest X-ray.

First the parents' body postures. Are they 'open' or 'closed'—that is, legs crossed, arms folded? Are they looking around nervously, or idly leafing through a magazine? Is the baby or infant in a stroller or clutched to Mum's chest? Is the pre-school child clinging to their parent or off glueing stars on paper with the play therapist? Does the older child sit confidently close to the anaesthetist and answer all questions independently or do they choose to maintain a safe distance, deferring all questions to the parents? Physical closeness often denotes higher levels of anxiety—for example, a child burying her head into the mother's lap. Finally, any reaction to the anaesthetist's approach and engagement can be observed. Observation is key when exploring a child's interests. Even the most non-communicative adolescent will light up when discussing their true interest.

Clinicians need to be aware of the non-verbal messages they may be conveying.[1] For example, clinician posture can affect perceived empathy.[1] Sitting down with patients at eye level sends the message that the clinician is interested in the patient and has time for them. Vertical distance between the clinician and the patient is particularly important in paediatrics. Assuming a dominant posture can make people appear physically larger and more threatening.[1] The anaesthetist should avoid looking down on children while interacting with them. Kneeling on the floor, while younger children are seated or standing, can facilitate engagement at their level. Clinician tone affects perceived empathy. A warm and caring tone correlates with no litigation history whereas a dominant tone correlates with malpractice claims.[1] There is a positive correlation between a doctor's affective behaviour and parental satisfaction and compliance.[6]

The 'GREAT' template for structuring an interaction (Chapter 2) can be utilized in the pre-anaesthesia consultation.

Greeting

Parent and clinician behaviour during a medical interview can either enhance or restrict the child's participation in the encounter. Speaking to the child first recognizes their autonomy, and places them at the centre of the encounter from the outset. The child is thus encouraged to participate in information gathering and decision-making instead of remaining a bystander.[8]

After introducing yourself, it is important to confirm the status of the child's carer to avoid calling a 'parent' '*Mum*' when in fact they are sister, grandmother, or even a close friend or guardian! Identify yourself including explaining your role in the child's journey. Provide an agenda for the meeting. This need only be one or two sentences explaining what will be discussed during the assessment and emphasizing to both child and parent that there will be an opportunity for them to voice any concerns or ask questions. Commenting in a positive way on what children are doing or wearing can be useful—for example, '*Lovely pink shoes!*'

Rapport

No matter what the child's age is or what activity they appear to be deeply engaged in, they will hear the anaesthetist–parent discussion and take on board what is said. Every opportunity should be taken to seed positive suggestions and to avoid nocebo.

A confident approach can increase rapport as patient safety and comfort are both explicitly and implicitly implied. The child's response to some non-anaesthetic questions can provide valuable information that can increase rapport and be utilized later. For example: *'What is the favourite thing in the whole wide world you like doing'?'* or *'What is your favourite colour?/food?/drink?'* For the older child *'Do you have any hobbies or sports that you like?'* or for adolescents, *'Do you like shopping?'*

Older children can be included in the medical interview with questions they will easily be able to answer; *'Do you need to take any medicines or inhalers?'* *'Are there any medicines you can't take for any reason such as allergy?'* This recognizes their emerging autonomy and can also take the conversation in unexpected but informative directions (see Case study 1). If a child appears pressured or uncomfortable, it may be preferable to redirect questions to the parents.

The use of slang serves to give young people a sense of identity and belonging. Trying to copy this language can risk alienating some young people[9] and requires ongoing medical education as adolescent communication changes with the seasons. Use humour or teen language if you are at ease with it but remember that no child expects (or wants!) an adult to be familiar with the latest lingo. If you convey that you are listening, attentive, and responsive to their needs, it is okay to be less than cool.

As the anaesthetist moves on to physical examination, they tend to learn more from the child's response to examination than the stethoscope tells them about cardiac status. Many children, especially if they have been examined before, will simply lift up a T-shirt or dress for auscultation. Others will require a more subtle approach. Never just place a stethoscope on the child's chest, or otherwise examine him or her, without permission. If the initial approach leads to a withdrawal response, it is time to reflect and change tack. Trust needs to be earned either directly, or through the parent. The anaesthetist will need to demonstrate that nothing will happen without warning. Pre-verbal children frequently find a direct approach frightening. Slow, careful, indirect movements will invariably succeed when more direct ones fail. Whatever the technique—and there are as many techniques as there are anaesthetists—providing the child is engaged in a friendly and playful way, the interaction is likely to be successful.

Pharmacological premedication may be useful for some children who are unresponsive to attempts at gaining rapport. Others will have had a premedication previously and the parents and/or the child may ask for the same thing again. Children 6 years old and above can be given the opportunity to choose. Offering a choice gives the child a sense of control and enhances their self-efficacy. Children who choose not to have the premedication are usually cooperative at induction of anaesthesia. If there are clinical reasons that premedication is not the best option, it can be suggested that *'Now the child is getting older, we often find things go a lot smoother whether a premed is given or not.'*

Expectations

The pre-anaesthesia consultation is the ideal time to seed positive expectancy in children and their parents about the procedure and recovery. Understanding the reasons for surgery from their perspective allows the anaesthetist to utilize their response in a positive way. For example, if the child says that they are having adeno-tonsillectomy because of recurrent infection, the anaesthetist can emphasize how good it will feel knowing that the throat will be so much more comfortable in the future. Indirect suggestions are useful—for example, *'Most children find that they recover quickly after this procedure and can eat and drink as soon as they feel like it.'* The importance of avoiding negative suggestions cannot be overemphasized. If, following questions from parents, you go into detail about the rest of the anaesthetic, be aware that little ears will be listening. Sometimes it is easier to send the child off to play. Otherwise you can end up with a child declaring, *'I don't want a tube in my throat.'*

'You will be asleep. You won't know about it.'

'I don't want to go to sleep ...' (tears).

Planting the seeds for induction can begin with enquiries such as *'What is your favourite colour?'* or *'What is your favourite food?'* The answer will give a starting point for conversation with the child in theatre and confirms that the anaesthetist has listened and understood.

Children can be shown the T-piece and mask, and encouraged to play with it, take it apart and put it back together, developing a sense of ownership. They can also be reassured that they can take their favourite toy into theatre, if they wish. Dual choices of comparable alternatives can be offered, allowing the child to feel in control (see section on *double-binds* in Chapter 4). For example, *'Would you like to breathe in the pink magic gas or blow it away?'* If one of these choices is made, the anaesthetist has been *'informed'* that the child will probably cooperate with an inhalational induction. The older or more cooperative child can be offered a more cognitive choice—for example, *'There are two options for getting off to sleep; the "sleepy wind" or a "plastic straw" in the back of the hand.'* If the child cannot decide at the time, the anaesthetist can explain about the 'numbing cream' and draw smiley faces on the back of the child's hands to indicate to the nurses where to put the cream—perhaps saying, *'We can decide when you get to theatre.'*

Addressing concerns

The anaesthetic visit can be equally effective as premedication when concerns are addressed and questions answered.[10] Furthermore, reducing parental anxiety is associated with a reduction in child anxiety.[11] Listening, observing, and accepting the parent's or child's expressions of anxiety are vital components in gaining rapport. It is then easier to address specific concerns as these are raised, being careful not to dismiss them even if they seem silly. For example, if a 9-year-old asks whether anything will be felt, the anaesthetist could say *'No!'* or *'Yes!'* Alternatively, the anaesthetist could use the child's words and acknowledge that something may be *'felt'* or whatever is *'felt'* will probably *'feel okay'* or *'feel as comfortable as possible'* (see Chapters 2–4 and 22). If an IV induction is planned: *'Some children say they feel something as the plastic straw or drip is positioned'*—or, for inhalational: *'Some children **feel** the magic wind over the mouth or nose as they blow it away, but most find that once we get started, before they know it, they are in the waking up room, surprised things went a little bit easier than they thought.'*

There are two common concerns of older children; that they may wake up during the anaesthetic, or they may not wake up at the end of the procedure. The anaesthetist can casually say to the parent, in earshot of the child, '*I will be with him at all times to make sure he is safely asleep during the operation and wakes up safely at the end.*'

Tacit agreement

The pre-anaesthesia consultation in some countries concludes with a symbolic signing of papers—an acknowledgement of a bilateral exchange of information and a contract of care arrived at through mutual decision-making and an understanding—that is, *informed consent* (see Chapter 7).

The journey to theatre

The anaesthetist may not have much involvement in the physical voyage to the operating room but has already been integral to the start of this metaphorical journey (see Chapter 5). The physical surroundings of the journey can be utilized to develop a focus of attention, engagement, and the development of a '*yes set*' (see Chapter 4). Children can be encouraged to walk or pedal to theatre. The anaesthetist can seed what is expected along the way with comments such as '*Do you want to climb on to the bed all by yourself or get Mum to lift you up?*'—another double bind. One can use the child's natural curiosity to engage them, '*Can you see the fish swimming towards the MRI submarine?*' '*We are in theatre number 5; can you see the signs and help us find the way?*' or '*When you are ready you can press the magic button to open the doors.*' This engages the child who generally wishes to be helpful and facilitates cooperation when the child reaches the operating theatre. Although the primary focus is the child, humour also may be helpful for the anxious parent.

Induction of anaesthesia

Be prepared for the child arriving in the theatre or the induction room. Children are often hypervigilant when stressed. Drawing up drugs in their presence can be frightening and prolongs the period of induction, known to be the time of greatest stress. In all age groups, positioning of the child, parent, and anaesthetist is important. Research shows that children are less fearful and distressed when positioned for medical procedures in a sitting position, rather than supine.[12]

Upon arrival, the child can be introduced to the theatre team. For example, '*Lizzie, this is John, he goes to St Mary's school*', or '*Lizzie, this is John, he has asked for the strawberry flavour in the mask.*' This introduces your assistant to the parent and shows you were listening and have made the effort to personalize the child's anaesthetic. Children, however, are in danger of being overwhelmed by 'helpful' staff who want to say 'hello'. An induction room can be invaluable in minimizing outside distractions. Where inductions occur in theatre, it can be explained politely—preferably before the patient enters the operating room—that it would be appreciated if other staff go quietly about their business in the background. ('Below ten'; see Chapter 17.)

The management of the induction has as many possibilities as there are parents, children, anaesthetists, and anaesthetic assistants. The primary concerns of comfort and safety will be accomplished by allowing parents and their child to have a sense of control as much as possible during this stressful time. The presence of only one parent helps the child focus their attention rather than splitting it between the two. Minimizing the number of people talking can be helpful. Whatever happens, the need for flexibility is essential as the anaesthetist engages with patient and parent as the induction of anaesthesia progresses. The following are helpful communication strategies.

Inducing the clingy 2–4-year-old

Sometimes the focus of attention is intensely physical, with the child 'glued' to the parent and head tucked down. This can be accepted by sitting the parent on a chair with the child facing them, one leg on either side of their waist, snuggled into the parent's chest. For an intravenous induction, one of the child's hands can go over the parent's shoulder or under their arm. The anaesthetist is then positioned behind the parent where the IV can be placed, out of sight. For a mask induction, the anaesthetist can stand behind the child and bring the mask around from behind the child's head. If the child leans forwards towards their parent, they lean into the mask. If they throw their head back the anaesthetist can support it and apply the face mask. This is a non-verbal communication accepting all responses, be they positive or negative, and utilizing them further. The parent, anaesthetic assistant, or anaesthetist can be the primary communicator during induction, depending on circumstance. It is best not to request a response from either parent or child as this can divide the focus between them.

If induction of anaesthesia proceeds with the child in the parent's lap, it is important to provide clear instructions on how transfer to the bed will be coordinated.

The inquisitive 3–5-year-old

The child in this age group may walk into the theatre with toy in one hand and parent's hand in the other. Some will prefer to sit on their parent's lap while others will tolerate lying on the bed with the parent nearby. The child can fit the mask and T-piece together themselves or place the pulse oximeter probe on their finger, promoting a sense of autonomy. Some anaesthetists encourage the child to paint the inside of the mask with a flavoured lip gloss of their choice. Others may give the mask either to their own face and pretend to breathe in, or to the parent. Unfortunately, some parents grimace at this, giving the child the subconscious cue that something smelly and bad is in the mask. An alternative strategy is to offer, in order, the choice of anaesthetist, child, or parent to hold the mask. Invariably, the child will choose the parent and will thereby have indicated an intention to cooperate with the induction.

Balloon blowing technique

The balloon blowing technique is useful for inhalational induction—'*When you blow in the mask, the balloon will get bigger and bigger and bigger.*' Many children will happily help the anaesthetist by holding on to their own mask, with a little direction on how to obtain a good seal. With the mask in place, the anaesthetist engages the child, re-enforcing blowing up the balloon by encouraging suggestions—for example, '*Well done, that's a really good breath, that's the biggest balloon so far.*' Alternatively, the focus can be away from breathing, allowing anaesthetists to display their singing talents with a favourite nursery rhyme.

Storytelling technique

Storytelling is an effective means of engaging pre-school children. A story can become even more engaging if the child's name is incorporated into the story. Repetition and rhythm create a calming effect for smaller children in the same way that a lullaby or a bedtime story does. Older children can be engaged by adding vivid imagery, sound, and movement. If the story is about a rocket ship, ask the child if they can smell the rocket fuel. If the story is about a rainbow, ask the child if they can see the rainbow or perhaps tell you the colours they see.

Counting as a focus of attention

A different technique is to focus attention using counting: '*We will count your breaths up to the number 20 as you blow the balloon up. When I get to the number 20, two things happen. First, the balloon will change to your favourite colour. The second thing you will notice is waking up in the recovery room with the operation finished and soon back with Mum.*' The implicit suggestion is that the child is focused on getting to the number 20. It is therefore important not to get to '20' before the child is unconscious as focus may be lost at this point. If for some reason the child is still awake at 16, then continue counting more slowly or in fractions, such as 16 and ¼, 16 and a ½. The number the child is asked to focus on—in this case '20'—acts as a symbolic representation of an end-point of focus. The actual induction involves letting the child practice blowing for 30 seconds or so (with an N_2O/O_2 mixture), before starting the count and with each counted breath turning the inhalational agent up a notch until it is at maximum on approximately the eighth counted breath.

If an IV induction agent is preferred, a similar range of focusing techniques can be used such as storytelling, or nursery rhymes. A *lived-in imagination* technique—guided imagery—can be used, such as asking the child to pretend to draw a picture. Asking what colour crayon the child is using, what part of the animal the child is colouring and so on. If the child responds as if actually doing the activity, it is very likely the insertion of the cannula will not be noticed. It is still important to inform children that they may or may not feel something and, if it bothers them, to take a deep breath, without suggesting what to feel.

As mentioned previously, children fear a loss of control, so rather than say,

'You will start feeling sleepy',

one could say,

'If you feel a bit sleepy you can relax back into the pillow.'

Direct suggestion may enable reinterpretation of unknown sensations as pleasant. For example,

'This sleepy medicine may look like milk, but sometimes it feels cool, like snow. If you feel that, you know it is working well.'

Alternatively, the *'sleep'* word can be avoided altogether, and a child reassured that he or she will be back with Mum or Dad very soon.

Once the child is anaesthetized, it should be remembered to reassure the parent. Saying *'Would you like to kiss your child goodbye?'* can indirectly imply death.[13,14]

An alternative statement might be,

'Thank you for your help. Would you like to give him a kiss? We will take care of him and get him back to you as soon as he is awake.'

This implies that the child will wake up and soon be back with the parent.

Children behaving badly

When things do not appear to be going well it is useful to stop and reconsider. Explanation and encouragement usually facilitate cooperation, even if tears continue. Children with previous anaesthetic experience can be provided with control by holding the mask themselves or being allowed to tell the anaesthetist when they are ready—**not** for the IV cannula to be inserted—but for the insertion to be **finished** with! If the child is crying and fighting the mask before an inhalational induction has commenced, IV cannula insertion can be offered as a less distressing alternative. Similarly, an apparently stoic adolescent who bursts into tears, at the thought of a needle can be offered an inhalational induction if finishing positioning the drip is uncomfortable. The anaesthetist should be aware that a good experience of having a comfortable IV cannulation can be an opportunity to build resilience rather than reinforce avoidance behaviours that may make future injections or anaesthetics even more stressful (see Chapter 15).

If the child refuses to allow the anaesthetist to proceed, a considered, flexible response is required. Sometimes, leaving the room to allow parent and child some space to discuss the situation, resolves the difficulty. Oral or intranasal pharmacological support can also be offered. On occasion it may be appropriate to postpone or even cancel the procedure (see Case study 1).

The anaesthetist's expectations can sometimes get in the way of flexibility, especially if the child has been labelled as difficult. Appreciating that there are always other choices and ways of doing things will usually help to avoid a battle of wills or an exercise in authority.

Case studies

Case studies to show how communicating effectively with children has enhanced their care.

Case study 1—The child refusing surgery—a lesson in competence, autonomy, and control

An 8-year-old girl presented for adeno-tonsillectomy. She seemed cooperative and answered all the anaesthetist's questions appropriately and readily allowed auscultation of the chest. Her father seemed to have an easy relationship with the child.

On arrival at the anaesthetic room, the child allowed an IV cannula to be inserted. As the anaesthetist picked up the syringe of propofol, the child stated that she did not want the surgery. The anaesthetist asked the child '*Why not?*' and she replied that she had '*not had an infection for the past three months and didn't need the operation anymore.*'

The father then insisted that the anaesthetist proceed. The child then stated to her father, '*Dad, you are not listening. Look at me! I don't need the operation!*' On discussion with the surgeon it was decided not to proceed and the child was reviewed six weeks later and no further surgery was thought to be indicated. This case emphasizes the importance of listening to young children who can, on occasion, demonstrate an ability to make logical, autonomous decisions regarding their care.

Case study 2—The child with intellectual disability saying she didn't want the needle or the mask

A 10-year-old girl with Apert's syndrome presented to the pre-anaesthetic clinic prior to her MRI scan. Her mother stated that the anaesthetist '*wouldn't get near her daughter with a mask or needle.*' The anaesthetist asked the child what she liked doing and her favourite colour. She said, '*watching SpongeBob Squarepants*' and her chosen colour was '*green*'. The anaesthetist told her that he had a '*magic balloon*' that could change colour to green as he counted her breaths blowing it up. On arrival at the MRI suite, the child was very apprehensive and refusing to come into the room.

The anaesthetist then asked about SpongeBob and whether there were any of his friends that she liked. She was then given a 'double bind' and asked whether she wanted to get Mum to lift her onto the bed or whether she wanted to climb up all by herself now she was '*getting so grown up*'. She climbed on the bed and was pushing the mask away with both hands outstretched as the anaesthetist asked, '*What is SpongeBob doing now?*' aiming to engage the child's imagination.

> **Patient:** '*He is cooking hamburgers.*'
> **Anaesthetist:** '*And is there any sauce while the hamburger is cooking?*'
> **Patient:** '*Tomato sauce.*'
> **Anaesthetist:** '*I wonder which hand is going to rest comfortably on your tummy first ... is it going to be this one or this one?*' As the left hand relaxed its grip the anaesthetist encouraged its movement by saying, '*That's right, well done! There it goes, well done, all on its own, all by itself resting comfortably on the tummy ... And I wonder when the next hand will follow its friend just like SpongeBob's hands, resting comfortably on his tummy while the hamburger is cooking.*'

Sevoflurane was then added to the gas mixture as the mask was moved in small increments nearer the child's face. As the mask was moved closer, the anaesthetist repeated how well the hamburger was cooking as SpongeBob blew the balloon up.

The child was induced smoothly, and during the induction it was emphasized to both the child and mother how cooperative the child was. In the above case, focus of attention was utilized initially by engaging with the child about her favourite cartoon character. Guided imagery was then utilized to encourage '*Lived-in imagination*' where the child was asked what SpongeBob was doing, the child's response was that he was '*cooking hamburger*'. This indicated that the child was fully engaged in this fantasy as if it was real. The anaesthetist then indirectly suggested that her arms could move to her abdomen to encourage the child's arm away from pushing against the mask. The mask was reframed as something to blow in to, so that the balloon could change to her favourite colour (see also Chapters 2, 4, and 23).

Case study 3—The child left with a bad taste in her mouth

A 10-year-old girl presented for laparotomy and central line insertion. When asked if she had any problems with her previous anaesthesia, she replied that she always woke up with a really bad taste in her mouth. She was then asked by the anaesthetist what her favourite food was and what she liked to eat when she was feeling well.

Patient: '*Strawberries.*'
Anaesthetist: '*Interestingly, when children who like strawberries pretend to eat them before their operation they often wake up with a really delicious taste in their mouth.*'

This is an indirect suggestion that if other children who like strawberries can wake up with a pleasant taste, so can she.

Anaesthetist: '*When I catch up with you later, I'll show you how you can look forward to having a really good taste and feel like eating and drinking after the operation.*'

This statement creates a positive expectancy and seeds future communications that are likely to function as positive suggestions. In the operating theatre an hour later while the IV cannula was being inserted, the child was asked if it would be okay to start imagining eating some strawberries and ice cream. Following an affirmative response, and a further 30 seconds, she was asked whether she had eaten the whole strawberry or whether she had only had a bite.

Patient: '*Just a bite.*'
Anaesthetist: '*Is there any ice cream with it or is it just the strawberry on its own?*'
Patient: '*Both.*'

The anaesthetist is encouraging a '*lived-in imagination*' technique using the present tense '*Is there any ice cream?*' rather than asking whether the child is '*imagining any ice cream?*'

Anaesthetist: '*You can carry on eating them throughout the surgery and when you wake up in recovery you'll be looking forward to eating and drinking as soon as you feel like it.*'

The anaesthetist has given an anti-emesis positive suggestion. Note, the anaesthetist did not say '*You won't feel sick or have a bad taste*' as this would be a suggestion 'to be sick' and 'have a bad taste'.

The child woke up in the recovery room and made an uneventful recovery. When questioned on the ward postoperatively, both parents and child voiced surprise at how well she had recovered after surgery, without unusual or unpleasant tastes.

Case study 4—Utilizing 'concrete' thinking

Dr Marion Andrew provides the following case example. A 7-year-old child on the operating table was asked by the anaesthetist as part of the pre-induction communication:

Anaesthetist: *'Do you know how to go to sleep?'*

Child: *'Close my eyes and stop talking!'*

This is a '*concrete*' interpretation of a previous communication from a parent.

Anaesthetist: *'That's clever! Would you like to learn a different way of going to sleep?'*

This utilizes previously expressed ability, accepting that going to sleep is a skill. It also differentiates the sleep at home as being something different.

Child: *'Yes.'*

The child appears pleased at being praised as '*clever*', and an uneventful inhalational induction follows.

Key points

1. Simple communication techniques can help the anaesthetist care for children in ways that are likely to make their journey easier.

2. Difficult behaviours are usually temporary, and there is always another way to engage the child.

3. Flexibility in approach is of the utmost importance.

4. The child's communication will guide the anaesthetist on how to communicate effectively.

5. A belief that the child can do more than he, his parents, or the anaesthetist thinks he can, will frequently engender surprisingly useful responses that facilitate anaesthetic care.

6. Respecting the child's autonomy and need for control will usually facilitate cooperation.

References

1. Riess H, Kraft-Todd G (2014). E.M.P.A.T.H.Y.: a tool to enhance nonverbal communication between clinicians and their patients. *Acad Med*, **89**(8), 1108–12.

2. Kain ZN, Caldwell-Andrews AA (2005). Preoperative psychological preparation of the child for surgery: an update. *Anesthesiol Clin North Am*, **23**(4), 597–614, vii.

3. Kuttner L (2012). Pediatric hypnosis: pre-, peri-, and post-anesthesia. *Paediatr Anaesth*, **22**(6), 573–7.

4. Lask B (1992). Talking with children. *Br J Hosp Med*, **47**(9), 688–90.

5. Levetown M, American Academy of Pediatrics Committee on B (2008). Communicating with children and families: from everyday interactions to skill in conveying distressing information. *Pediatrics*, **121**(5), e1441–60.

6. Tates K, Meeuwesen L (2001). Doctor-parent-child communication. A (re)view of the literature. *Soc Sci Med*, **52**(6), 839–51.

7. Claus LE, Links AR, Amos J, DiCarlo H, Jelin E, Koka R, et al. (2021). Parent experience of communication about children's surgery: a qualitative analysis. *Pediatr Qual Saf*, **6**(3), e403.

8. Clemente I, Heritage J, Meldrum ML, Tsao JC, Zeltzer LK (2012). Preserving the child as a respondent: initiating patient-centered interviews in a US outpatient tertiary care pediatric pain clinic. *Commun Med*, **9**(3), 203–13.

9. White B, Viner RM (2012). Improving communication with adolescents. *Arch Dis Child Educ Pract Ed*, **97**(3), 93–7.

10. Lindemann H (2014). Why families matter. *Pediatrics*, **134** Suppl 2, S97–103.

11. Manyande A, Cyna AM, Yip P, Chooi C, Middleton P (2015). Non-pharmacological interventions for assisting the induction of anaesthesia in children. *Cochrane Database Syst Rev*, **7**, CD006447.

12. Committee on Hospital C, Child Life C (2014). Child life services. *Pediatrics*, **133**(5), e1471–8.

13. Carlyle AV, Ching PC, Cyna AM (2008). Communication during induction of paediatric anaesthesia: an observational study. *Anaesth Intensive Care*, **36**(2), 180–4.

14. Cyna AM, Andrew MI, Tan SG (2009). Communication skills for the anaesthetist. *Anaesthesia*, **64**(6), 658–65.

Chapter 12

Critical care

Daniel Nethercott and Maire Shelley

'The problem in the world today is communication.
Too much communication!'
Homer Simpson

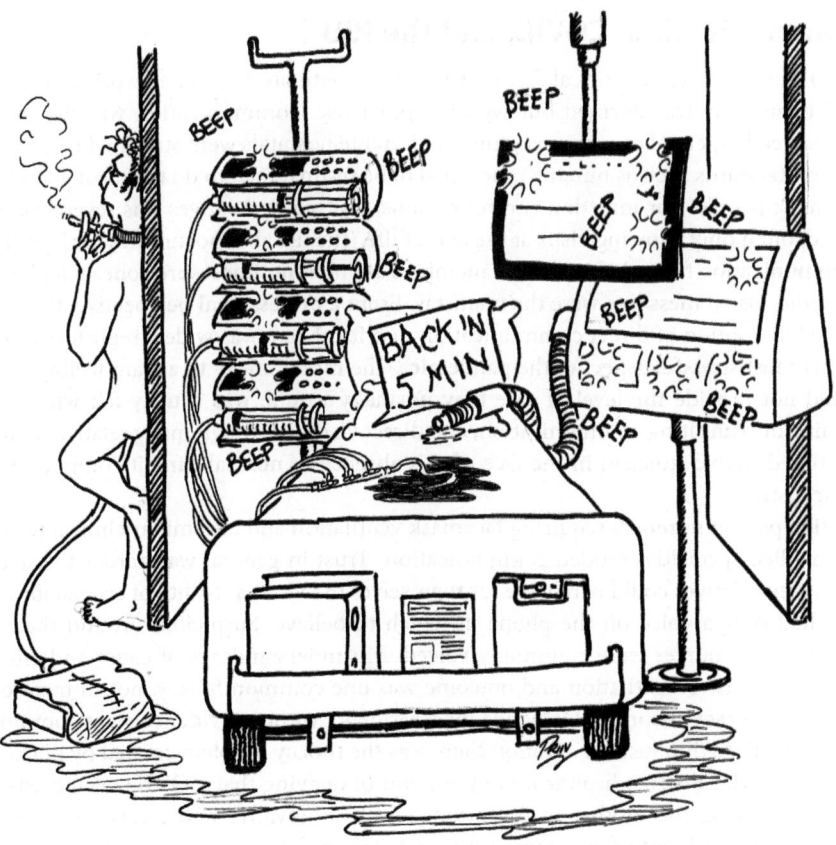

What this chapter is about

Communication, COVID, and the ICU

In 2019, the delivery of critical care for COVID-19 patients dominated world attention and completely transformed our working practices. Communication was the most widespread aspect of care that was impacted. Acute hospitals were stretched to a point where standards such as nursing ratios, had to be re-imagined to do the most good for the most people. For infection control reasons, visiting by relatives was severely curtailed, often only allowing visits at the end of life. The usual opportunities for layering communication from different team members at different times were gone. Telephone or audio-visual messages were the mainstay. From a professional perspective, this enforced disruption of direct communication in critical care was widely reported as the single most stressful aspect of the pandemic.[1] The moral injury to a team feeling they could not provide the level of care they normally would, was acutely felt when rationing or truncating communication, and direct visits. Although many relatives demonstrated heroic stoicism in the face of this absence of normal care, it compounded their distress.

High patient numbers requiring facemask ventilation and unfamiliar clinical teams from allied specialties eroded communication. Trust in general was harder to establish when relatives could barely see for themselves the visceral reality of critical illness and had only a voice on the phone in which to believe. Suspicions around the rationing of resources were commonly voiced. Misunderstandings of cause and effect between invasive ventilation and outcome was one common fallacy, not to mention overt conspiracy theorists. Demands for treatments without evidence were common and difficult to disabuse. In addition there was the thorny problem created by pockets of society who distrust healthcare to the point of denying that COVID even existed. Necessity being the mother of invention, several innovative and creative solutions emerged to ameliorate the communication problems.[2] However, of the many things these dreadful conditions proved, the vital role of communication in critical care was highlighted by its absence.

It is well recognized that errors of communication are associated with harm to patients on the intensive care unit.[3] This chapter presents a patient-based narrative in order to focus attention on useful communication skills.

Communication needs to convey a message that sits within its own context. For instance, the way that proxy decisions are made for patients who lack capacity varies with both culture and region. Resources are variable, and this includes the time that can be allocated to communication. Although beyond the scope of this chapter to offer guidance on exactly what information should be given to patients and their relatives, we aim to highlight useful ways of making the communication of that information more effective.

Communicating with teams in crisis situations

See Chapter 17.

> 03:00 in a district general hospital emergency department. The on-call intensive care doctor is fast-bleeped to the resuscitation bay to see a 35-year-old man called Stephen, who has been brought in by ambulance from a roadside accident. He is conscious but distressed with significant injuries to both legs and thorax. A 'trauma team' of doctors is assembled, plus the delivering paramedics, accident and emergency qualified nurses, and health care assistants.

Communicating with teams in time-critical situations presents a clear challenge. Team members can be unknown to each other with a variable skill mix. Clinical problems are undefined, different personnel have different and sometimes conflicting motives and goals, with clinical priorities that can shift over time. Within a medical team, hierarchy gradients will always exist to some extent, and they will sometimes need to be reversed in a crisis.

Under stress, most team members will respond well to someone else taking the lead. They will usually do as asked if they understand the instructions, are competent, and are not overloaded with other tasks. Closed-loop communication is a good way to keep communication efficient: *'Someone get me a tube!'* can be misunderstood or ignored by most of the team.

'Sarah, I want you to get a size 8 endotracheal tube from the trolley and test the cuff for me. Do you know how to do that?' is specific, directed to a named individual, and asks for them to confirm their understanding and competence to complete the task.

'Yes, I'll get you a size 8 tube' closes the communication loop.

Some trauma teams use jackets which clearly identify the team members' roles, but this is not universal. It can save time and promote clarity to ask all members of the team to have their name badges visible during a resuscitation scenario. Some trauma teams assemble with specifically labelled garments on to make the roles very obvious and reduce errors of delegation.

Although the default should be to communicate to identified individuals, sometimes addressing the whole group is required. This needs authority expressed through tone of voice, clarity of speech, and effective volume. The anaesthetist may become aware of an impending crisis before the rest of the team. The aim is to re-focus the team to the acute change. Guidelines from the Difficult Airway Society (UK) emphasize the importance of communication with the assistant if the airway management strategy has failed.[4] This allows them to prepare to change strategy. Another example in a resuscitation scenario might be '*I think she is about to arrest! Prepare for CPR!*' The situational awareness of the individual is spread to the team.

When leading a team, your communication should be modulated to match the clinical situation. Keeping communication quiet, calm, and encouraging while things are proceeding as expected allows for the contrast in volume and urgency when a crisis is encountered. Communication which is continuously at crisis pitch quickly becomes background noise and loses impact. Similarly, a running commentary from the team leader *can* be successful in helping the team act cohesively with focused goals and priorities but beware the commentary that becomes either repetitive or verbose. This style of communication can dominate the team and discourage other members from expressing themselves.

Debriefing teams is important after critical incidents. (See Chapters 13 and 17.)

Prioritizing communication

Emergency situations require tasks to be effectively prioritized and this includes communication. No communication is wasted but on occasions can distract from other more important tasks or generate damaging emotional responses in the clinician, which once recognized, can be stopped and re-directed.

For example, the junior surgeon wishing to insert a urinary catheter while the anaesthetist is attempting laryngoscopy and intubation. One approach is to show that the behaviour is unwanted by stressing the emotional effect it is having and then proposing an alternative.

> '*Talking about the catheter with you like this makes me worried that I can't concentrate on intubating this patient safely. Can we please talk about it in a few minutes when I have finished?*'

Another approach using the 'LAURS' framework:

> **Anaesthetist:** '*I think the catheter can wait until we've got the airway sorted out.*'
> **Junior surgeon:** '*But we need to assess his urine output.*'
> **Anaesthetist:** '*That's important* (Listening and Acceptance) *and you can do it once we've got him asleep and his airway is secure.*'
> **Junior surgeon:** '*We need to know how well we've resuscitated him. I think I should put in a catheter now.*'
> **Anaesthetist:** '*Okay* (Listening and Acceptance) *I agree we need to know how well we are resuscitating him* (Utilization). *Why don't you go and wash your hands and put some gloves on* (Suggestion), *by which time the patient's airway should be secure.*'
> **Junior surgeon:** '*Okay.*'

Listening to the surgeon allows us to accept her reality even if we don't agree with it. It can then be utilized by giving her something to do that can allow her to move towards her goal of catheterizing the patient while at the same time allowing the anaesthetist to secure the airway uninterrupted.

Handover

Stephen is stabilized in the emergency department. Bilateral chest drains are inserted, he is intubated and ventilated, and then taken for a CT scan. This shows lung contusions and splenic injury. He is taken to theatre where he undergoes splenectomy and open reduction and internal fixation of a femoral fracture, and compound tibial fracture. He requires a massive blood transfusion and is admitted to the intensive care unit (ICU) postoperatively. Stephen remains ventilated and sedated, and the theatre team hand over to the intensive care team.

Handover should be considered a risky procedure that poses a threat to the patient. The more handovers, the greater the likelihood of information being altered or omitted. Inadequate or incorrect information can have serious consequences and direct patient harm is not uncommon.[3]

The handover should be respected as an important but vulnerable process (see Chapters 17 and 18). There should be minimal interruptions or distractions, and it should not be cut short for the sake of expediency. Sometimes handovers between medical teams can lose focus and actually become de-briefing sessions or storytelling (Chapter 5). Debriefing has an important role, but it should not subvert the function of the handover, which is to communicate the information needed to continue patient care.

Meetings with relatives

Stephen's family is waiting in the intensive care relatives' room to be spoken to by the on-call doctor. Present are his mother and father, his sister, and three of his friends, one of whom was involved in the accident but was relatively unharmed.

There is very little advice from professional bodies on how much to say to the relatives of patients who lack the capacity to decide to whom they wish medical details be disclosed. It is a fair assumption that most people, if critically ill and temporarily lacking mental capacity to consent to providing information to their relatives, would wish for this communication to go ahead. Unless there is a specific reason to believe otherwise then healthcare professionals are probably on safe medico-legal grounds for such communication to be the default position. It is generally the case that communicating with relatives can be viewed as acting in the patient's best interests, in that it is likely to accord with the wishes of the majority of people (see Chapter 7).

Judgements must be made in individual cases with regard to the principle of maintaining patient confidentiality. Certain issues which might objectively be considered trivial, or non-sensitive, may not be so to the patient nor to their family. The overall seriousness of the clinical circumstances combined with relationship to the patient usually informs how much information should be given. This will vary and must be adapted to culturally accepted norms. Whether to communicate information remotely (e.g. by telephone) can generate a dilemma, but the same principles apply. Reasonably balancing the observance of *confidentiality* with a pragmatic perspective on the patient's *best interests* necessitates some degree of disclosure to close relations that will serve all but the most unusual circumstances.

Maintaining confidentiality for the critically ill patient with a temporary lack of mental capacity is even more tricky when social media intrudes. Beyond advising relatives on the importance of confidentiality, it is unlikely that healthcare professionals have a genuine duty to intervene if relatives share information unwisely (see Chapter 22). Navigating this territory is an evolving area of our practice and should be approached cautiously. A truly structured approach to these meetings can be difficult as the clinician has to respond to the unfolding communication fluently and instinctively.

It is common to be faced with a room full of relatives, some of whom may not have a close relationship to the patient or to each other, and it is difficult (if not impossible) to tease out the exact nature of every relationship. When faced with large groups it is probably advisable to err on the side of non-disclosure of all but the most basic of information so as to respect patient confidentiality. You should be confident to take an authoritative position and if required then make the group smaller. Establishing chosen representatives to receive information can resolve this issue. Close relatives can then make judgements on how best to disseminate information to the wider group. However, beware warring factions within families. Group dynamics can be highly variable: Sometimes one member occupies all the roles of leader, emotional responder, information giver and receiver. At other times each role is taken by a separate individual. Attending to a group dynamic in this way means the clinician will likely generate rapport with the most effective member of the group at each stage, and communication is optimized. Talking to large groups can be a daunting prospect, but the needs of the whole group can be met by communicating with each role player individually, and thus the clinician feels less like a lecturer addressing an audience.

Using 'GREAT' to structure an ICU interaction

Greeting

Introductions will give immediate clues to the dynamics. Often, individuals introduce themselves but occasionally there is an introducer and, if so, this is a useful sign they are appointing themselves as '**leader**' for the group.

Rapport

Consultation is not just about giving information, but also about understanding and acknowledging the emotional response to the information.

'*How do you feel about this?*' is a very direct way to elicit an emotional response.

Less direct alternative statements such as, '*I imagine this has come as a shock!*' perform the same function (also see section 'Silence and empathy'). Another important group member can present themselves here; the **emotional responder** who will express emotion for the group. Often other group members will comfort, collude with, or deny this individual. The group might find it difficult to move to the next stage until this person's emotions are under control.

Expectations

This is the '*What do you know so far?*' stage.

The first responder to this question often emerges as the primary **information giver**. Others may then fill in details or even present an alternative story. This is an important stage for developing rapport and further establishing the group roles. This stage also presents the answer to '*How much do you want to know?*' In groups, each member may have a different answer to this question, and it is often easy to identify the primary **information receiver** at this point. The amount of information can then be calibrated as you go through to the next stage.

Addressing concerns

Information can be presented to the '**information receiver**' though it is important to scan the entire group to check understanding. It is particularly important to check that the '**information giver**' understands, as it is most likely to be this person who disseminates information to others.

Tacit agreement

This is where the conversation is summarized and the next steps are explained. All group members should be involved in this, particularly the '**information receiver**' to ensure conversation structure is maintained. The final element is ending the conversation with a brief summary of what has been discussed, and where to go from here.

Recording and relaying communication

Good medical records are as vital to good continuing communication as they are to continuing patient care. The medico-legal importance of full contemporaneous records of communication is self-evident.

Communicating important issues with families is more effective if it is unhurried and allows more time for them to talk.[5] Creating a full transcript of any discussion is unrealistic in normal clinical practice. Formal audio recording of meetings is becoming commonplace. In the context of complaints or legal action, this is neither pragmatic nor desirable for day-to-day clinical work. Nevertheless, key messages and themes, including the levels of understanding, should be recorded and assessed. Verbatim quotes are helpful to highlight important moments in the meeting.

Continuity of message is important. Some ICUs use specific communication forms in the patient notes with spaces for separate themes or messages, equivalent to system-based daily intensive care review forms for patients. These notes can prompt the recording of information which might be forgotten, such as exactly who was spoken to, and what their subjective level of understanding was. Different messages from different members of staff can increase stress in family members. Figure 12.1 shows an

```
┌─────────────────────────────────────────────────────────────┐
│              Intensive Care Unit Communication Sheet          │
│                                                               │
│  Date: 11/4/09                          Time: 08:30           │
│                                                               │
│  Patient Name: Stephen Smith     Hospital number: 234567      │
│                                                               │
│  Present:                                                     │
│  M. Smith (mother), D. Smith (father), F. Smith (sister), J. ?Clements │
│  (friend, in the car), 2 other friends (?names), R. Pandit (Nurse, ICU). │
│  Dr Evans (Cons), Dr Hussein (Registrar)                     │
│                                                               │
│  Information given:                                          │
│  Punctured lung, damaged spleen, broken leg, long/combined operation. │
│  Now sedated, try to wake up later depending on lungs/oxygen levels. │
│                                                               │
│  Level of understanding:                                     │
│  Good understanding of injuries and operation.               │
│  Probably underestimating extent of injury/speed of recovery. │
│  Friend also involved upset++                                │
│                                                               │
│  Conclusions/Comments/Problems:                              │
│  Updates PRN, No major issues.                               │
│                                                               │
│  Signed:    R. Evans, 11/4/9                                 │
└─────────────────────────────────────────────────────────────┘
```

Fig. 12.1 Communication sheet.

example of an ICU communication template that can be used as an aid to continuity and consistency of message when communicating with patients and their relatives.

It can be useful to have one clinician to act as lead communicator to minimize situations where communication becomes very difficult between staff and relatives, for instance, conflict over plans of management with major clinical consequences.

The perception, *'They don't know what they are doing!'* that results from discordant inter-physician messages can be decreased. It is also useful to pre-empt confusion about the fact that the clinical condition of critically ill patients can change very quickly and that a different message from one moment to the next does not mean a difference of opinion.

Silence and empathy

Silence can feel uncomfortable to the **lead communicator** in a dialogue, but families need time to absorb messages. Critical illness is neither planned nor welcome. What they are hearing usually represents a major life event, something shocking and tragic they will likely never forget. For the clinician, however, the same meeting is part of the working day. Most doctors will have experienced some family encounters that affected them emotionally more than others. There is always an 'emotion gap' between the relatives and the doctor. Expressions of empathy are important to relatives, but must be well-judged to avoid inappropriate intimacy, and maintain professionalism. A well-observed silence after the communication of serious, life-changing news is a good way to express empathy. It marks the gravity of what has just been said and it can be an effective way of drawing speech from others. The perception of time is altered in states of high emotion and what the doctor feels to be a long silence will seem shorter to relatives (see Chapter 4—time distortion).

When actively expressing empathy, many doctors fear appearing glib and might adopt a more clinical manner to avoid this. Of course, it is important to be true to one's own nature. A forced or sentimental statement will be at best awkward, and at worst insulting. One method to strike an acceptable balance is to use empathic words in an indirect context.

> '*I'm sorry for what has happened to Stephen*', which is a direct expression of empathy,
> '*I'm sorry to have to be so blunt with the facts of what has happened*', contains the subtext '*I'm sorry*', but is slightly more oblique.

Although medical professionals fully accept that people without medical training or experience are probably not fluent in common medical parlance, it can require deliberate focus to weed out the jargon and translate medical language effectively. The level of understanding in the general population of even basic facts of human biology or medical treatments is surprisingly low.[6,7] Aiming low with the technical concepts you use in your communication and working upwards might be a stronger tactic than aiming high and missing altogether.

'*Do you have any questions?*' is not a very useful substitution for failing to target the right level of understanding. Consider the following paraphrased communication:

> '*Hello, I am Dr Evans ... information, information, information, percentage, information, ratio, information, information, uncertainty, information, likelihood, unknown word, confusing metaphor, information, information ... Do you have any questions?*'

The answer invariably is '*No*', probably because it is quite a challenging phrase. It carries the undertone of being a test of the listener. The answer, '*Yes, I do have a question*' is either an accusation that the message has been poorly communicated or that the listener has failed to listen properly, neither of which wants to be admitted. '*Do you have any questions*' is also heard as a conclusion and implies that the process of information giving has finished.

It is important to check the understanding of the listener in some way to find out what they have heard and so correct any misinterpretation. This can be done more effectively by a phrase simply designed to let them speak. Rather than the challenge of '*Do you have any questions?*', eliciting an emotional response to the information and acknowledging that the information itself is complex, gives a more welcome space for the listener to articulate.

> '*This must be a terrible shock*'; '*I'm sure this is all very confusing*';
> '*That's a lot of information to take in isn't it?*'; '*I can see that what I've said is not what you expected, Were you expecting me to say something different?*'

'*Do you have any questions?*' can work as part of the conclusion or summary of the conversation, but it is not likely to be successful while an emotional reaction is still forthcoming.

Talking to the ICU patient with a tracheostomy

Stephen has been on the ICU for eleven days. He has developed an acute lung injury after his initial operation and associated blood transfusion. Respiratory weaning has been slow and his progress has been hampered by poor tolerance of the oro-tracheal tube. A tracheostomy tube is sited, allowing the sedation to be stopped and consciousness to fully return.

One of the advantages of tracheostomy in the management of intensive care patients is to allow for reduced sedation, making communication more likely. Tracheostomy interferes with vocalization. There is a common subconscious bias that means when someone cannot speak, they are less likely to be spoken to. Perhaps communication is avoided simply because it is difficult.

Not being able to vocalize is tremendously frustrating and writing messages down, using communication boards or electronic systems, is a poor substitute for speech. A sad but common sight is the patient who gives up after the clinician, trying to lip-read has repeatedly mistaken the words. In this situation a closed question will often get to the point more quickly than an open one:

> '*Is the pain worse when you're being turned?*' allows a nod or a thumbs up, rather than '*Tell me about the pain?*'

The limiting effect on communication of tracheostomies can be very burdensome for patients. It is important to emphasize that it will be removed as soon as possible or changed for one that allows speech. There is a risk that patients become demotivated and a downward spiral of non-communication develops. In the meantime, acknowledge the frustration, use non-verbal adjuncts, and avoid the bias that '*Can't speak*' equals '*Can't hear*' by making deliberate efforts to regularly communicate simple and routine information about their progress. Techniques to bring the point of successful phonation forward in the patient's recovery include '*above cuff vocalization*' and the expertise of allied specialists in speech and language can be very valuable.[8]

Talking about withdrawing life-prolonging treatment

Stephen has been on intensive care for 26 days. Weaning from the ventilator has been prolonged and he has lost much of his muscle mass. He develops pneumonia and despite antibiotics this progresses to severe sepsis. He soon becomes unresponsive to high doses of vasopressors. Oliguric renal failure and thrombocytopenia develop. The next day he is noted to have fixed and dilated pupils. A CT scan reveals a haemorrhage in the midbrain. There is a consensus reached amongst the treating team that limitation of therapeutic effort and progression to end-of-life care is appropriate.

Personalizing communication

The patient should always be the centre of the communication. Referring to them by name or specific status (e.g. '*your son*') helps confirm this.

The ICU is renowned for being a busy place with high demand on its resources, and families may easily be aware of bed-status issues. The doctor should quickly and assuredly dissipate any misapprehension that the process of withdrawal is because of lack of beds or the rationing of any other resource, or indeed that subsequent organ donation has any influence on the decision. In fact, it is paramount that consideration of potential organ donation is clearly separated from issues such as withdrawal of care and resource management.

Active listening should be employed to allow the family to tell you about their loved one who is near death. The doctor is the expert on the condition of the patient and their treatment, but the relative is the expert on the patient before they became a patient.

As well as seeking out narrow information, such as pre-existing attitudes to intensive care or pre-morbid exercise tolerance, it can be fruitful to ask open questions.

'*What was he like before all this happened?*' can open up a torrent of heartfelt anecdotes about the patient's sense of humour, kindness, free spirit, and independence. The conclusion that '*This isn't what he would have wanted*' often spontaneously follows. Small insights into the patient's life can raise empathy in the doctor and empathic body language is a common progenitor of rapport. A family that feels listened to will have more faith in the strength of the doctor's judgement. Actively eliciting and listening to these stories is usually time well spent.

Communicating the withdrawal of therapeutic effort is not the only discussion that is important on the ICU, but it can be a complex message and so is a good example to take. The principles involved can be translated to meetings with other themes. Although this often takes the form of '**breaking bad news**', one should recognize that it might not always be perceived as '**bad news**'. Relatives can express great relief that the time has come for palliation.

The response to the message can vary greatly, which makes the '*check of understanding*' or '*evaluation phase*' paramount. Certainly, it is a failure of communication if the relatives don't understand that death is inevitable. A common misunderstanding is that the option being presented is between life and death, rather than the true option being the optimal management of inevitable progression toward the end of life.

Of course, the limitation of therapeutic effort should only be decided on a patient's behalf when they cannot make that decision themselves and when there is enough certainty that death is indeed inevitable. This degree of certainty should be communicated explicitly, that all avenues have been explored and all opinions sought. If the decision to withdraw therapy ultimately rests with the physician then this should be conveyed. Relatives should not be left believing that they alone are making a proxy decision on this issue.

At the first consultation, a lack of understanding of even fundamental issues is common in the relatives of intensive care patients.[9] The clinician should strive for absolute clarity on the underlying message. If the message is, '*He is going to die, regardless of what we are doing for him*', then this should include unequivocal words.

A consultant in emergency medicine once told the friend of a man who had suffered an out-of-hospital cardiac arrest that the patient had '*passed away*', to then be immediately asked, '*Do you think there's any hope for him, doctor?*' The terms '*Death*', '*Die*', or '*Dying*' are clear and once understood, softer more sensitive phrases such as '*passed away*' or '*passed on*' can be substituted.

Being positive in a bleak situation

When explaining withdrawal of therapy, some clinicians feel it very important to be explicit on the details of withholding cardio-pulmonary resuscitation. This can be unhelpful and even confusing to relatives and so great care should be taken.

'*If his heart stops then we don't think it's right to jump up and down on his chest or give him any electric shocks*', was said by a senior trainee in intensive care to a patient's wife, who seemed to have no idea that this referred to the process of advanced life support and was clearly non-plussed. It seemed bizarre to have described such a strange process with no reference to its aim, and then be told that this process '*will not*' be applied to your loved one.

Explaining that medical treatment is considered futile and that extreme measures are not appropriate should always pave the way for talk of what '*will*' be done. Withdrawal of treatment is often conveyed with a negative pitch which is natural in the context, but positive themes can still be brought to the fore when discussing death. An unsolicited list of all the things that are sometimes done with the aim of organ support, such as mechanical ventilation, haemofiltration, inotropic therapy, etc. but thought futile, and therefore not to be continued nor embarked upon, can build up a picture of impenetrable hopelessness. Many relatives have no idea what such therapies involve or achieve. Raising the potential for a therapy by explaining it only to snatch it away, by telling them that it is futile, can lead the meeting into a bleak landscape. Some relatives may have specific queries about treatments. These should be addressed. The technicality of providing critical care is important and interesting to the practitioner; it is rarely so to the relative.

Attempting to cover yourself by explaining every possible option of medical management does not automatically result in a relative being 'informed'. Indeed, the opposite is more likely. Sometimes we run through the options for medical management and the reasons why they will not be effective as a way of openly affirming the decision to withdraw. This can become a process of self-soothing for the doctor but leaves the relative confused.

Positivity and hope may seem perverse when death is deemed inevitable, but the communication can be done with positive language and hopeful messages. Hope in the face of calamity is a fundamental human quality. To completely crush the natural hope of the family in crisis threatens their trust and belief in the doctor. Honesty and clarity about the negligible chance of survival are vital, but hope can be re-directed. False hope for a miracle cure can be maladaptive and distract relatives from psychological preparation for the impending death. If re-directed towards hoping for an achievable goal, then hope itself is maintained.

Good-quality palliative care is by no means universal in intensive care, but it is certainly an achievable goal. The negative instruction '*Do Not Resuscitate*' is being replaced in some areas with the more neutral phrase '*Allow Natural Death*'. Discharging patients directly from critical care to their own home to die is logistically challenging, but can bring a positive and valued outcome.[10]

Non-abandonment

Non-abandonment is a crucial concept to convey to relatives. It means that although **certain** *treatments* might be withheld or withdrawn, *care* certainly is not. When this is turned into a positive aspect of the communication of withdrawal it serves as a good conclusion to the meeting. The emphasis on comfort and dignity suggests that care will still continue and that the family are an important part of any decision-making. The decision in itself is important; it has been made on the patient's behalf and it will result in positive things happening.

The decision to withdraw life-sustaining therapy from Stephen is explained to his family by the intensive care consultant. The discussion is concluded:

> *'This is a really important decision, but now that everyone who is caring for Stephen is clear that we can't get him better, we will be really focused on keeping him as comfortable as we can, and letting his death be as dignified as possible, with whoever he might wish to be near him there if they want.'*

The fear of abandonment is commonly expressed when approaching the end of life. Evidence from the analysis of recorded family conferences suggests doctors use three modes of expressing non-abandonment.[11]

'We will not abandon your relative' is rarely stated explicitly. The description of maintaining comfort by treating pain and agitation properly implies that care will continue. The promise to the family of continuing accessibility implies that the patient is not being forgotten. *'We're here 24 hours a day, there's always a nurse by the bed, and the doctors working on the ICU are close at hand.'*

The offer to make sure that relatives can be with the patient if they wish, either at a point of deterioration or death, *'Have we got your contact details up to date, so we can call you if there's any change?'* carries the message that the family is still valued and that they are not being abandoned either.

Patients for whom curative and supportive treatment is being withdrawn with the move to end-of-life care are sometimes discharged to ward areas rather than cared for on the ICU, usually for clinical and organizational reasons. These can both be given as a positive presentation regardless of the patient's destination.

> *'Intensive care is a good place for him to be. He's got his own nurse and there are always doctors on hand to make sure he gets any medication he might need.'*
> *'He's got a bed on the ward, which will be quieter for the family, less noise, and a bit more privacy, too. We'll hand over to the ward doctors, so they know how we've been treating his discomfort.'*

This might seem too much like 'political spin' on two opposing policies, but both statements can be true and delivered with sincerity. Although the message of non-abandonment is implicit, it is clear even with discharge from the unit.

Bereavement interviews

Very often contact with relatives of patients ends when the patient has been discharged or dies. Bereavement interviews should perhaps be considered part of the normal process of communication. Although personal experience suggests that many relatives do not take up the offer of a bereavement interview, for those that do, fundamental misunderstandings can be cleared up quickly. Explanations can be given, such as the details of the death certificate. Distressing concerns, such as perhaps the patient could have survived if something else had been done, or that they died in pain, can be explored. Those relatives who attend often give feedback on the care their loved one received which is good for staff morale. Occasionally improvements are recommended.

Unintended communication

Although we often worry that patients and relatives aren't getting the message, too often they are getting messages, but these are messages we did not intend to give, and what is being said has no relevance to the patient. An awake, agitated, and mildly hypoxic patient is having a central venous catheter placed by a doctor, with another doctor observing.

> **Doctor 1** (observing): '*... there has been a lot of staff sickness this week.*'
> **Doctor 2** (inserting line): '*I know, I was doing a vascular list yesterday and there was no trainee with me, which was a real shame.*'
> **Patient:** '*You haven't had any vascular training! Do you know what you're doing?*'

Clearly there is a misinterpretation of the conversation. Acute psychological distress can result in hypervigilance with enhanced sensory sensitivity and heightened attention to environmental threats. This can lead to a state of paranoia—not paranoia in a persecutory sense, but in its true meaning of believing that everything in the world pertains to oneself. It would be natural to think that the doctor who is treating you is talking about you and when further distorted through the fog of critical illness, an aberrant reception of what is being communicated is almost inevitable.

This phenomenon can also affect the family. The stress of having a critically ill relative is considerable, and it does not necessarily reduce over time. Watch the way that the relatives by the bedside react acutely to the persistently chiming alarms that are merrily ignored by staff. Anxiety correlates with cognitive biases such as tending to interpret neutral information as negative and increasing attention toward threatening or negative perceptions. These biases occur at a subconscious level via an automatic evaluation mechanism that registers emotionally significant cues.[12] Attentional vigilance increases exponentially in high anxiety states.[13]

Staff members should have a mind to this. Relatives and awake patients often feel starved of information, and they pick up any scraps available. Messages which are objectively neutral or insignificant can be perceived as significant and negative. Body language and tone of voice are particularly important at the end of the bed. Communication cannot simply be delivered in neat aliquots when it suits staff, who should consider themselves to be communicating all the time by the bedside. Discussion of other patients, disparaging remarks about colleagues, and dressing down of juniors within earshot all erode trust and respect. An attitude of thoughtfulness, diligence, and care provides indirect but positive communication, and these are basic components of professionalism.

The practice of intensive care medicine requires effective communication in several distinct areas. Multidisciplinary teams and critically ill patients and their relatives need different styles of communication at different times. Experience, self-reflection, and feedback from others are all fundamental to making the skill of communication more successful.

Acknowledgements

This chapter was originally written by Daniel Nethercott and Maire Shelly in the first edition. It was reviewed and updated by Daniel Nethercott in the second edition.

Key points

1. Emergency situations require tasks to be effectively prioritized and this includes communication.

2. Handovers are risky procedures and there should be minimal interruptions or distractions.

3. When talking to relatives avoid the temptation to respond to confusion by giving more and more information.

4. Differing messages from different members of staff increase stress in family members.

5. A well-observed silence after the communication of serious news is a good way to express empathy without risking insincerity.

6. We should consider ourselves to be communicating all the time by the bedside.

7. We communicate our professionalism by being professional.

References

1. Shale S (2020). Moral injury and the COVID-19 pandemic: reframing what it is, who it affects and how care leaders can manage it. *BMJ Leader*, **4**(4), 224–7.

2. Chua CKZ (2022). New strategies to improve communication in the intensive care unit during the COVID-19 pandemic. *Crit Care*, **26**(1), 191.

3. Reader TW, Flin R, Cuthbertson BH (2007). Communication skills and error in the intensive care unit. *Curr Opin Crit Care*, **13**(6), 732–6.

4. Frerk C, Mitchell VS, McNarry AF, et al. (2015). Difficult Airway Society 2015 guidelines for management of unanticipated difficult intubation in adults†. *BJA: British Journal of Anaesthesia*, **115**(6), 827–48.

5. Curtis JR, White DB (2008). Practical guidance for evidence-based ICU family conferences. *Chest*, **134**(4), 835–43.

6. Napadow V, Li A, Loggia ML, et al. (2015). The imagined itch: brain circuitry supporting nocebo-induced itch in atopic dermatitis patients. *Allergy*, **70**(11), 1485–92.

7. Babitu UQ, Cyna AM (2010). Patients' understanding of technical terms used during the pre-anaesthetic consultation. *Anaesth Intensive Care*, **38**(2), 349–53.

8. McGrath B, Lynch J, Wilson M, Nicholson L, Wallace S (2016). Above cuff vocalisation: a novel technique for communication in the ventilator-dependent tracheostomy patient. *J Intensive Care Soc*, **17**(1), 19–26.

9. Shaw DJ, Davidson JE, Smilde RI, Sondoozi T, Agan D (2014). Multidisciplinary team training to enhance family communication in the ICU. *Crit Care Med*, **42**(2), 265–71.

10. Battle E, Bates L, Liderth E, et al. (2014). Enabling ICU patients to die at home. *Nurs Stand*, **29**(5), 46–9.

11. West HF, Engelberg RA, Wenrich MD, Curtis JR (2005). Expressions of nonabandonment during the intensive care unit family conference. *J Palliat Med*, **8**(4), 797–807.

12. Arrow K, Burgoyne LL, Cyna AM (2022). Implications of nocebo in anaesthesia care. *Anaesthesia*, 77 **Suppl 1**, 11–20.

13. Mathews A, Mackintosh B, Fulcher EP (1997). Cognitive biases in anxiety and attention to threat. *Trends Cogn Sci*, **1**(9), 340–5.

Chapter 13

When bad things happen

Diana C. Strange Khursandi and
Suyin G.M. Tan

'Though it be honest, it is never good to bring bad news.'
William Shakespeare

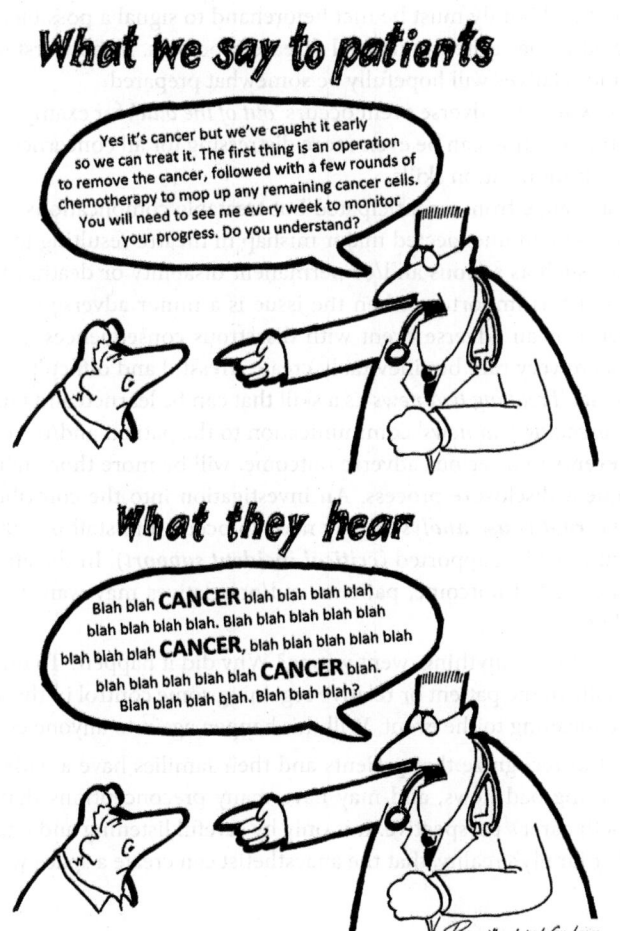

What this chapter is about

Breaking bad news using 'LAURS'

When bad things happen, good communication skills and honesty are of supreme importance. Breaking bad news to patients, relatives, or staff is never easy. Anaesthetists are most familiar with imparting bad news when they are working in critical care, where the possibility of bad news is implicit (see Chapter 12). The necessity to do so in anaesthetic practice arises relatively infrequently.

When, prior to surgery, patients are acutely unwell, elderly, frail, or otherwise high risk, the patient and family must be met beforehand to signal a possible, or probable, unfavourable outcome related to natural disease processes. If the worst does happen, the patients and relatives will hopefully be somewhat prepared.

In situations where an adverse event occurs '*out of the blue*', for example death due to anaphylaxis, the situation can be even more distressing for all concerned and requires considerable communication skills.

Incidents can range from unanticipated but treatable complications—for example, dural puncture—to an unexpected major mishap in theatre resulting in a serious adverse outcome, such as serious and/or permanent disability or death. Effective communication is just as important when the issue is a minor adverse outcome or side effect, as when it is an adverse event with disastrous consequences. Major mishaps in anaesthesia are very rare but inevitably create stressful and difficult situations. The good news is that '*breaking bad news*' is a skill that can be learned and taught.

The initial '*breaking bad news*' communication to the patient and/or relatives about the series of events in a serious adverse outcome, will be more thoroughly explained in the subsequent disclosure process. An investigation into the contributing factors in such events (***root cause analysis***) may need to occur, and staff members involved in the incident must be supported (***critical incident support***). In the aftermath of an adverse or unexpected outcome, patients and/or relatives may want to know many things including:

◆ The truth—what, if anything, went wrong? Why did it happen? To understand the '**Why?**' results in the patient or relative regaining some control in the situation and gives some meaning to the event. Will this happen again to anyone else?

It is important to recognize that patients and their families have a wide range of responses to hearing bad news, and may have many preconceptions that are at odds with their health carer's perspective. It is only by careful listening and engaging in the patient's and or family's reality, that the anaesthetist can create a space where they can express emotions, ask questions, and feel that their concerns have been heard and responded to in a caring and compassionate manner.

'LAURS' provides a useful underlying philosophy to guide the clinician in communication in challenging circumstances such as *breaking bad news*, or managing an adverse event or complaint. The word 'person' is used interchangeably in the following text and applies to patients, family members, and significant others.

Listen

This is the key activity that underpins all interactions. At times the anaesthetist who has to break bad news can be so overwhelmed by emotion that listening and focusing on the person's need is overlooked. The interaction can then become dominated by the clinician's need to '*deliver the package*' (i.e. break the bad news rather than engage in a human connection with the person). In such circumstances, it becomes easy for the clinician to be seen as uncaring, rushed, or overly focused on technical aspects. Conversely, some anaesthetists may be so apprehensive about breaking bad news that they may '*beat about the bush*', which can stress both themselves and the person. Asking open-ended questions helps create space for the person to talk, and guides the anaesthetist into a better understanding of where the person is in their own reality. Checking what the person already knows or thinks will allow a better assessment of the situation, will gain some rapport, and will gauge how much information the person may **want** to know. Some people will need every detail—others will need an outline, or very little information.

The anaesthetist can ask,

> '*Can you tell me what you know?*'
> '*What's your understanding of what's happened?*'
> '*Did you think something serious was going on?*'

Even if the interview has been arranged as soon as possible, it is often unclear how much information may have been acquired before the breaking bad news interview. The patient and family members may have had discussions with nurses or other personnel to find out what has happened, may have no information, a little or incorrect information, or may have misinterpreted what others have said.

Important information can be gained about the patient's or relative's emotional state. This is of great value in framing the communication. Uninterrupted listening is important—see Chapter 2. There is a natural tendency to plan what to say next, rather than listen to what the patient or relative is saying. This temptation should be avoided where possible so that the patient or relatives feel, and see that they are being taken seriously, being listened to, and that concerns are being heard, understood, and addressed.

Attentive, uninterrupted listening is the most effective strategy to clarify the person's understanding, and allows a clinician to tailor the communication to the individual. It is a very different task to break bad news to someone who has long expected it, than to a family who had absolutely no inkling that something calamitous has happened.

Acceptance

The emotional response to the grief of hearing bad news can range from disbelief, anger, sadness, desolation, and wailing, to resignation—the last especially, if the information has been expected for some time. It is important to acknowledge and encourage expressions of emotion.

For example:

> 'I can see you are really angry about this incident.'
> 'I can see that this is very upsetting for you.'

It is also helpful for the bearer of bad news to recognize that, in these situations, anger is a common response of the patient or relatives and is the hardest one to deal with. It is important to recognize, acknowledge, and validate this response. Without blaming an individual where an adverse event has occurred, an apology should be made for any harm incurred, and reassurance given that the incident is being investigated so that it will not happen again. This may help to defuse the anger.

In response to the patient's or relative's hostility, the anaesthetist may be tempted to show frustration, irritation, or defensiveness, or may blame others for what went wrong. Awareness of, and insight into these possible responses will allow unhelpful emotions and behaviours to be kept in check. The focus should be on recognizing and accepting the person's present emotional state, thoughts, and beliefs, however challenging or irrational they may appear. This is particularly true when responding to complaints which may appear vexatious, trivial, or incomprehensible to the clinician. Being able to, at least temporarily, accept and engage in another person's reality is the foundation for establishing rapport and moving forward into the next phase of communication.

Utilization

Having carefully listened to the person and gauged where they are in terms of understanding and perception of the situation, and having accepted that person's reality in terms of their emotions, thoughts, and beliefs, it is now time to utilize that information in a constructive and therapeutic way.

For example, the mother of a 24-year-old son is distraught at hearing of his sudden death due to anaphylaxis. She is anxiously demanding that someone go round to the house to look after her son's dog. While some doctors might be of the opinion that this is not a major priority at the moment and respond with a comment such as,

> 'I think that's the least of your worries right now!'

Or even ignore what has been said, it is vitally important that the person is heard and responded to.

An alternative response might be,

> 'Okay, Mrs Lassie—I can see that you are worried about your son's dog. How about we find someone such as a neighbour who can help with this?'

This demonstrates that the person has been heard and that the anaesthetist has engaged with the person's concerns and responded in a caring supportive manner. This also helps to allay anxiety and allows progression onto other issues.

Most of the time, anaesthetists instinctively utilize what is communicated, but at times of stress it is important to be particularly mindful of using what is actually being presented as opposed to defaulting to what is believed should be happening.

Reframing

Reframing is a high-level, sophisticated, communication skill which is most often practiced intuitively by skilled communicators. However, like all communication skills, it can be learned and improved with practice. It may seem insensitive to consider positively reframing experiences such as death or serious adverse outcomes, but reframing can be used to direct a person towards a more productive or therapeutic path.

For example, in the above case, Mrs Lassie's concern for her son's dog can be reframed into concern for her own welfare.

> 'It's lovely to see that you care so much for your son's dog. It's also really important that we take care of you. How can we best help you at this time?'

Suggestion

Listening, accepting, and actively utilizing the information that is presented, inevitably promotes engagement and rapport. This, in turn, allows the person to be more responsive to suggestion. Generally in a *breaking bad news* situation, therapeutic communication is directed towards providing not only factual information but also support and empathy, including managing distressing emotions such as anger. Potentially useful suggestions encompass encouraging the person to consider ongoing emotional support.

> 'Our social worker is available if you would like to see him?
> Perhaps you should get some rest now.'

A practical guide to breaking bad news using the 'GREAT' approach

After a serious adverse event, the anaesthetist and other key staff involved, including, for example, the surgeon, should meet as soon as possible to plan the debrief interview with the patient and/or relatives.

The first thing to consider is which staff member is going to do the talking. The team need to be on the same page so that the patient or relatives hear a consistent account of what has happened—the **when, where, how,** and **why** the adverse event occurred.

If there is dissension within the team, consideration should be given to delaying the meeting until this has been resolved or at least the key individuals are in agreement on how to proceed. While it is important to send a clear and consistent message, it is equally important to be open and honest. Many patients feel that medical staff may be 'hiding something' or 'covering up a mistake' so all communication must be based on factual information where available, along with open acknowledgement of doubt and uncertainty.

The 'breaking bad news' interview should take place at a time to be negotiated, but as promptly as practicable. It is important that all staff members relay consistent information of known events. The interview should take place in private. The anaesthetist, even if not new to breaking bad news, will need to think about what will be said to the patient.

The persons conducting the interview should ensure that their pagers and mobile phones are turned off. The number of people in the interview room may range from two to several. Frequently there will be at least four persons—the patient or relative, a support person, the doctor and the doctor's support person. It may be that the anaesthetist involved in the incident is too upset, in the immediate aftermath, to meet the patient or family. However, it is advisable that the anaesthetist does speak to the patient or relatives at some stage. This allows patients or relatives to talk directly to the person who was there at the time of the incident, who can provide the most accurate factual information. This strategy will convey implicitly that an open process is occurring. The presence of the whole team, as suggested by Bacon,[1] may be overwhelming for the patient or relatives, or may be perceived as 'closing ranks'.

The planning of the 'breaking bad news' interview must include weighing up these considerations with regard to individual circumstances, and choosing the most appropriate staff members for the interview. A senior anaesthetist should be present for advice and expertise, as well as offering support to a trainee if involved in the incident. If the patient has died or is in intensive care, it is the relatives who are receiving the bad news. An interview with these relatives should be arranged in consultation with the other healthcare workers involved. The relatives may also wish to have a support person present—perhaps the family doctor, social worker, or religious representative. The relatives should be asked,

'Is there someone you want to bring with you?'

Greeting

At the start of the interview, a simple introduction of the hospital staff in the room will help increase rapport. This can be followed by identification of the patient or the relatives with whom it is intended to talk. Don't assume that the person by the patient's bed is the spouse, a parent, or son/daughter. Asking the persons present how they wish to be addressed demonstrates respect and helps build rapport.

Rapport

While breaking bad news is hardly an occasion for small talk, it is very important to establish some degree of rapport. This is easier if the anaesthetist has already met the patient or family previously, but if this is the first encounter then simply acknowledging that it is a difficult situation, and asking if they need anything (e.g. a drink) is a simple way of showing care and concern.

Expectations

Communication of bad news to patients and relatives is about giving information in a caring, supportive, and genuine way.[2] It is likely that the patients or relatives will be anticipating bad news to be communicated in the interview. Emotions will be running high. To expect bad news is different from actually hearing it! It is helpful for the anaesthetist to have thought about how to signal that bad news is coming before it is actually delivered. This tactic is called 'firing a warning shot'.

> 'I'm afraid I have bad news.'
> 'I am sad to have to tell you that your father is seriously ill.'
> 'Unfortunately I am here to tell you about an accident.'
> 'I am very sad to tell you that something unexpected has happened in theatre.'
> 'I am really sad to have to tell you some bad news ...'

Information is delivered or confirmed, and, not infrequently, misinformation corrected. The aim should be to build on what the patient or relative already knows, to deliver the information in small bites, and to ensure that no jargon is used. A check for understanding is necessary since people vary in how much information they can take in, and in their ability to understand what is being said.

It is important to emphasize that the facts as communicated are those known at the time of the interview, to restrict the discussion of what happened to the facts currently known, and to avoid any speculation about cause or blame directed towards the hospital or colleagues. In situations where there has been a critical incident resulting in an adverse event, rather than a natural death or adverse outcome, patients and relatives often want to know whether changes in policies and procedures have been implemented that will reduce or abolish the chance of a similar incident happening again. This may be their primary concern. If the **Why?** is unknown, patients and relatives can be informed that the hospital is investigating the incident, outlining the process of root cause analysis, and that they will be informed of the results of any enquiry as soon as these become available.

> 'We will look at our processes to see if anything can be changed to ensure that this accident will never happen to another patient.'

Since it is unlikely that all the answers will be available at the breaking bad news interview, the recipients can be informed that after further investigation, during the root cause analysis process, more information will be available.

Addressing concerns

The stress of hearing bad news can significantly reduce the ability to process information. Pauses should be allowed for the news to sink in. In many cases patients or relatives will be hearing the worst news they have ever had. Everyone takes time to digest momentous new information. So, giving too much information at once should be avoided. See also Chapter 12.

> 'Can you tell me if you have understood what I am saying, or would you like me to repeat something?'

It is very important to allow time for the recipients to understand what has happened, and then allow time for them to frame questions.

It is vitally important to communicate bad news with empathy and acknowledgement of the emotions that are arising. It is also appropriate to acknowledge one's own emotions in an honest way—either to oneself, one's colleagues, and even the person.

> *'I am really sorry to have to be the bearer of such tragic news.'*
> *'I know how upsetting this news must be for you.'*
> *'Obviously, this is terrible news ... '*

Anger, denial, and disbelief are common initial responses. People need time and space to absorb the information and adding even more information, or attempting to argue back, is frequently unhelpful and may inflame matters. Even if, at this stage, emotions are running high, the anaesthetist should avoid calling hospital security. Nevertheless, be mindful of personal safety. Sometimes it may help to offer *time out* to allow emotions to settle and then reconvene after a short break. If a person appears too distraught to continue, support should be offered and the meeting rescheduled.

Ongoing acknowledgement and support in allowing the person to air their distress is usually the optimal course. Be mindful that anger can resurface at any time—if so, return to attentive, uninterrupted listening, and again acknowledge the emotion with an empathic remark.

> *'I can see that this makes you angry.'*

When the bad news has been relayed, empathy expressed, and emotions acknowledged, it is then possible to move on to ask if there are any other concerns.

It is particularly helpful for the anaesthetist to allow time for questions, and to avoid rushing the interview. If the anaesthetist appears to want to get things over with, this attitude can be interpreted as uncaring. The anaesthetist may have to ask for questions more than once during the *breaking bad news* interview, as new concerns may surface at any time. Useful statements might include:

> *'Have you any other particular concerns at the moment?'*
> *'Do you wish to tell me any other thoughts or worries?'*
> *'Is there anything else that is troubling you about the situation?'*
> *'Do you feel I have covered all your concerns for now?'*

Tacit agreement

There will be a need to check that the patient or relatives have understood the information including follow-up arrangements. Receiving bad news can put all other thoughts to one side, so the topic may need to be returned to more than once. An appointment with a psychologist, or a minister of religion, can be offered and arranged where appropriate.

> *'Would you like me to arrange an appointment with someone who can help you deal with this tragic situation?'*
> *'Would you like to talk to the social worker, or someone else who could help you?'*

Ongoing support is frequently appreciated by patients and relatives, and demonstrates genuine concern and care on the part of the anaesthetist:

'Perhaps we should meet again, to answer any further questions.'
'If you would like to come to talk to me any time in the future, please contact me on this phone number.'
'We can arrange another appointment at a mutually convenient time.'

Important considerations

Documentation

It is vital to document immediately afterwards what information was covered in the debriefing interview, as well as who was present. To enable this to happen, one of the interviewers should take notes at the time, or document the information at the earliest opportunity after the interview. It is important to document the facts only, regardless of one's own personal opinions, thoughts, or feelings, and resist the temptation to opine on causation, assign blame to any member of the team concerned, or express judgements on an individual's actions.

The salient details should be documented in the patient's records. It may be necessary in the future to provide this account in court or to a medical defence organization (MDO). Therefore, it is wise to retain a personal copy of the document, and to supply another copy to the MDO if required. During the crisis it is often impossible to document what happened. The account in the patient's record of what happened must often be written after the episode has been brought under control. The record must clearly indicate that it has been written following the acute episode. Any subsequent conversations should also be documented contemporaneously in the medical record.

Patient perceptions

In difficult communication situations, hospital staff are likely to feel uncomfortable, edgy, or embarrassed, and may want to get the whole process over with quickly. Such feelings tend to translate into behaviour that may be perceived by the patient or relatives as uncaring or insensitive. Creating this perception must be strenuously avoided, as it may cause mistrust. It can also generate unnecessary distress, interfere with good communication, and may increase the likelihood of long-term adverse consequences. Recognition, acceptance and even admission of these uncomfortable feelings may allow the anaesthetist to behave in a more genuine way.

Stress/Burn-out

Anaesthesia is, by its nature, a specialty where the need to break bad news is infrequent. Therefore, no matter how experienced the individual, the process is always stressful to some degree. Knowledge, training, practice, and shared experiences of the skills required when breaking bad news can reduce stress to the doctor. Support in the workplace is an important factor in minimizing the development of **burn-out**.[3,4] Addressing both individual and workplace issues are required for there to be a comprehensive solution.[5] If the patient or relative concerns are not addressed or emotions acknowledged, they may suffer long-term distress, especially if the amount of information given is not tailored specifically to them. That is, too much or too little information. Time taken to ensure that emotions are recognized and validated is time well spent.

Litigation

Patients and relatives are more likely to proceed to litigation if:

♦ they feel that the breaking bad news interview has gone badly; or
♦ the doctor was uncaring or insensitive;
♦ they were not given enough information;
♦ they were not being told the truth in a timely fashion;
♦ concerns were not being heard and dealt with.

Critical incidents

Critical incidents are those where a patient or staff member has experienced an adverse event or just avoided an adverse event (i.e. a *near miss*).

What might constitute an adverse event?

♦ Death
♦ Paraplegia
♦ Loss of limb
♦ Trauma or anaesthetic incident resulting in brain death
♦ Staff suicide or drug overdose

What processes need to be followed after any one of these events?

♦ **Breaking bad news** to the patient and/or the family (see earlier).
♦ **Critical incident support** involves providing support for the anaesthetist(s) and other staff involved with the adverse event—the *'second victim'*. For example, the young anaesthetist whose patient has died on the operating table, as well as support for all other staff involved in the incident. Many employers have staff counselling services available and anaesthesia colleges also provide support services.
♦ **Root cause analysis**. This process is an investigation into possible causes or contributing factors leading to the incident. It is important for relatives to know that an investigation has been started. Whatever the institution, there should always be a risk management process initiated after a serious adverse event. Root cause analysis aims to examine and analyse likely factors which have contributed to a serious adverse event. This culminates in a report highlighting what can be done to avoid or mitigate future errors in similar circumstances. Implementation of the recommendations arising from the root cause analysis will hopefully result in improvements in the healthcare process.
♦ **Open disclosure** is defined as the frank discussion of incidents that result in unintended harm to a patient while receiving healthcare, as well as the associated

investigation and recommendations for the improvement of practice.[6] The definition of open disclosure in different countries is not exactly the same, but most emphasize open and honest communication with patients and their families after an adverse incident. The initial breaking bad news interview, which needs to occur immediately after the incident, is the start of an open disclosure process.

The 'second victim'

The 'second victim' is the anaesthetist or other person involved in the adverse event. Many doctors feel that they are directly to blame for an adverse incident occurring to one of their patients, even when the causes are not the doctor's fault in any way.[7] More often than not it is a team responsibility, and system errors are frequently uncovered.

The **perception** of self-blame by the doctor involved '*at the sharp end*', even when no fault can be attributed, may result in major personal stress. It can cause depression or other mental illness, including the potential for adjustment disorder and post-traumatic shock disorder (PTSD). Tragically it has occasionally resulted in suicide. It is thus of extreme importance to offer practical and emotional support to those involved. The guilt felt by the individuals involved is worse if:

- the incident was potentially avoidable;
- the patient is young;
- the anaesthetist is inexperienced;
- the anaesthetist thinks the case was mishandled;
- the case was an emergency;
- a junior anaesthetist was unsupervised;
- there was no support from colleagues;
- the anaesthetist was not working in the usual team or a familiar environment (e.g. when acting as a locum);
- a member of staff is the patient.

As experienced by the '*second victim*', the stages of distress at the event can be likened to those of bereavement or other traumatic event—denial, isolation, anger, bargaining, depression and, finally, acceptance.[8]

If litigation follows from the adverse event, then these feelings are likely to be exaggerated, and the stress can continue for several years. The chances of doctor suicide are greatly increased by the inevitably prolonged medicolegal process.[9–12]

In the immediate post-incident period, the person responsible for critical incident support, perhaps a designated senior anaesthetist, as suggested above, should contact the '*second victim*' to offer comfort, support, and relief from duties.

A confidential interview in private should be suggested.

> '*I've just heard what happened, would you like to come to talk about it with me?*
> *I have arranged for someone else to take over your list. If you need time off work,*
> *this can be arranged.*'

The individual involved should be encouraged to reflect on the episode, and talk about it. Any expression of blame should be avoided. At a later stage, when the doctor is ready to write down the facts, a mentor can offer help with this document. Empathy for the person involved can be shown by validating the experience—perhaps with examples from personal experience.

I had a similar thing happen to me some years ago—and I found it very difficult to come to terms with—I was enormously helped by ...

In some centres the *'second victim'* will be informed that a root cause analysis will take place. The support person should emphasize that there are usually several contributing factors in any adverse incident, and that system errors are frequently uncovered. Knowing that deficiencies in the system may be identified can help the anaesthetist come to terms with what has happened. It is appropriate to ask if the anaesthetist would like access to professional help—for example, a psychologist, counsellor, or a religious representative.

'Would you like me to contact anyone to help you? For instance, someone to talk it through with you?'
'Would you like me to let your partner or family know what's happened?'

Ongoing support can be offered:

'My door is always open if you need to talk further, or explore anything else you might be feeling later down the track.'

Where a trainee is involved and is to rotate to another anaesthetic department or hospital, it is essential to ensure ongoing support by communicating the incident to the trainee's next supervisor. Some individuals can deal with adverse events without external support, although this may depend on the nature of the incident and indeed the individual concerned. If the anaesthetist initially refuses help, or says *'I'm okay—I can deal with it'*, the support person will need to continue to check, on a daily basis, with the person involved. This will be particularly important during the root cause analysis or medico-legal processes, which may continue for some time after the incident, and are sources of continued stress for the doctor(s) concerned.

What should the 'second victim' do?

The anaesthetist should expect to be offered support. If this does not happen, they should contact the department head, the on-duty anaesthetist, or a mentor. It is often hard to persuade young doctors to seek outside help—the stigma of mental health problems remains strong. Some may be able to cope alone with the help of family and friends,[13] although the capacity to deal with feelings may depend on the nature and severity of the incident. The need for outside professional help from, for example, a psychologist or another appropriate person, may not be recognized initially. However, the mentor can emphasize that these professionals are better able to give impartial and supportive advice. If litigation is a possibility, the incident has the potential to cause distress for several years, and there is an increased danger of consequences as noted above—depression, PTSD, adjustment disorder, or at the very worst, suicide.

> ## Key points
>
> Breaking bad news and the management of critical incidents require:
>
> 1. acceptance that **bad things happen**, through disease processes, system factors, and inevitably, human error;
> 2. anaesthetists to communicate with patients and relatives with empathy and care in a planned interview, including attentive uninterrupted listening;
> 3. follow-up to be offered to the patient and relatives;
> 4. support to those involved in the incident—*critical incident support*.

References

1. Bacon AK (1989). Death on the table. *Anaesthesia*, **44**, 245–8.
2. Buckman R (1992). *How to break bad news: a guide for health professionals*. Baltimore, MD: The Johns Hopkins University Press.
3. Afonso AM, Cadwell JB, Staffa SJ, Zurakowski D, Vinson AE (2021). Burnout rate and risk factors among anesthesiologists in the United States. *Anesthesiology*, **134**(5), 683–96.
4. Hyman SA (2021). Burnout: the 'other' pandemic. *Anesthesiology*, **134**(5), 673–5.
5. Baile WF, Buckman R, Lenzi R, Glober G, Beale EA, Kudelka AP (2000). SPIKES—a six-step protocol for delivering bad news: application to the patient with cancer. *Oncologist*, **5**, 302–11.
6. Iedema RA, Mallock NA, Sorensen RJ, et al (2008). The National Open Disclosure Pilot: evaluation of a policy implementation initiative. *Med J Aust*, **188**(7), 397–400.
7. McCawley D, Cyna AM, Prineas S, Tan S (2017). A survey of the sequelae of memorable anaesthetic drug errors from the anaesthetist's perspective. *Anaesth Int Care*, **45**(5), 624–30.
8. Kubler-Ross E (1997). *On death and dying*. New York, NY: Scribner.
9. Martin CA, Wilson JF, Fiebelman ND 3rd, Gurley DN, Miller TW (1991). Physicians' psychologic reactions to malpractice litigation. *South Med J*, **84**(11), 1300–4.
10. Charles SC, Wilbert JR, Franke KJ (1985). Sued and non-sued physicians' self-reported reactions to malpractice litigation. *Am J Psychiatry*, **142**, 437–40.
11. Birmingham PK, Ward RJ (1985). A high-risk suicide group: the anesthesiologist involved in litigation. *Am J Psychiatry*, **142**(10), 1225–6.
12. Wilbert JR, Charles SC, Warnecke RB, Lichtenberg R (1987). Coping with the stress of malpractice litigation. *Ill Med J*, **171**(1), 23–7.
13. Raphael B, Meldrum L, McFarlane AC (1995). Does debriefing after psychological trauma work? *BMJ*, **310**, 1479–80.

Chapter 14

Other challenges

Gillian M. Hood and Suyin G.M. Tan

'A man has the right to look down on somebody, only when he is helping him to get up.'
Gabriel Garcia Marquez

What this chapter is about

Patients with complex communication needs

Most anaesthetists recognize that there are specific groups of patients with whom communication is especially difficult due to issues relating to language. These groups are patients in whom a disease process interferes with communication—for example, intellectual disability or hearing impairment, those with whom we do not share a common tongue, and those patients whose cultural background differs from ours.

Patients with communication difficulties are disproportionately represented in the hospital population for a variety of reasons. The elderly form the bulk of hospital in-patients and are much more likely to have problems such as deafness, dementia, confusion, sedation, and dysphasia.

It is important to be cognisant of the issues that may arise with patients who have communication problems and, in addition to being aware of these problems, it helps to have a structured way of approaching the issue.

Recognize and define the communication issue

Reading the patient's notes prior to consultation gives advance warning of issues such as dementia or hearing impairment and allows communication to be tailored to the patients' needs. Sometimes the patient's understanding of language may be difficult to assess on first meeting—anaesthetists have all encountered patients who answer questions with a smiling 'Yes' or 'No', only to subsequently discover their comprehension has been minimal. Enquiring of relatives, friends, and staff helps to give a picture of a patient's ability to communicate in the chosen language. Similarly, enquiring of the patient how communication can be facilitated, is helpful.

'It says in your notes that you have trouble finding words since your stroke—is there anything I can do to make it easier for you to speak?'

Once the communication problem has been delineated it makes it easier to move on to the next step.

Orientation

Having orientated oneself to the patient's particular problems with communication, it is also important to orientate the staff with whom one is working.

'Rob, we are going to see Mr Smith now. He's had problems with alcohol withdrawal over the last few days and he is still a bit confused. It is probably best if just one of us does the talking—are you happy to do that?'

Not:

'I wish you wouldn't contradict me when I'm talking to patients ...'

Having made an effort to identify the barriers to communication in the patient, anaesthetists need to be mindful of the barriers to communication in themselves. Is the mind focused on the conversation or are thoughts straying to the '*difficult*' patient on the afternoon list? Are we becoming irritated, angry, frustrated, or simply bored by the patient's concerns or demands?

Identifying their own emotional responses can help anaesthetists recognize that patients have emotional responses too, and that acknowledging and accepting these are key elements in improving communication skills. For example, the anaesthetist may become increasingly annoyed by the ex-IV drug user, who is angry, sarcastic, and demanding whenever he is visited on the pain round. Recognizing that the patient has poorly controlled pain, is scared of the disfigurement caused by his accident, and lacks social skills to communicate appropriately helps the anaesthetist to view the patient dispassionately and to acknowledge any frustrations over the lack of progress, or prejudices about patients with drug use issues.

Using 'GREAT' to structure the interaction

Greeting

Anaesthetists should ensure that they are close enough to be seen and heard. It may be useful to show patients an ID badge so that the name and position of the anaesthetist can be read, especially if the patients are hearing impaired. Patients who are confused or demented may need to be reminded if they have met you before—for example,

'I'm Dr Thompson—I looked after you when you had your hip operation last Tuesday.'

Rapport

Establishing rapport with these patients usually requires some lateral thinking and being mindful of particular patient needs. Reducing background noise is a valuable asset. Turning the television off helps to focus attention and reinforces the importance of the interaction between anaesthetist and patient. Other helpful tactics include, where necessary, ensuring hearing aids are on and working, or organizing an interpreter to be present, or finding the patient's false teeth. Sitting on a chair sends a strong non-verbal signal that the anaesthetist is interested and engaged with the patient.

The anaesthetist should be mindful that women in general and especially from some cultures may feel intimidated by the close proximity of an unfamiliar male. It may be useful to consult colleagues who share a similar cultural background to glean further knowledge. An awareness of the medical issues affecting the patient aids effective communication. For example, patients who have recently been sedated for a procedure are unlikely to be able to communicate. It may be appropriate to return at a later time.

The presence of a nurse or relative who is familiar with the patient is useful in facilitating communication and provides the opportunity for the message to be conveyed in a way that works for the patient and can be reinforced by repetition later. If the issue to be discussed is complex or sensitive, or an extended therapeutic intervention is intended, it may not be appropriate to have a huge entourage of medical students and trainees. While it is entirely appropriate that trainees are exposed to difficult communication scenarios, this is often best done as a one-to-one teaching session rather than as a group, to avoid embarrassment, distress, or confusion.

Expectations

It is important to have in your own mind the essence of what you want the interaction to achieve, be it a preoperative assessment or a discussion with the patient about weaning their patient-controlled analgesia (PCA).

The goal of the interaction can then be explained.

'Do you know why you are seeing an anaesthetist today?' or *'I have come to talk to you about the anaesthetic for your operation tomorrow, Is that your understanding?'.* The main content of the consultation should be as short and simple as possible while allowing the patient the opportunity to express any concerns or queries. This is especially true when a patient has very marked cognitive impairment—for example, severe dementia or the inability to verbalize. Rather than a technical discussion of postoperative complications, the use of metaphor, analogy, or story-telling is often helpful in assisting patients' understanding as it allows meaning to be conveyed in simple language which is easy to recall—for example,

'Recovering from an operation is like a journey—sometimes it is short and easy, sometimes we end up taking a more twisting, turning route but in the end we reach the same destination. Sometimes we hit a bump in the road—for example, a wound infection . . . '

Patients with memory problems, or from a non-English-speaking background, often benefit from written information that they or their relatives can refer to after the consultation—for instance, a list of their medications and their indications.

Addressing concerns

Allow time for the patients and their relatives to absorb the meaning of what is being said, and check understanding by asking questions. Open questions require an extended answer rather than closed questions and are a better way of ensuring patients have understood the issues. *'Tell me how you use the PCA button'*, rather than *'Do you understand how to use it?'*

At the end of the interaction offer the opportunity for patients to ask questions. Often the type and quality of questions give an indication of the patients' understanding of the issues and highlight their particular concerns.

Tacit agreement

The interaction is terminated with thanks and an explicit or tacit agreement as to the nature of future care.

Patients with intellectual and behavioural disability

Communication abilities may be compromised by intellectual disability or by social and language development difficulties. Down's syndrome or trisomy 21 is the most commonly encountered congenital syndrome of intellectual disability, occurring in approximately 1 in 800 births.[1] With improved healthcare, people with Down's syndrome are living longer and are likely to be *'frequent flyers'* in primary and specialist healthcare areas.

Cooperation may be severely affected by multiple previous bad experiences, and it is highly desirable for patients and carers that effective communication creates a positive experience. Up to 10% of children and adults with Down's syndrome may also have a diagnosis of autism, necessitating a different communication style. For most people with Down's syndrome, receptive language development follows a 'normal', if slower, course than other developing children. Almost all children with Down's syndrome have an impairment of verbal expressive language development. Many have poor articulation and a number will have speech motor mapping problems with dyspraxia.[2] Thus, the gulf between receptive and verbal expressive language may be large. Hearing loss is common. Auditory processing may be impaired and short-term memory poor, especially with advancing age.

Pre-operative consultation and transfer to the operating theatre

Prior to anaesthesia, speaking with a carer or parent of the patient is invariably helpful. Other than obtaining a medical history and a history of communication abilities, likes, and dislikes can also be noted. Information about past experiences from patients themselves, their carers, or from the case-notes, can assist with planning and utilization.

Parents and carers of people with handicaps or rare syndromes or diseases may often be extremely knowledgeable about their wards' conditions. The rarer the syndrome, the more likely parents' or carers' knowledge will exceed that of the anaesthesia team looking after them. That well-worn cliché, '*Right or wrong, the customer is always right*' is worth bearing in mind under these circumstances. An open question such as, '*Can you tell me about your child's communication skills?*' is more likely to bring forth more information than, '*Can he talk?*' It is vital to ensure that patients are not bypassed because there may be communication difficulties, and patients ought not to be talked about as if they are not present.

All initial greetings should be directed first to the patient, accompanied by an appropriate welcoming gesture—the ubiquitous '*High Five*' appears to work well in a wide age range. An additional amount of time should also be allowed for a response before repeating a statement or question. Listening to and observing the responses will give clues for induction planning. Only if there is no response or an inadequate response should redirecting the communication to the carer be considered. Asking permission by way of, '*Is it okay if I ask your Mum some questions?*' is more respectful of the patient's autonomy than just turning away.

The preoperative discussion with the patient can follow similar pathways to those described in Chapters 6 and 11, with age-appropriate utilization of the person's imagination skills. Anecdotally, this age-labelling of people with intellectual handicap is disliked by parents, particularly if the gap is large between this and the chronological age. As children with Down's syndrome may also have hearing deficits and are good visual learners, the additional use of picture communication devices and sign language or gestures may be helpful.

Transferring the patient to the operating theatre should be conducted in such a way as to allow for a maximum sense of control by the patient.

Case study 1—A suboptimal transfer to theatre

A 15-year-old girl with Down's syndrome attended a day-procedure hospital for elective dental treatment under general anaesthesia. Although nervous, she was absorbed in drawing some pictures, and her mother said that it was one of the girl's favourite activities. The pre-anaesthetic consultation ended with an agreement that she could '*keep on drawing*' up to the time she would blow up some balloons in theatre. Some time was spent with the patient's mother rehearsing this plan so that she would remember the sequence of events. However, when the patient was brought to theatre she was very distressed. Her paper and crayons had been left in the admission area. In a short debrief, the nurse that brought her to theatre reported that she had gone to collect the patient and had told her, '*Put your crayons down now, we're going to theatre!*' as she was unaware of the anaesthetist's plan. The lesson to be learned was that despite the anaesthetist spending time orientating the patient to a future successful outcome, the plan had failed due to a simple lack of communication.

A double bind (see Chapter 4) at the time of transfer, '*Would you like to take your crayons and paper with you or leave them here while we go to theatre?*' might have been more effective. Interrupting what the patient was enjoying, and removing control from her, was a lost opportunity to utilize her coping strategy of drawing pictures. Even when plans are derailed, it is always possible to restore the patient's perception of control by redirecting the conversation back to a new, modified plan—in this case, one of balloon-blowing. A debrief with other team members can provide valuable education for future encounters. Regaining control can also include the use of double binds,

'*Would you like to climb up on the bed from this side or that side?*'
Whichever side she chooses will likely result in her being on the bed.

Case study 2—Optimizing cooperation by promoting autonomy

A 13-year-old girl presented for examination under anaesthesia. A chat with her mother revealed she loved helping at home. She chose '*banana sleepy gas*' (sevoflurane) for an inhalational induction. A discussion about what she was going to listen to when her ears were clear and what she was going to have to eat after the operation created a positive expectancy for recovery.

The way to theatre was assisted with questions like '*Which one is theatre 3? ... Thank you, you're very helpful*'—utilization of her '*helpful*' nature. Once in theatre, she chose which side of the bed Mum would sit while she lay down on the bed. She also decided which finger the oximeter probe fitted best (both double bind and maintaining control). The mask was placed near her mouth.

> **Anaesthetist:** '*Now it was banana flavour, wasn't it? ... Isn't that the best banana you have ever had?*' (Girl nodded) '*That's 1% banana, what's next?*'
> **Patient:** '*2!*' (Meanwhile, the anaesthetic assistant took this as his cue to increase the percentage of sevoflurane!)
> **Anaesthetist:** '*That's right, 2% banana, I'm so glad you're here to help me ... and what's next?*'
> **Patient:** '*3!*'
> **Anaesthetist:** '*That's right, 3% banana, I'm so glad you're here to help me ... and what's next?*'

Utilization and repetition were continued until the girl was anaesthetised.

Autism and related pervasive developmental disorders

This is a diverse group of conditions with a reported incidence 1.5% in developed countries.[3] None of the linguistic or behavioural characteristics is unique to, or diagnostic of, autism and may also be present in others with developmental delay. Patients' language development may be affected in a wide range of ways and to varying degrees from no verbal expressive language to difficulty with idioms, sarcasm, and humour. Some patients use communication devices such as PECS (picture exchange communication system) cards and sign language. Those with savant skills may have distinct abilities in one or more areas—for instance, musical ability.

Those who do talk may produce a bewildering array of words and phrases with many possible interpretations. Echolalia is the repetition of vocalizations heard immediately or in the past and may be due to failure to comprehend.[4]

For example, saying '*Can you take off your shoes, please?*' is likely to elicit a response, whereas '*Can you remove your footwear, please?*' is likely to be repeated back to the person. The anaesthetist should use immediate echolalia as both an indication of level of comprehension and a cue to modify or simplify their language. There may be other communication impairments (both receptive and expressive), and difficulty in relating to people, objects, and events. Emotional responses may be non-existent or inappropriate—for example, laughing when a sad event occurs.

Delayed echolalia is the term used when the person repeats a statement heard in the past, anything from a few minutes to many years ago, and can be an indication of high emotions—either negative or positive. Phrases uttered may have scant or no obvious relevance to current events, although a parent or carer may be able to explain a connection. When echolalia is accompanied by some acceleration of maladaptive behaviours, the likelihood is that it's time to reduce sensory input to the patient (see next).

Joint attention is a pre-verbal mechanism for directing the listener to an object or other person.[5] Statements, for example indicating moving to another location, should be specific.

'*We're going to theatre through the sliding doors next to the elephant picture*' may be more effective than, '*We're going to theatre through that door*' and pointing.

In people with intellectual delay and in children with autism, the use of multiple adjectives may be confusing. Asking '*Would you like to blow up the big balloon or the little balloon?*' may be understood better than '*Would you like to blow up the big green balloon or the little blue balloon?*'

Preoperative preparation

The parent or carer may provide valuable insights into communication strategies. Particular likes and dislikes can be identified and stressors that may trigger out-of-control behaviours can be noted. The parent should be encouraged to bring with them whatever they think may help to calm the patient. On arrival, it may be more calming for all to conduct the interview with the patient in a private room, away from excessive stimulation. At all times, the anaesthetist should look for increased frequency of maladaptive behaviours and use these indications to change or modify the direction the communication is taking. For example, a person who initially seems to be coping with a story being told starts to cover his ears. This is a cue to stop, modify, or finish the narrative.

People with high-functioning autism, despite superficially demonstrating good language skills, may have difficulty with humour and idioms. For example, a statement like '*Let's get the ball rolling*' is likely to have the person looking around the room for the ball!

Patients with autism and other disabilities often have difficulties with changing tasks or changing locations. Time should always be taken, and permission should always be obtained, before proceeding to the next phase of the process of anaesthesia. People with autism may struggle with making choices, thus increasing their stress levels. This may limit the use of the 'double bind' strategy which works well in many other areas.

Case study 3—Utilization of patient skills and motivations

A 28-year-old man who attended for colonoscopy had a diagnosis of autism with savant skills. His carer described his skill as his '*party piece*' and '*obsession*'. This was the ability to calculate the day of the week that an event had occurred—for example, the day of the week that a person was born. He disliked being touched. During the pre-anaesthetic consultation, he repeatedly asked the anaesthetist: '*When were you born?*' Having already established via the carer that this was his skill, it was then utilized with the phrase '*Okay, I'll tell you once the drip is in*'—something he was reluctant to accept initially. In theatre he continued to ask all the nurses the same question but, with the staff educated about the bargaining tool, they all repeated the anaesthetist's plan. He was so motivated to perform his party piece that he allowed all the necessary monitoring devices to be applied, as well as the intravenous line. Each time he allowed something to happen he was 'rewarded' with a team member's date of birth. The speed of his responses was astonishing. The transition from pre-anaesthetic consultation to induction was greatly facilitated by the utilization of his unique ability while seeking permission at all stages.

Minimizing and managing maladaptive responses

A meltdown in a person with autism can be of sudden onset, may be triggered by a seemingly trivial event and to the observer will manifest as an extreme version of a toddler tantrum. It may be preceded by acceleration in self-stimulating behaviours such as rocking or hand flapping. A person covering his ears may be indicating sensory overload. Self-injurious behaviour, such as head slapping, head banging, or self-biting may also precede a meltdown. In contrast to a toddler tantrum, the person will not necessarily look for or care about a reaction to the behaviour. As there appears to be no clear age limit to this behaviour in people with autism, there are risks of injury to the patient, carers, onlookers, and property. Such extreme behaviours are most likely to occur when these patients are under stress, while feeling unwell and out of their normal routines.[6] It would seem, therefore, that the hospital environment is the perfect location to trigger a meltdown!

Strategies to defuse a meltdown include the following:

- **Identify the triggers** beforehand.
- **Reduce sensory input** by decreasing the number of people in the room, dimming the lights, and speaking quietly.
- **Distract**—if the patient really wants to pull all the rubber gloves out of the boxes there may be something equally distracting but less destructive. Nevertheless, pick your battles! The carer or parent may also have a 'calming toy' with them.
- If all else fails and meltdown occurs, **move the person out of harm's way** and ride it out. Continue to use a controlled voice and continue to use language suggesting '*calm*', '*time-out*', and '*control*'.

Communicating with children and adults with a diagnosis on the autistic spectrum can be as rewarding as it is exhausting. As with other fields of practice within anaesthesia, it is important to build a repertoire of skills—for example, finding different ways to say a single phrase when at first you are not understood.

Listen and look for triggers to both calming and heightening behavioural responses. Avoid idioms and complex syntax. Double binds may be ineffective as making choices may heighten stress. Environmental stimuli should be minimized to match the person's coping strategies. Finally, sometimes things will not go to plan and this should be accepted. To paraphrase Rudyard Kipling, '*Keep your head even when all about you are losing theirs*'.

Trauma-informed communication

The past decade has seen much cultural change in society's understanding of psychological trauma and its lasting effects on people's mental health and behaviours. Adverse developmental experience (ADE) in childhood including physical, sexual and emotional abuse is distressingly common and is a significant risk factor for not only mental health and substance use issues but also increased rates of physical disease.[7] ADE also compromises normal psychological development and predisposes to problems such as post-traumatic stress syndrome (PTSD), personality disorders, risk-taking behaviours, maladaptive social skills, and chaotic lifestyles.[8]

It is therefore inevitable that people with psychological trauma experience are commonly encountered as patients. Such patients often struggle in the hospital environment and end up in conflict with the nursing, medical, and other staff. Similarly, some patients have been traumatized by early childhood or even adult experiences in hospital and may be hospital-phobic or needle-phobic (see Chapter 15) and have difficulty engaging in care. It is not uncommon for a patient's trauma to be undisclosed, unrecognized or undocumented which makes it hard for clinicians to identify patients with specific care needs and prepare appropriately. Creating a psychologically safe environment which promotes trust, autonomy, and engagement is paramount in building a therapeutic relationship in order to provide patient centred care.[9]

The 'LAURS' framework is a useful way to approach these challenging communication issues.

Listen

The ability to actively listen is vitally important in establishing a connection with patients whose trust has often been violated and who often feel unheard. Taking the time to '*hear the person out*' is the foundation stone of communication.

Accept

Many clinicians struggle to remain dispassionate in the face of what they perceive to be poor lifestyle choices and self-inflicted problems. Patients may present many challenging behaviours including aggression. Maintaining a calm, compassionate, and non-judgemental attitude requires practice and focus. This does not mean that you endorse the behaviour, rather that it is seen as a transient phenomenon which can be modified.

Similarly, patients who have been abused may have great difficulty with intimate examinations such as endoscopy and exhibit high levels of fear and anxiety. Well intended comments such as '*There's nothing to be afraid of*' are not helpful to someone who is being overwhelmed by uncontrollable emotions, memories, and sensations which feel just as real as the original trauma. Accepting and validating the patient provides support and improves compliance—'*It's perfectly understandable that you feel the way you do. Is there anything I can do to help you deal with this? I want you to know I will stay here and look after you until your procedure is finished'*. Traumatized patients are often afraid that they will be abandoned so it is important to ensure they feel secure.

Utilize

Virtually every patient who has come through traumatic experience has inner strengths and abilities developed in adversity and many are very highly functioning. Moving the focus of the interaction away from what they can't do towards what they can, allows the clinician to utilize the patient's strengths to respond to the stressful situation in a more positive way.

Asking the patient what their special talent is or favourite pastime provides a segue into a discussion about where they would rather be or what they would rather be doing. The patient can then be encouraged to enter *'a lived-in imagination'* experience instead of being stressed in the present situation or given permission to *'Zone out and be somewhere else'*.

Similarly helping the patient to identify their goals and their previous successes helps support and motivate them towards recovery and discharge home (e.g. *'So now you've told me how well you went with your first knee replacement I'm confident you'll be even better with this one—you've done this before so you know you can do it!'*).

Reframe

Patients with trauma have often had multiple bad experiences and frequently have negative expectations of hospitals and staff. They may catastrophize with comments such as *'I've been here dozens of times ... they always treat me like a junkie. I'm in the too-hard basket—the staff hate me'*. Reframing comments such as this takes practice and involves reflective listening and generating a yes set by echoing the patient's words *'So you've been here dozens of times ... the staff treat you like a junkie'*. Then reframing the *'too-hard basket'* into something more positive by suggesting, *'So perhaps it's time to put you in a **different basket'*** This then opens a discussion of what could be done differently this time.

Suggestion

Most hospital patients experience a degree of anxiety and this can be intensely magnified in patients with PTSD. The overwhelming emotions suppress cognitive rational brain function and renders them highly suggestible. Particular care should be taken to avoid nocebo type suggestions (see Chapter 3) such as *'This will sting a bit'*. Conversely the use of positive suggestion can be very powerful in these patients.

Working with interpreters

Communities worldwide are becoming increasingly diverse and there is a growing need to use interpreters with our patients. The use of a third party to facilitate communication can be a blessing or fraught with difficulty depending on circumstance.

A well-briefed, experienced interpreter who has good communication skills and is able to establish rapport with both health professional and patient is a great ally. An interpreter who is time-pressured, poorly understands the clinical scenario, and has poor communication skills can be a liability.

Many health services now mandate the use of official interpreters to avoid family, friends or members of staff from being drawn into the complexity of translating difficult concepts, especially around consent and end-of-life care. However, there is still a place for family and staff to assist in translating for daily care and minor procedures. Some hospitals provide phone interpreters which increases the availability of interpreters but significantly reduces the quality of the communication in all but the most straightforward of situations. Common drawbacks of interpretation include lack of availability especially out of hours, lack of fidelity to the intended message (lost in translation!), exclusion of family members who may wish to be involved in communicating with the patient and cultural nuances which may escape the attention of the health professional.[10]

Tips for success

1. Get trained in how to work with an interpreter if there is a course available.
2. Ensure the environment is set up with adequate privacy, space, and quiet.
3. Brief the interpreter before seeing the patient family so they understand the purpose of the consultation and the main points to be covered.
4. Keep the dialogue brief to avoid overload for the interpreter and patient.
5. Direct communication to the patient rather than the interpreter and confirm understanding.
6. Use diagrams/visual aids to help get the message across.

Overcoming the mask barrier

The COVID-19 pandemic has once again made mask-wearing mandatory in most healthcare environments as well as in some social contexts (see also Chapter 12). There is a lack of research to inform us as to the impact of mask-wearing on communication but the empirical evidence is that mask-wearing complicates communication. This is due to a combination of factors—masks tend to muffle speech especially in the presence of background noise, masks also remove the visual cues of body language such as smiling as well as making identification of the individual more difficult.

There are a variety of strategies to help overcome these barriers, for example, reducing background noise, facing the person, and increasing the volume of your speech and wearing your name and role on your hat. Some patients may feel uncomfortable with being cared for by people they have never actually seen and in some cases it may be appropriate to remove your mask to allow a patient to see who is caring for them. Mask-wearing increases the requirement for excellent communication skills to help generate trust, rapport, and understanding.[11]

Key points

1. People have diverse needs and may be challenging to look after.

2. Key strategies for patients with special needs (e.g. autism) are to listen, observe, investigate likes and dislikes, enlist the help of the parents or carers, and focus on abilities and utilize them.

3. The potential gulf between receptive and verbal expressive language should be remembered. The anaesthetist needs to be prepared to allow extra time for communication.

4. Working with interpreters and mask-wearing pose additional challenges in communication which can be overcome with forethought and organization.

References

1. Irving C, Basu A, Richmond S, Burn J, Wren C (2008). Twenty-year trends in prevalence and survival of Down syndrome. *Eur J Hum Genet*, **16**(11), 1336–40.

2. Roberts JE, Price J, Malkin C (2007). Language and communication development in down syndrome. *Ment Retard Dev Disabil Res Rev*, **13**(1), 26–35.

3. Lyall K, Croen L, Daniels J, et al. (2017). The changing epidemiology of autism spectrum disorders. *Annu Rev Public Health*, **38**, 81–102.

4. Neely LC, Gerow S, Rispoli M, Lang RB, Pullen N (2016). Treatment of echolalia in individuals with autism spectrum disorder: a systematic review. *Rev J Autism Dev Disord*, **3**, 82–91.

5. Meindl JN, Cannella-Malone HI (2011). Initiating and responding to joint attention bids in children with autism: a review of the literature. *Res Dev Disabil*, **32**(5), 1441–54.

6. Taghizadeh N, Davidson A, Williams K, Story D (2015). Autism spectrum disorder (ASD) and its perioperative management. *Pediatr Anesth*, **25**(11), 1076–84.

7. Felitti VJ, Anda RF, Nordenberg D, et al. (1998). Relationship of childhood abuse and household dysfunction to many of the leading causes of death in adults. The Adverse Childhood Experiences (ACE) Study. *Am J Prev Med*, **14**(4), 245–58.

8. Lancaster CL, Teeters JB, Gros DF, Back SE (2016). Posttraumatic stress disorder: overview of evidence-based assessment and treatment. *J Clin Med*, **5**(11), 105.

9. Edmondson AC, Lei Z (2014). Psychological safety: the history, renaissance, and future of an interpersonal construct. *Ann Rev Organ Psychol Organ Behav*, **1**(1), 23–43.

10. Shapeton A, O'Donoghue M, VanderWielen B, Barnett SR (2017). Anesthesia lost in translation: perspective and comprehension. *J Educ Perioper Med*, **19**(1), E505.

11. Marler H, Ditton A (2021). 'I'm smiling back at you': exploring the impact of mask wearing on communication in healthcare. *Int J Lang Commun Disord*, **56**(1), 205–14.

Chapter 15

Needle phobia

Allan M. Cyna and Marion I. Andrew

'Every problem has a gift for you in its hands.'
Richard Bach, Illusions: The Adventures of a Reluctant Messiah (1977)

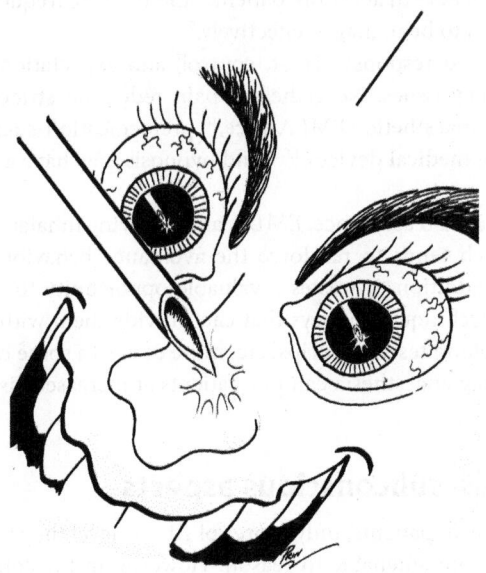

don't **WORRY** – **THERE WILL BE** no **PAIN** –
there'll be no **NEED To SCREAM** –

What this chapter is about

Setting the scene

Needle phobia describes an anticipatory fear of needle insertion,[1] and is a well-recognized clinical entity of particular relevance to the anaesthetist.[2,3] It may affect up to 10% of the general population, and is more common in women[4] and the young.[5] Avoidance behaviours are common[6] and needle phobia can prevent patients from seeking medical care such as immunizations.[7] The development of trust, a perception of control, and an understanding of the conscious–subconscious aspects of the problem can help manage these patients.[8] In addition, patience and time are frequently needed if this distressing problem is to be managed effectively.[9]

Needle phobia is usually a learned response. Trust, control, and expectation rather than the pain itself are the key issues. Nevertheless, pain reduction strategies such as eutectic mixture of local anaesthetic (EMLA), ice,[10] premedication such as dexometomidine,[11] stress-reducing medical devices,[12,13] and hypnosis may have a role in management.[14–16]

Anaesthetists have traditionally used reassurance, EMLA, and by giving inhalational inductions. However, this approach tends to reinforce the avoidance behaviour of both patient and anaesthetist! In addition, it wastes a valuable opportunity to educate and equip patients to utilize techniques in ways that can provide them with the necessary skills to manage future blood tests and drips, etc. more easily. In some cases avoiding IV access prior to inducing anaesthesia can put patients at increased risk of complications.[7,17]

Understanding conscious–subconscious aspects

Patients with needle phobia are like all patients, only more so! At one level they function consciously and logically and are amenable to reason. However, in the context of hospital procedures subconscious responses take over. These patients often verbalize their behaviour as '*Silly*', '*Illogical*', or '*Crazy*', but find that they just can't help themselves. They may describe their predicament as being in '*two minds about it*' or

Table 15.1 Nocebo communications commonly used with patients suffering from needle phobia

Unhelpful communication	Therapeutic alternative
'It's only a small needle'	*'We will position the drip as safely and comfortably as possible'*
'We're just about to start'	*'We're just about to finish'*
'Your tattoos and body piercings would have been much more painful than anything we are doing'	*'I can't imagine how difficult this is for you'*
'Don't be such a baby'	*'Can you tell me what has been helpful to you previously'*
'Sting coming!'	*'Just numbing the skin to allow us to finish as comfortably as possible'*

'beside themselves'. This mindset illustrates probably more clearly than any other, the conscious–subconscious basis of the problem.

To help engage with sufferers of needle phobia, it is helpful to consider the anxiety response of the patient to needles as the **subconscious** *response*, and the desire to be able to have a drip or blood test as the logical **conscious** *decision* to obtain optimal medical care. The inability to comply with the treatment, despite logically recognizing the need for it, is brought about by the subconsciously generated fear. This anxiety response is typically expressed as sweating, shaking, *'knots in the stomach'*, hyperventilation, and vaso-vagal episodes.

Patients often describe the needle in emotive, kinaesthetic language such as, *'a red hot poker'* or a *'molten sword piercing my skin'* or in visual terms (e.g. as a *'horse needle'*). Sometimes it is difficult to empathize with these patients, especially if they present with tongue studs, body piercings, and tattoos. However, the fears are very real.

Context is everything, as even patients with severe needle phobia may be able to tolerate body piercing with little difficulty, and yet generate a huge anxiety response to a blood test. The patient's 'reality' usually has nothing to do with the sensation of an injection, but everything to do with the perception, meaning, context, and associated imagery. Needle-phobic patients are usually highly responsive to suggestion (see Chapters 3, 4, and 23). If they weren't, they wouldn't be needle-phobic in the first place! This gives clues to effective treatment strategies. Patients frequently receive negative suggestions from well-meaning hospital staff, escalating the problem. Table 15.1 shows the types of unhelpful phrases used with possible alternatives.

Appreciating the origin of the problem

Many patients are unaware of the origin of their problem. The initial sensitizing event usually occurs in early childhood—especially when patients say they have had needle phobia *'as far back as I can remember'*. The emotional response is often reinforced by repeated bad experiences in hospital and successful avoidance behaviours. Irrespective of the source of the problem, the phobia needs acceptance as a very real experience before it can be managed. Dismissive or belittling attitudes such as, '*It's only a small needle*', '*what's the fuss*', or '*You are behaving like a baby!*' only serve to escalate the problem at hand.

'LAURS'

'LAURS' and the use of metaphor can be helpful (see Chapters 2 and 5).

Listen reflectively: This is always of value as the patient's description of symptoms can be utilized later (see Chapter 9).

Acceptance: The development of trust and rapport is facilitated when the patient's behaviour and perceptions are accepted dispassionately no matter how bizarre they may appear.

Utilization: The anaesthetist can utilize the patient's language to communicate in a way that implicitly and explicitly recognizes that the patient is in control. The anaesthetist reinforces trust and builds confidence, by checking in at each stage and asking permission frequently as each step in the process is achieved.

Reframing: This may be useful on occasion, although suggestion is usually of far more value in these patients.

Suggestion: Positive expectancy can be seeded by using positive suggestion, which can also alter perceptions and even induce arm anaesthesia.

Utilizing metaphor to promote patient rapport

Patient rapport and trust can be established by accepting the patient's reality and demonstrating to the patient that the anaesthetist understands that the problem is real. Metaphor can also be useful. The '*plank of wood*' metaphor involves asking the patient if there would be any problem walking across a plank of wood lying on the floor when it is one metre wide and six metres in length. The patient usually responds with a '*No*'.

The question can then be asked,

> '*What if exactly the same plank of wood was over a precipice with a 300-metre drop and you had to walk across it? It is identical in every other way to the plank of wood lying on the floor. How would you feel?*'

Patients usually respond with words such as '*Terrified!*' or '*Anxious!*'

The anaesthetist's response to this could be,

> '*That is good because if you didn't have that response to dangerous situations, you would constantly be putting your life and well-being at unnecessary risk. Anxiety regarding walking across the plank in this situation is not only useful but potentially lifesaving. Unfortunately, people with needle phobia have a part of their mind that thinks that they need protecting ... It is as if the plank is over a 300-metre precipice, even though it is consciously recognized as being on the floor.*'

This tends to explain why the patient's anxiety response to needles is generated.

This metaphor frequently facilitates rapid patient rapport as it becomes clear that the matter is being taken seriously and not being dismissed as trivial. The patient's reality is being accepted in a non-judgemental way. Patients normally smile spontaneously and acknowledge being understood. If this does not happen, alternative metaphors can be used, as may the use of suggestions.

Using repetition frequently reinforces the message.

Anaesthetist: *'It is very common to be in two minds about this. You know in one part of your mind at some level knows that the plank of wood is on the floor, yet another part of your mind still thinks you need protecting for some reason.'*

Useful suggestions

1. *'Fortunately, there are lots of well-recognized strategies that people can learn, allowing them to have blood tests and drips much more easily than they might think.'*

   'Lots of well-recognized strategies' tells the patient that there is a range of solutions that could be helpful to them. *'People can learn'* is an indirect suggestion that implies that the patient too can learn.

2. *'We usually show people with needle phobia how they can feel more in control and feel more comfortable than they might have anticipated'* is an indirect suggestion that the patient too can experience this.

3. *'Patients with needle phobia can usually gain a sense of control by focusing their gaze on that spot on the ceiling. They can then notice that each time they take a deep breath they feel stronger and more in control and each time they breathe out they feel themselves relax. As they relax, the arm relaxes outstretched too. This allows the drip to be placed much more comfortably than previously thought.'* This is an indirect suggestion for relaxation, control, and 'arm anaesthesia'

It should be remembered that one of the most effective ways of promoting a sense of control is by obtaining the patient's permission at each stage, thereby letting the patient know that they are in the driving seat.

A 'GREAT' interaction

Greeting

'Hello, I'm Dr Sharpe, I'm told you like to be called Tyson. I've come to help you get your cannula placed as comfortably as possible.'

Rapport

Seeking permission using a *'Yes-set'* and indirect suggestion.

Anaesthetist: *'I show a lot of people who are nervous about drips and injections, strategies that they can use to experience things in an easier way than they might have anticipated. Is it okay to talk about how we usually show people different ways of feeling more in control and comfortable?'*

Expectation

More anxious patients will need more time to develop trust and a perception of control. In the case of mild needle phobia, it may be simply a matter of acknowledging the problem and suggesting confidence, calm, and competence in performing the task comfortably. In a very anxious patient, it may be advisable initially to wait at the door of the room when greeting the patient and begin developing rapport there, asking for permission to approach when the patient is ready.

> Anaesthetist: 'Is it okay if I come over to the bed to talk ... ?'

This emphasizes that the patient can say when they are ready for the next step in the process.

> Anaesthetist: 'I normally tell patients that I will not do anything without their permission. Is that okay?'

Addressing concerns

This involves managing any other concerns not yet addressed and how these can be resolved when the patient is ready.

> Patient: 'Can you only go where the cream is?' or 'Don't do it without letting me know!'

> Anaesthetist: 'I'll only go where it's going to be most comfortable for you and will only finish up when you are ready. Is that okay?'

Tacit agreement

> Anaesthetist: 'You can let me know when you are ready for it to be finished.'

After the cannulation, 'Thanks for allowing me to show how you can do this more easily in the future.'

Strategies to consider

The anaesthetist can ask a series of questions checking in with the patient at each stage.

> Anaesthetist: 'Is it okay to come a little closer?' 'Is it okay to stand next to the bed?' 'Is it okay to look at the arm?' 'Is it okay to look at the back of the hand?' 'Is it okay to place the tourniquet around the arm?' 'Is it okay to tap the back of the hand to allow things to be more comfortable for you?' 'Is it okay to wipe away some of the sensations with some antiseptic to clean the skin?' 'Is it okay to finish up?'

It is not uncommon to have to wait before a request is accepted. It is important that the patient has time to comply and consent to each request.

Suggestions can be useful. '*In a moment the arm can straighten as if it is relaxing all on its own without you thinking about it.*'

Immediately prior to needle insertion it is important to inform the patient—but not to give a negative suggestion or use the negatively valenced words, '*Needle*', '*Sharp*', or '*Scratch*'.

> '*If you feel anything at all that bothers you, a cough, wriggling the toes, or a deep breath can all help this to be completed as comfortably and as safely as possible for you*'.
>
> **Not**
>
> '*Sharp **needle** and a **BEE STING** coming now!*'[18]

If the patient is so overwhelmed they cannot verbalize consent, they might find it easier to communicate non-verbally. This can be utilized by the anaesthetist to gain final permission from the patient for cannula placement.

> **Anaesthetist:** '*You can nod your head when you are ready for us to finish*'.

At this stage the severely phobic patient is either highly focused and quiet, or very anxious, trembling, and crying. If the patient is trembling, this can be utilized.

> **Anaesthetist:** '*You can shake off some of those concerns and worries just now. In a moment, as you shake off those unwanted feelings, things will just seem to settle down as the arm starts to relax and feel sleepy and comfortable*.'

Use of the words '*Try*' and '*Not*' therapeutically (see Chapter 4),

> **Anaesthetist:** '*If you prefer, you can **try not to relax** and then **find yourself relaxing** all on your own without you thinking about it*.'

The verbal procedure can be completed with a double bind and a focus on success of finishing the cannula insertion rather than starting to insert the drip. '*When you are ready for this to finish you will find that you can just nod your head or let me know with an "okay" as soon as you are ready!*'

Reinforcing success

At the end of the procedure, it is very important not to waste any success that has been achieved. Each step that went well can be re-enforced followed by a post-hypnotic suggestion. Patients are frequently in a trance-like state when having needle procedures.

> **Anaesthetist:** '*As with anything—for instance, learning to drive—when we practise new skills things become easier and feel more straightforward. Most people find that before very long they are surprised that things that would previously bother them for some reason are no longer a concern and we don't even have to know why. In future any time a blood test or drip is required people find that once they have achieved the success you have had today, they build on that success knowing things will be easier should anything similar be required.*'

This statement combines the use of positive suggestion, re-enforcement, and repetition.

Hypno-communication techniques

Awake suggestions for *arm anaesthesia* in IV access

'Is it okay for you to go to a favourite place in your mind?' … *'a holiday place'* … *'or somewhere you can relax and feel comfortable?'* … *'notice the sights, the sounds'* … pause, *'the tastes'* … pause, *'the smells'* … pause, *'the humidity'* … *'now, while one part of your mind is on holiday another part of your mind can allow the left arm to relax'* … *'in a moment'* … *'but not yet, I am going to ask you to straighten the arm'* … In response to the arm moving say, *'Well done'* or *'That's right, excellent, That's good'* … *'Is it ok to place the tourniquet on the arm keeping it loose'* … *'Is it okay to tighten the tourniquet so the at the arm changes sensation'* … *'Perhaps a tingly feeling'* … *'Perhaps a sleepy feeling'* … *'Perhaps an anaesthetic feeling* … Is it okay to tap the back of the hand so that it can feel sleepier than it is already?'* … *'Is it okay if I wipe some of the sensation away with the antiseptic?'* … *'Is it okay to finish?'*

Emergency management

A 35-year-old woman presenting for emergency surgery started shouting at the anaesthetist approaching her with a 16 G intravenous (IV) cannula for IV access to facilitate a rapid sequence induction of anaesthesia.

> **Patient:** *'If you come near me with that needle, I'll **die**!'*
>
> **Anaesthetist:** *'Well, that's **okay**. Just let **the arm die** for a **moment**.'*

The patient's left arm rapidly became limp and relaxed, allowing the 14 G IV cannula to be inserted comfortably without local anaesthetic. A second or two later the patient realized the drip was in place. She had experienced this quite comfortably and was surprised how straightforward it had been.

The explanation of how '**LAURS**' was utilized in this case is detailed next:

Listening—The anaesthetist listened to the words the patient used; *'**I'll die**!'*

Acceptance of the patient's reality involved accepting her belief by saying '**Okay**'. This was essential to engage with the patient and develop rapid rapport; no attempt was made to contradict the patient's irrational belief by saying for instance, *'Of course you are not going to die—it's just a little needle!'*

Utilization involved using the patient's words to facilitate the subconscious response to the suggestion that only the arm will '**die**' and for only a '**moment**';

Reframe—The patient's own words were reframed in a new context so that the '**dying**' can be for just '**the arm**' and not the whole body;

And that the arm would go '**dead**' only for '**a moment**';

Suggestion—Using the words '**the** arm' rather than '**your** arm' also encouraged dissociation of the arm from the rest of the body to facilitate arm anaesthesia.

Effectively managing patients with needle phobia requires a patient's trust and confidence. Rapport building through a 'LAURS' approach promotes autonomy; empowers the patient and increases a sense of control. Such techniques frequently succeed when logic, cajoling, or 'jollying along' has failed.

Lived in imagination and awake suggestions

A lived-in imagination technique (Chapter 23) can be helpful in needle-phobic adult patients and involves engaging the patient in a favourite activity like hiking or eating a favourite food (e.g. raspberry cheesecake) and asking questions of the patient as if they are actually doing the activity (see Videos 15.1–15.3, linked to this chapter).

> **Anaesthetist:** '*When you are ready to do some cooking in your mind allow the eyes to close*'. After the eyes have closed: '*Where are you?*'
> **Patient:** '*In the kitchen.*'
> **Anaesthetist:** '*Have you started eating the cheesecake yet?*'
> **Patient:** '*No.*'
> **Anaesthetist:** '*Let me know when you have taken the first bite?*'
> **Patient:** '*Okay.*'
> **Anaesthetist:** '*Is it room temperature?*'
> **Patient:** '*No, it's just out the fridge.*'
> **Anaesthetist:** '*Are you using a fork or a spoon?*'
> **Patient:** '*A fork.*'
> **Anaesthetist:** '*While one part of your mind is eating cheesecake,* (conscious) *another part of your mind* (subconscious) *can allow the arm to relax and change sensation as the tourniquet tightens.*'
> **Patient:** (Nods)

Switch-wire imagery

This technique is optimally used in in young children between the ages of 5 and 10 and described in detail elsewhere[16] and can be viewed in the video linked to this chapter.

Key points

1. The specific conscious and subconscious aspects of the problem need to be recognized.
2. The 'LAURS' concept can be effective in establishing patient rapport and trust.
3. Metaphor may help the anaesthetist express empathy with the patient's apprehension.
4. Positive expectancy is generated by a confident, calm approach with a clear expectation of success.
5. It is vital to ask permission at each stage, since control and trust are critical.
6. It is important to reinforce any success achieved.

Additional video content

Discover additional video content demonstrating various communication techniques that assist the development of hypnotic arm anaesthesia.by searching for this book's title or ISBN (9780198858669) at academic.oup.com/oxford-medicine-online. If you would like access to the whole book, or are interested in accessing other titles, you can recommend it to your librarian.

References

1. Thurgate C, Heppell S (2005). Needle phobia—changing venepuncture practice in ambulatory care. *Paediatr Nurs*, **17**(9), 15–18.

2. Rice LJ (1993). Needle phobia: an anesthesiologist's perspective. *J Pediatr*, **122**(5 Pt 2), S9–13.

3. Bamgbade OA (2007). Severe needle phobia in the perianesthesia setting. *J Perianesth Nurs*, **22**(5), 322–9.

4. McLenon J, Rogers MAM (2019). The fear of needles: a systematic review and meta-analysis. *J Adv Nurs*, **75**(1), 30–42.

5. Veerkamp JS, Majstorovic M (2006). [Dental anxiety and needle phobia in children. A relationship?]. *Ned Tijdschr Tandheelkd*, **113**(6), 226–9.

6. Alsbrooks K, Hoerauf K (2022). Prevalence, causes, impacts, and management of needle phobia: an international survey of a general adult population. *PloS One*, **17**(11), e0276814.

7. Simon GR, Wilkins CJ, Smith I (2002). Sevoflurane induction for emergency caesarean section: two case reports in women with needle phobia. *Int J Obstet Anesth*, **11**(4), 296–300.

8. Searing K, Baukus M, Stark MA, Morin KH, Rudell B (2006). Needle phobia during pregnancy. *J Obstet Gynecol Neonatal Nurs*, **35**(5), 592–8.

9. Cyna AM, Andrew MI, Tan SG (2009). Communication skills for the anaesthetist. *Anaesthesia*, **64**(6), 658–65.

10. Sarifakioglu N, Sarifakioglu E (2004). Evaluating the effects of ice application on the pain felt during botulinum toxin type-A injections: a prospective, randomized, single-blind controlled trial. *Ann Plast Surg*, **53**(6), 543–6.

11. Nafiu OO, Srinivasan A, Ravanbakht J, Wu B, Lau WC (2008). Dexmedetomidine sedation in a patient with superior vena cava syndrome and extreme needle phobia. *J Cardiothorac Vasc Anesth*, **22**(4), 581–3.

12. Kettwich SC, Sibbitt WL, Jr., Brandt JR, Johnson CR, Wong CS, Bankhurst AD (2007). Needle phobia and stress-reducing medical devices in pediatric and adult chemotherapy patients. *J Pediatr Oncol Nurs*, **24**(1), 20–8.

13. Kettwich SC, Sibbett WL, Kettwich LG, Palmer CJ, Draeger HT, Bankhurst AD (2006). Patients with needle phobia? Try stress-reducing medical devices. *J Fam Pract*, **55**(8), 697–700.

14. Morse DR, Cohen BB (1983). Desensitization using meditation-hypnosis to control 'needle' phobia in two dental patients. *Anesth Prog*, **30**(3), 83–5.

15. Dash J (1981). Rapid hypno-behavioral treatment of a needle phobia in a five-year-old cardiac patient. *J Pediatr Psychol*, **6**(1), 37–42.

16. Cyna AM, Tomkins D, Maddock T, Barker D (2007). Brief hypnosis for severe needle phobia using switch-wire imagery in a 5-year old. *Paediatr Anaesth*, **17**(8), 800–4.

17. Sehgal A, Mendonca C, Stacey MR (2001). Needle phobia in a patient for urgent caesarean section. *Int J Obstet Anesth*, **10**(4), 333–4.

18. Varelmann D, Pancaro C, Cappiello E, Camann W (2010). Nocebo-induced hyperalgesia during local anesthetic injection. *Anesthesia & Analgesia*, **110**(3), 868–70.

19. Cyna AM (2019). The Laurs of hypnotic communication and the 'lived in imagination' technique in medical practice. *Int J Clin Exp Hypn*, **67**(3), 247–61.

Chapter 16

Intraoperative awareness

Christel J. Bejenke and Suyin G.M. Tan

'To sleep perchance to dream: ay, there's the rub ...'
William Shakespeare

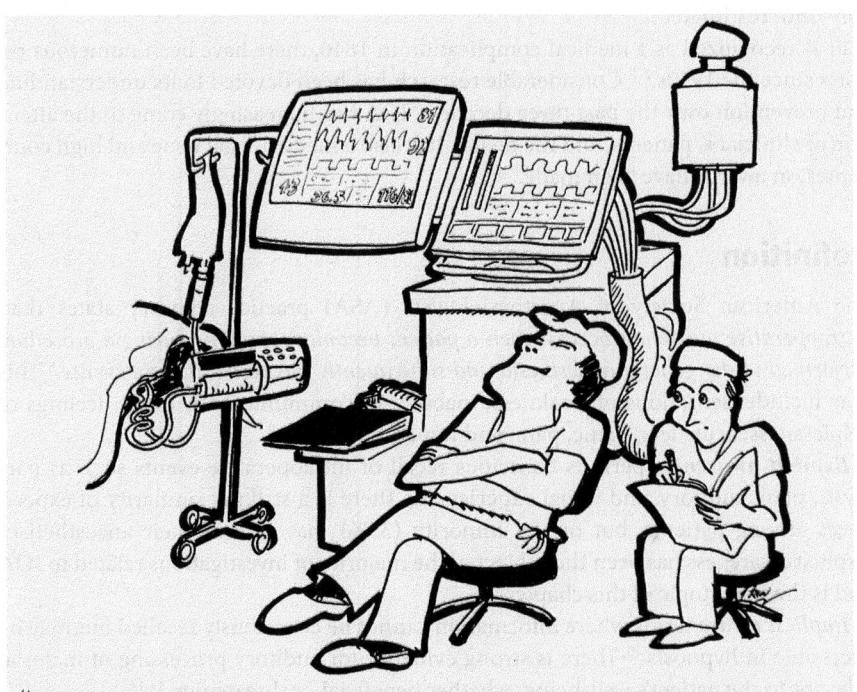

"Remember- always try to be more conscious than the patient..."

What this chapter is about

Intraoperative awareness (IOA) represents a range of heterogeneous experiences and is a topic of considerable relevance, not only to anaesthetists, but to all theatre staff. This chapter focuses on communications that the anaesthetist may find helpful in ameliorating or preventing adverse sequelae associated with IOA. This is a well-described, infrequent complication of general anaesthesia[1] with a reported incidence of between 0.1 and 0.9%. However, the true incidence of recall is probably underestimated.

First recognized as a medical complication in 1846, there have been numerous reports since the 1950s.[2–5] Considerable research has been devoted to its understanding and prevention over the past three decades.[6] IOA has increasingly come to the attention of clinicians, patients, and the media. It is also a medico-legal issue and high compensation awards have been made.[7]

Definition

The American Society of Anesthesiologists (ASA) practice advisory states that, *'Intraoperative awareness occurs when a patient becomes conscious during a procedure performed under general anaesthesia and subsequently has recall of these events'.*[8] This may include: sensations of weakness; inability to communicate or move; feelings of helplessness; acute fear, panic, pain, and impending death.[9]

Explicit awareness permits conscious recall of intraoperative events such as paralysis, pain, auditory, and visual experiences. There is a striking similarity of experiences among patients, but only a minority (35%) may inform their anaesthetist.[6] Explicit awareness has been the subject of the majority of investigations related to IOA and is the main topic of this chapter.

Implicit awareness is where information cannot be consciously recalled but may be accessible in hypnosis.[10] There is strong evidence for auditory processing of material relevant to the patient's well-being, whether beneficial or threatening.[11,12]

Risk factors

Risk factors include light anaesthesia, a history of awareness, chronic use of central nervous system depressants, younger age, obesity, anaesthesia delivery problems, total intravenous anaesthesia (TIVA) and neuromuscular blockade.[13]

Adverse sequelae

The trauma experienced by some patients has been well documented and *'may lead to ... intense emotional states which interfere with the ability to develop a narrative of the events ... memories may gradually emerge over time'.*[14] Moerman found that 70% of patients report sleep disturbances, nightmares, fear of future anaesthetics, or daytime anxiety. Symptoms may be aggravated when patients are not taken seriously by physicians or family and are told that they were *'making it up'* or *'are crazy'.*[6] Late psychological symptoms may lead to post-traumatic stress disorder (PTSD).[15] PTSD is characterized by re-experiencing the traumatic event, hyperarousal, nightmares, flashbacks, and avoidance behaviour. Patients with the most severe symptoms are severely impacted and may be unable to engage in healthcare especially involving surgical procedures.[9] However, simply suffering pain and hearing voices or noises does not cause late psychological symptoms. In fact, wide-awake patients who suffer greatly during the procedure may have fewer traumatic symptoms afterwards than obtunded patients, perhaps because what happens is not in doubt when awake.

Recommended preventive measures

BIS (bispectral index) monitoring—considered the standard of care by the ASA and by most researchers—was expected to reliably identify the depth of anaesthesia, function as an index of consciousness and ensure the prevention of awareness. However, recently Avidan reported that *'awareness occurred even when BIS values were within the target ranges',* and that BIS *'could give anaesthetists a false sense of security'* as borne out by the B-aware study.[3,16]

Recommended clinical measures are:

1. Use of multiple modalities to monitor depth of anaesthesia, including clinical vigilance and conventional monitoring systems.
2. Avoiding total paralysis by limiting the use of neuromuscular blocking drugs.[1]

Neither scopolamine nor benzodiazepines reliably reduce the incidence of recall.[4]

Mitigating the adverse effects of awareness

While the anaesthetist usually does not consider communication skills to be a part of the management and prevention of the serious consequences of IOA, specific approaches are proposed below. The goal is to ameliorate the acute experience of awareness; to lessen or prevent long-term sequelae; to facilitate management of patients who have experienced awareness in the past; and to facilitate preoperative preparation of patients who previously experienced IOA. Finally, effective communication may obviate litigation.

Aspects of communication to consider include:

♦ Preoperative preparation;

♦ Intraoperative communication;

♦ Communicating with the theatre team;

♦ Management of patients who report having just experienced awareness;

♦ Management of patients who have previously experienced awareness and may suffer from PTSD.

Preoperative preparation

Information is essential. It establishes rapport and confidence in the anaesthetist's competence and commitment. A description of the sequence of events from admission through to the recovery room is an essential part of anaesthesia care in general. Specific issues are the induction, emergence, and extubation. Patients can be reassured that the first priority is always *safety*.[17]

The expectation that unconsciousness is an absolutely necessary component of successful, safe anaesthesia should be revised. Patients can be reassured that, while complete unconsciousness cannot always be guaranteed, every effort will be made to provide effective analgesia, and that becoming aware of touch, lights, sounds, and conversation can be a normal aspect of anaesthesia care. In cases where awareness and pain may occur for reasons of safety such as high-risk patients, appropriate explanations should be given preoperatively.

By using a metaphor of ' ... *the surface of water*', the anaesthetist can explain that '*depth of anaesthesia*' varies, '*Sometimes patients come up slightly above the surface ... that's when they may hear or feel something ... and then drift down again ...*' (see Chapter 5).

Strategies for communicating with the anaesthetist in the event of awareness can be discussed.

> ' ... *from time to time you may feel me squeezing your hand ... and if you feel like it ... you can squeeze back ...* '

Preoperatively this simple statement conveys a sense of control to the patient and is perceived as empowering. Even during muscle relaxation, residual muscle power may allow the patient '*to squeeze back*' and an aware patient is apt to do so. If appropriate, anaesthesia can be deepened; if it is contraindicated, the anaesthetist can explain that ' ... *it will be just another few moments ... before it is the right time ... to give you more medicine ...* '. Even when experiencing pain, just hearing such a statement can be comforting to the patient. It should be noted that conscious recall of such events is unlikely as demonstrated by Tunstall's use of the *isolated forearm* technique, where patients only rarely remember responding to commands under GA.[18]

Patients can be informed in a way that is factual, supportive, and generates positive expectation and if at increased risk of IOA, then this awareness is only a slight possibility with comfort and safety still foremost. While such information could function as a negative suggestion (see Chapters 3 and 23), whether it actually does or not depends upon how this information is communicated. If IOA is addressed, it should be done without being defensive or apologetic in advance.

Because the induction of anaesthesia is one of the most likely periods for awareness, explaining intubation and the endotracheal tube as '*normal and safe*' may reduce the fear and psychological trauma of assuming that 'something went wrong', should the patient experience awareness and recall.

> '*Once you are relaxed, the anaesthetist will put a breathing tube through your mouth (nose) into your windpipe ... which makes breathing extra **safe** during the operation ... and is a part of **safe** anaesthesia.*'

As with all patient–anaesthetist interactions, the anaesthetist should avoid false re-assurance and be prepared to be held to any promises made. Patients can be reassured that the anaesthetist is committed to scrupulous vigilance in protecting them. Positive suggestions can be included with every item of information, during all interactions, including induction (see also Chapters 4, 8, and 23). The patient can also be advised of the possibility that another anaesthetist may take over intraoperatively. An example of information provided during preoperative preparation to a high-risk patient for cardiac surgery is given:

> '*As you know, anaesthesia has to do with* **comfort and safety**—*and most of the time we can provide both. But, every once in a while we must decide which is more important ... There may be a time when we want to (***not** '**have** to*') be extra* **careful** *... and extra* **gentle** *... to keep your heart as strong ... and working as well as possible. Sometimes it is best to have less anaesthesia and that may be the time when you might hear or feel some of the work going on ... And just as soon as I know ... that your heart is strong enough to take a little more anaesthesia ... I will give it to you right away.*'

The administration of muscle relaxant effects can also be addressed.

> '*It is also important that your surgeons have the best possible conditions to work under ... So, I will give you a special medicine that makes all your muscles com-pletely loose and relaxed ... That will make it much easier for your surgeons ... to do the best possible job ... This feeling may be different from anything you felt be-fore ... but you will know that I am watching everything very closely ... and taking good care of you ... so that* **you will be completely safe**.'

The patient has been given factual information with positive connotations. Possible awareness and paralysis are equated with '*doing the best for your heart*'. The anaesthe-tist should note that:

1 the patient acts as a 'partner in care', rather than a passive recipient of medical tech-nology, which can be very empowering;

2 statements such as those above can be reassuring both preoperatively and intraoperatively should consciousness, pain, and/or paralysis be experienced;

3 explaining the beneficial purpose of paralysis and preparing the patient for this for-eign and otherwise frightening sensation is helpful;

4 '*You are safe*' is one of the most important statements a patient can hear pre-, intra- and postoperatively.

Intraoperative communication

It is important that the anaesthetist is cognisant that awareness can occur and to treat patients as if they are awake under regional or nerve block. Signs of pain or distress should be looked for: movement, hypertension, tachycardia, tearing, pupil size changes, or sweating. As always, optimal analgesia is desirable pre-emptively and intraoperatively. Apart from pharmacotherapy, speaking to patients in simple language—avoiding the use of technical terms and 'jargon'—may be helpful when clinical observations suggest they might be 'light': '*I am giving you a little more medicine right now to help you feel more comfortable*'. Word choice is important as patients tend to interpret communications literally under these conditions.

Reassuring, situation-specific comments, and occasional 'progress reports', can reduce patients' fear, if aware, and enhance recovery. The surgical and theatre team can be educated to avoid careless comments. When negative comments occur, corrective statements can be made with realistic positive connotations.

Surgeon: '*He's full of cancer!*'

Anaesthetist: '*Well—now that we know what the problem is*' ... '*the most effective treatment can be instigated!*'

This is not a false promise, nor an empty platitude like '*You're going to be okay*'.

Touch reassures the patient that someone is there—watching. Arms or blankets can be readjusted, a hand placed on the patient's shoulder, hands, or feet—whatever happens to be accessible.

Communicating with the theatre team

Theatre staff have a strong expectation that general anaesthesia involves complete unconsciousness from start to finish. They may find direct communications with patients under general anaesthesia challenging and may question the anaesthetist's competence in providing adequate anaesthesia. This presents the anaesthetist with an opportunity to inform the operating team of current research on awareness and the role their speech may play. It may improve operating room decorum and etiquette for the patient's protection, particularly avoidance of conversations with negative connotations or content—even when referring to other patients. See also Chapter 18.

Patients who report having just experienced awareness

Practice will vary as to whether to check routinely for awareness during the postoperative review. When awareness is suspected (e.g. intraoperative inadvertent TIVA disconnection or postoperative patient reports) a careful debrief usually clarifies what was experienced or recalled. Care must be taken not to imply or suggest awareness. The timing and frequency of the interviews may be important, more than one interview may be needed to clarify events and the credibility of reports should always be verified. Awareness may be missed in some patients, especially when discharged from the hospital before an adequate assessment has been made.

Five questions are recommended that do not suggest awareness:

1. What was the last thing you remember before you went to sleep?
2. What was the first thing you remember when you woke up?
3. Can you remember anything in between these periods?
4. Did you dream during your operation?
5. What was the worst thing about your operation? Or alternatively '*What could we have done better?*'

Using 'GREAT' in awareness

A 35-year-old electrician has had a partial lung resection for recurrent bullae. A thoracic epidural had been placed preoperatively and TIVA used for induction and maintenance of anaesthesia. During the procedure, the TIVA was inadvertently disconnected for approximately 30 minutes. The patient was reviewed postoperatively to check for awareness.

Greeting

Dr A: *'Hello, Mr Wake, I am Dr A. I was your anaesthetist yesterday and I am here to check that everything is okay with you.'*

This is an open question without automatically suggesting that anything untoward has happened.

Mr W: *'Well, I was wondering what a "rib spreader" was ... ?'*

Rapport

Dr A: *'Where did you hear about a rib spreader?'*
Mr W: *'Well, yesterday during my operation, after the surgeon had talked about his golf lesson he asked for a rib spreader and I was a bit unsure what that might be.'*
Dr A: *'So you remember some discussion during the operation ... is that right?'*
Mr W: *'Yes, but I think I must have nodded off at some point 'cos I can't remember much else apart from someone telling me that they were going to give me some more sleeping medicine.'*
Dr A: *'How did you feel about that?'*
Mr W: *'Well I didn't feel any pain, if that's what you mean.'*

The first thing Dr A does is to listen to the patient and confirm whether awareness is a possibility or likely. The anaesthetist accepts the report by the patient and acknowledges the episode. The patient seems to have perceived awareness, and this needs to be dealt with honestly, objectively, conveying concern and empathy as appropriate. The anaesthetist can ensure that the patient realizes that his account is being taken seriously by documenting the account while explaining this to the patient. The anaesthetist's perspective of what happened can be discussed in the presence of the patient and explanations given, as appropriate. It is extremely important to avoid dismissing patient's concerns, even if they seem irrelevant.

Expectations

Dr A: *'It sounds like you were awake for some of your operation ... is that right?'*
Mr W: *'Yes, Doc.'*
Dr A: *'We know for a period of time during your surgery that the anaesthetic wasn't getting to you properly but we were unsure whether you would remember anything or not. We did give you extra anaesthetic as soon as we realized what had happened.'*
Mr W: *'Oh' ... 'That's why I got off to sleep then.'*

The anaesthetist confirms that the patient was aware during his operation and offers an explanation to the patient as to how this has happened (see Chapter 13). Also during the procedure the anaesthetist mitigated the potential for a negative experience by appropriate calm, confident communication that more anaesthetic was being administered.

Addressing concerns

Dr A: *'Do you have any concerns over what has happened?'*

Mr W: *'Yes, the surgeon says that I will probably need the other side done sometime soon—is this going to **happen** again?'*

Dr A: *'What has **happened** to you is a very uncommon event and for this to **happen** again with you is extremely unlikely. We will make a special note in your medical records so that any future anaesthetist will take particular care to stop this **happening**. Have you any other issues you wish me to address?'*

Mr W: *'No, I think I'm okay with that.'*

The anaesthetist has used the patient's own words in response to queries and, as the patient has not voiced the experience in a negative way, neither has the anaesthetist (see Chapters 3 and 4).

Tacit agreement

Dr A: *'I will pop back to see you in the next couple of days to see how you are going. Is that okay?'*

Mr W: *'Thanks—I'm hoping to get out by Friday!'*

The above case demonstrates that patients can be quite accepting of awareness providing they trust their doctors and have not had a painful or emotionally distressing experience. If awareness with pain and/or emotional distress has occurred, the principles of listening and acceptance are equally applicable (see also Chapter 13).

Patients benefit from a clear explanation of what has happened, and why—if this is known. If appropriate, an apology can be made. A frank discussion by the anaesthetist, whom the patient might view as the *'perpetrator of his suffering'* can be therapeutic but challenging. Effective communication in these circumstances can obviate the development of persistent psychopathology (such as PTSD), and legal action.

If patients appear traumatized, they should be referred early to a knowledgeable and skilled psychologist. Maintaining contact with the patient and therapist demonstrates concern and allows the anaesthetist to participate or intervene as appropriate.

Patients who have previously experienced awareness

Most anaesthetists will encounter patients who are nearly unmanageable due to extreme fear of anaesthesia or of hospitals. They have often postponed necessary operations for weeks, months, or even years. Normally rational and competent, they may not understand why they have been unsuccessful in willing themselves to set foot in a hospital. Many are even unable to visit hospitalized relatives or friends. These patients may have previously experienced explicit or implicit IOA, although they are often unaware of it as a cause of their fears and simply identify themselves as *'phobic'*.

Possible approaches include: listening; acknowledgement of the occurrence, and of any subsequent or continued suffering. If records are available these should be reviewed thoroughly with the patient. These patients yearn for information and every effort should be made to respond comprehensively to their numerous questions. Most important to the patient is trust, and ongoing support until resolution.

Case study

Natalie, scheduled for multi-level spinal fusions had had '*horrible experiences*' during two preceding operations a few days earlier. A 7-hour emergency surgery after a car crash (abdominal, thoracic, and orthopaedic injuries) was followed by an equally long second operation. During both operations she experienced full consciousness and '*excruciating pain*'.

> '*I felt exactly what they were doing ... I tried to let them know ... but I couldn't move. Then I figured out that I was paralysed ... I screamed inside . . . but they didn't hear me ... I thought I was dying ... and they had no idea ... I panicked ... I was completely powerless ... and there was nobody to protect me ... to help me.*'

She also recounted detailed conversations, comments, and exclamations by individuals whom she identified by name. '*Many words I didn't know.*' Later, while being ventilated in ICU, she again reported being fully awake, paralysed, and in excruciating pain '*For days ... I didn't know what was going on—I thought I was dying there too. That tube in my throat was killing me ... but nobody talked to me.*'

She was petrified of the upcoming operation and had hardly slept since the previous surgeries. The anaesthetist (who had not been involved in her previous care) communicated with her as described earlier, after which Natalie commented, '*For the first time, I am not afraid*'. In the morning she reported excitedly that she had slept soundly.

At the conclusion of the operation while still in the prone position, she suddenly lifted up her head, and reached towards the endotracheal tube. The anaesthetist restrained her arm and spoke calmly:

> '*Everything is going well for you ... **and you are safe**. You are feeling the tube in your mouth and windpipe—exactly as we had talked about ... and you know that this tube is helping you breathe **safely** ... so you **can feel very safe** .... I already gave you more medicine ... So you can go back into a deeper sleep.*'

Natalie was then resedated for transfer back into her bed.

Later on that day ...

Anaesthetist: '*Do you remember anything about this operation* (making sure NOT to suggest awareness) ... *you told me so much about your last ones?*'
Natalie: '*No, it was just so different and ... so nice.*'
Anaesthetist: '*Do you remember me speaking to you?*'
Natalie: '*Oh that! You mean when you were telling me about the tube in my throat? I was so glad you were there, I felt so safe. It all was so different from the other two operations.*'

This patient illustrates that despite our best efforts, awareness can still occur but it can be perceived and remembered differently depending on the expectations that are generated and the sense of rapport and trust that occurs between patient and anaesthetist. Awareness does not have to be a traumatic experience even when the patient is already 'primed' to expect it. Instead, effective preparation and intraoperative communication may have benefits both in the short and long term.

Acknowledgements

This chapter was originally written by Christel Bejenke in the first edition. It was reviewed and updated by Suyin G.M. Tan in the second edition.

Key points

1. Intraoperative awareness may occur in any patient during general anaesthesia.
2. Implicit awareness deserves greater attention.
3. The patient can be educated preoperatively that *safe* anaesthesia does not necessarily mean or require profound unconsciousness at all times.
4. Optimal analgesia should always be provided and, where possible, complete muscle relaxation avoided.
5. Signs of awareness should be looked for.
6. Theatre team education regarding awareness, being mindful of conversations in the operating theatre, is important.
7. Reassuring verbal and non-verbal communications to the patient pre- and intraoperatively may mitigate the adverse effects of awareness.
8. After an event, the patient needs to be believed and the evaluation discussed with the patient. Early referral for psychological counselling may be appropriate.
9. Consider remaining in contact with the patient and therapist.

References

1. Cook TM, Andrade J, Bogod DG, et al. (2014). 5th National Audit Project (NAP5) on accidental awareness during general anaesthesia: patient experiences, human factors, sedation, consent, and medicolegal issues. *Br J Anaesth*, **113**(4), 560–74.
2. Graff TD, Phillips OC (1959). Consciousness and Pain during apparent surgical anesthesia: report of a case. *J Am Med Assoc*, **170**(17), 2069–71.
3. Myles PS, Leslie K, McNeil J, Forbes A, Chan MT (2004). Bispectral index monitoring to prevent awareness during anaesthesia: the B-Aware randomised controlled trial. *Lancet*, **363**(9423), 1757–63.
4. Ghoneim M (2010). The trauma of awareness: history, clinical features, risk factors, and cost. *Anesth Analg*, **110**(3), 666–7.

5. Cheek DB (1964). Surgical memory and reaction to careless conversation. *Am J Clin Hypn*, **6**(3), 237–40.

6. Moerman N, Bonke B, Oosting J (1993). Awareness and recall during general anesthesia. Facts and feelings. *Anesthesiology*, **79**(3), 454–64.

7. Oglesby FC, Ray AG, Shurlock T, Mitra T, Cook TM (2022). Litigation related to anaesthesia: analysis of claims against the NHS in England 2008–2018 and comparison against previous claim patterns. *Anaesthesia*, **77**(5), 527–37.

8. (2006). Practice advisory for intraoperative awareness and brain function monitoring: a report by the American Society of Anesthesiologists Task Force on Intraoperative Awareness. *Anesthesiology*, **104**(4), 847–64.

9. Samuelsson P, Brudin L, Sandin RH (2007). Late psychological symptoms after awareness among consecutively included surgical patients. *Anesthesiology*, **106**(1), 26–32.

10. Bailey AR, Jones JG (1997). Patients' memories of events during general anaesthesia. *Anaesthesia*, **52**(5), 460–76.

11. Nowak H, Zech N, Asmussen S, et al. (2020). Effect of therapeutic suggestions during general anaesthesia on postoperative pain and opioid use: multicentre randomised controlled trial. *BMJ*, **371**, m4284.

12. Linassi F, Obert DP, Maran E, et al. (2021). Implicit memory and anesthesia: a systematic review and meta-analysis. *Life (Basel)*, **11**(8), 850.

13. Cook TM, Andrade J, Bogod DG, et al. (2014). The 5th National Audit Project (NAP5) on accidental awareness during general anaesthesia: patient experiences, human factors, sedation, consent and medicolegal issues. *Anaesthesia*, **69**(10), 1102–16.

14. Levinson BW (1965). States of awareness during general anaesthesia: preliminary communication. *Br J Anaesth*, **37**(7), 544–6.

15. Mashour GA (2010). Posttraumatic stress disorder after intraoperative awareness and high-risk surgery. *Anesthesia & Analgesia*, **110**(3), 668–70.

16. Avidan MS, Zhang L, Burnside BA, et al. (2008). Anesthesia awareness and the Bispectral Index. *N Engl J Med*, **358**(11), 1097–108.

17. Bejenke CJ (1996). Painful medical procedures. In: J B (ed.) *Hypnosis and suggestion in the treatment of pain: a clinical guide*, pp. 209–61. London: W.W. Norton.

18. Tunstall ME (1980). On being aware by request. A mother's unplanned request during the course of a Caesarean section under general anaesthesia. *Br J Anaesth*, **52**(10), 1049–51.

Section 4

Communication with colleagues

Chapter 17

Safety critical communication

Stavros Prineas

'Okay, Houston ... we've had a problem here.'
Apollo 13 crew

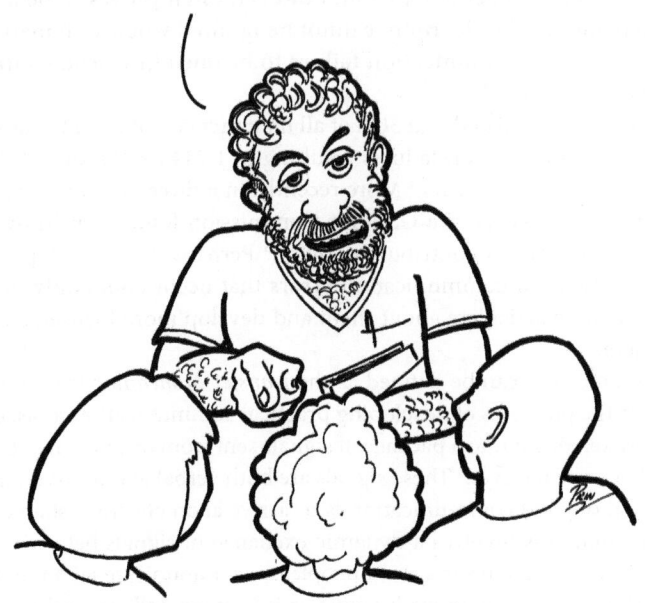

What this chapter is about

Communication errors—the mammoth in the room

In Chapter 1 we highlighted an example of failed handover in a tragic case report.[1] This example underscores the difficulty that doctors, as a craft group, often have when talking about communication problems. When trying to explain why an adverse event has occurred, we frequently invoke '*poor communication*' as a contributing factor and then retreat to the comforting realm of the technical, where the landscape is reassuringly familiar and the outlines are, for us, more clearly defined. Deeper discussion, however, often proves to be a woollier beast; and the mammoth in the room cannot be ignored when systematic scrutiny consistently reveals communication failure to be one of the lead contributors to serious adverse events.[2,3]

A 2016 study estimated that 30% of all malpractice claims in US hospitals were due in part to communication failures resulting in 1,744 deaths and $1.7 billion in malpractice costs over five years.[4] More recently, in a three-year review of 2,587 sentinel medical adverse events, the US Joint Commission found that in over 68% of cases communication was a contributing factor.[5] Perhaps if we develop a better vocabulary of the types of communication errors that occur commonly in the workplace, we can be more articulate about them and develop more focused strategies to overcome them.

Communication can be defined as the *transfer of meaning* from one person to another. For the purposes of developing practical communication tools, communication can be broken down into a package of signals sent from one person—the transmitter—to another—the receiver.[6] These signals are both verbal and non-verbal.

The goal of good communication is to arrive at an effective, shared understanding of a situation. This involves a dynamic exchange of signals between transmitter and receiver. We don't communicate *at* people, we communicate *with* them, so good communication is as much about *listening* as it is about *talking*, and as much about the dynamic conventions we use to arrive at an equilibrium of understanding. This is achieved by checking, as closely as possible, that what was '*heard*' matches what was '*said*' (see Chapter 2).

	Focus: Task	Focus: Power
'Stepping Up'	**Assertive**	**Aggressive**
'Stepping Back'	**Cooperative**	**Submissive**

Fig. 17.1 Communication styles.[10]
(Derived from the Qantas Model.)

Communication skills need to be seen in the context of other 'non-technical' or 'para-technical'* skills, such as situation awareness, task preparedness, team-working, and decision-making.[7] A number of practical tools are available to improve the fidelity of transfer of meaning between members of clinical teams.

Communication styles

The way we say things often reveals what is important to us. Even when it doesn't, others will try intuitively, rightly or wrongly, to infer this from the way we say things. In a workplace, some communication styles are more constructive than others. Trainee pilots are taught a useful matrix for categorizing communication styles[8] according to whether the person communicating is more focused on who will dominate in a conversation, rather than focus on the task at hand, and whether they are electing to lead ('stepping up') or follow ('stepping back'—see Figure 17.1).[9]

With an *aggressive* style, a person elects to **dominate** a conversation irrespective of whether or not this is in the interests of the task. This style is typified by a range of readily identifiable behaviours—from the use of demeaning and intimidating language, put-downs, snide remarks, intrusive body language, and stand-over tactics, to overt acts of violence and abuse.

....

* Author's note: while the term *non-technical skills* has become entrenched in prevailing literature, it is the author's contention that, as our understanding of and expertise in these important skills increases, this term may become a misnomer. Much research is being directed at developing practical tools, protocols, and techniques to hone communication and teamwork skills, supported by validated data—in other words, to '*technify*' the '*non-technical*'. One can foresee a time when communication techniques such as SBAR and graded assertiveness are as well-defined a part of an anaesthetist's technical armamentarium as the rapid sequence induction technique for emergency anaesthesia, or the primary survey technique for assessing trauma patients. Furthermore, there is a danger in assuming that these skills can be taught in *isolation* (dread the thought) *instead* of the technical skills with which they are meant to operate. Rather they should be seen as operating alongside these skills, and indeed intertwined with them. In this sense the term *paratechnical*, from the Greek *para-* meaning '*alongside*' or '*accompanying*', may better reflect their true relationship.

A *submissive* style is one where a person elects to **submit** to intimidation regardless of whether this is in the best interests of the patient. This style is typified by remaining silent, even when a situation is deteriorating by not speaking up nor escalating concern or, apologizing where no apology is required.

In a *cooperative* style, a person elects to **follow** the lead of another and to actively support another's plan, believing it to be in the best interests of the patient and the right plan for the situation. This style is typified by active feedback toward the achievement of the common goal, encouragement—'*Good idea!*' and acknowledgement—'*Thank you!*' '*Well done!*' and offering assistance.

An *assertive* style is one where a person elects to **articulate concerns** in the best interest of the patient, even in the face of a contrary point of view. This style differs from the aggressive style in that the language is not directed at intimidating others but framed purely around the task itself or the patient's interest, and around whatever actions need to be taken. In effect it's about articulating clearly a person's view of '*What*' is right, rather than '*Who*' is right. Elements of this style are detailed in greater depth later in this chapter.

In the vast majority of situations, a cooperative communication style, actively supporting and following an agreed plan, is all that is required. However, when a plan goes awry, or the plan seems unclear or wrong, staff must know when, and how, to speak up.

In healthcare environments, aggressive communication styles are commonplace, and they significantly impair team function.[11,12] They tend to polarize others into reacting in an aggressive or submissive way, and set the cultural tone for how others are expected to behave in order to survive in the workplace. Yet it may well be the prevalence of *submissive* communication styles that pose the more serious threat to patient safety. A UCLA study found that when faced with managing conflict, first-year US anaesthesiology residents were more likely to compromise by accepting that both parties' goals will only be partially met or accommodated, giving way to the other party at the expense of achieving one's own goals.[13] If that conflict is over a safety issue, it may directly subvert our '*duty of care*' to patients. In a pilot test of a multicentre simulation training programme for operating theatre teams, anaesthetists reported '*a greater need than surgeons to work on personal assertiveness*'.[14]

In any hierarchical training environment, there are significant implicit barriers to speaking up.[15] A survey of over 1,300 healthcare professionals found that 55% felt barriers to speaking up about patient safety concerns.[16] The survey uncovered a common fear of retaliation or negative feedback, fear of being wrong, or a sense of futility that nothing would change. Rather than assuming that staff will know when and how to assert themselves, healthcare organizations have an obligation to monitor and actively cultivate a work environment where personnel feel comfortable, safe, and supported when they wish to clarify instructions and escalate concern, and to provide adequate ongoing assertiveness training for all staff. This can be done through a range of tools.

Graded assertiveness

When things don't go to plan, or errors or mishaps occur, and patient safety comes under imminent threat, healthcare workers sometimes need to assert themselves clearly and, in a timely fashion. Graded assertiveness[17] (GrA) is a technique for escalating concern in a graded fashion until the person asserting is either dissuaded, put on hold, or overruled by the person being asserted to. Senior nursing staff will recognize this as a formalized variation of 'the *doctor–nurse* game'.[18,19]

The protocol has four levels.

- **Level 1: Observation** The asserter makes a neutral statement that relates to the concern. The statement could be as simple as stating a vital sign—for example, '*Her blood pressure is 80 systolic* or *Sats are 89%*'—or stating a relevant fact, '*I've never used remifentanil before*'.

- **Level 2: Suggestion** The asserter makes a positive alternative suggestion using a co-operative communication style. This can be in the form of a statement (e.g. '*Perhaps I can check the pharmacopoeia for the correct dose*') or a question ('*Would you like me to give some IV fluid?*')

- **Level 3: Challenge** The asserter directly questions the plan or decision, requesting a clarification or explanation. The name of the person and the word '*You*' are usually included to secure the attention of the listener. '*John, are you sure you want to give 40 mg of vitamin K?*' or '*Excuse me, Sarah, but why don't you want to call your consultant?*'

- **Level 4: Emergency** The asserter gives a direct order to deal with an emergency situation. It is used only when there is an immediate threat to life and limb. In aviation, the coded phrase always used in Level 4 assertions is '*Captain, you must listen*'. In healthcare, we can use the title of our colleague, followed by a coded phrase, followed by a direct instruction, and usually with some expression of the consequences of failing to follow the instruction. The actual words used are less important than having a standardized and readily recognizable phrase that is used throughout the organization. For example, '*Doctor, in the interests of this patient you must listen. I will not give the drug as you've prescribed it. Please revise the dose*'.

What happens after Level 4?

In aviation, '*Captain you must listen*' is code for the equivalent of '*Captain, if you don't return the plane to a safe condition now, I'm taking over control of the plane*'. This is because the person asserting is almost always a co-pilot, and therefore trained to take over. In a clinical emergency situation, where a person is empowered to take over, they should do so (see 'Prerequisites', next). Unfortunately, in healthcare the person asserting is often not in a position to assume the task they're concerned about. There are nevertheless a number of alternative actions staff can take:

- The most important action wherever possible is to get help—a senior supervisor, a colleague of the same rank, or indeed anyone that can help resolve the situation.

- Refuse to participate in the intervention, or to administer a prescribed drug.

- Withhold access to drugs or equipment.

- Document the Level 4 interaction in the patient record.

Refining Graded Assertiveness (GrA)—entry level escalation

It is recommended that where the situation allows, GrA is started at the lowest level of assertion, and escalated in a stepwise fashion until there is a resolution. In some situations, however—for example, in cardiac arrest resuscitation, there may be no time to step through the levels, and entry at Level 2, Level 3, or even Level 4 may be required. In other situations, there may not be an imminent threat to a patient's safety or there may be time to seek advice or a senior ruling outside the current conversation. In these cases, escalating beyond Level 2 may lead to needless confrontation. Like any skill, GrA requires practice to develop an intuition for when to step in and how far to step up.

Prerequisites to implementation of GrA training

Despite the absence of aggressive language, Level 3 and Level 4 assertions can be quite confronting, especially to senior personnel, who may feel that it is their authority overall which is being challenged, rather than their decision in this instance. Furthermore, it is not uncommon for the person asserting actually to be mistaken or misinformed, and that the other person has an entirely valid and appropriate explanation for their decision.

It is therefore important that certain conventions be in place to ensure the tool withstands the challenges posed by our work environment.[20]

1. GrA requires formal *managerial endorsement* from the highest levels of the organization, encouraging junior personnel to speak up and also informing senior personnel that this language is being used not as a personal challenge to their authority but as an impersonal safety technique.

2. A *standardized language and format* should be taught throughout the organization so that individuals, both junior and senior, can readily identify the tool and its intent when it is being deployed. Ideally, training should be mandatory for all personnel.

3. One must be able to assume that people are *acting in the best interests of the patient*. Thus the use of the tool to pursue mischievous ends, personal agendas, or 'point-scoring', undermines the credibility of the tool and must not be tolerated by the organization.

4. It follows from this that GrA works best in an environment where it is *integrated into regular in-service training* with other communication and teamwork tools.

5. It must be understood that the use of the assertiveness protocol is not rigid. But *can and must be adapted according to the circumstances*. Entry level rate of escalation, and the maximum assertiveness level, will vary according to the situation and the people involved. Developing an intuition for this flexibility requires practice.

6. Finally, invoking higher levels of assertiveness (Levels 3 and 4) should be *based on sound knowledge and awareness* of the situation and of a clear and imminent

threat to patient safety. Usually this means having clear evidence of concern. An exception to this is when it is evident that the team have not gathered the information needed to proceed safely with a critical task. This could be, for example, not knowing how a new drug might interact with a patient's concurrent medications. In this situation one can escalate concern not on the basis of facts, but based on the *absence* of requisite facts. The senior clinician can then decide whether there is time to get that information, consider alternatives, or proceed with a calculated risk assessment.

In aviation, the use of this tool has allowed both '*asserter*' and '*assertee*' to become sensitized to the various levels, so that all staff are attuned to responding to lower levels of assertiveness. This means that overt confrontation in day-to-day safety discussions is largely avoided, and that exchanges at higher, more confrontational, levels of assertiveness are less common. This cultural shift has occurred through the application of, and commitment to, the tool over time. Targeted assertiveness training during simulation sessions with anaesthesia trainees may have an important role in developing assertiveness behaviours.[21] Having said this, Raemer et al. suggest, based on their simulation study, that education interventions alone are ineffective.[22] Broader measures are required to better develop a culture of speaking up for safety.

Other assertiveness protocols exist. The Team STEPPS system advocates a three-step escalation process—'*I am concerned*'/'*I am uncomfortable*'/'*This is a safety issue*'.[23] Whatever system is employed, in-servicing of the technique should follow the prerequisite guidelines stated above, and it should be subject to ongoing audit and refinement.

Systematic handover and briefing techniques

Poor handovers and briefings prior to critical tasks are a well-recognized source of communication failures linked to adverse events.[24-26] Perioperative briefings are shown to be effective in improving group climate and work efficiency of surgical teams.[27] Over the last decade a number of formalized handover and briefing tools, derived loosely from models used in the military, have been developed for healthcare.

'SBAR'

A structured communication technique called SBAR was developed by the US Navy nuclear submarine industry for high-risk situations, and, for its versatility, has been adapted to healthcare.[28,29] SBAR is a simple tool for organizing and sharing information in a task-oriented way. The name is an abbreviation of its four basic elements—Situation, Background, Assessment, and Recommendation.

Situation

Two parts describe the situation. The first is a brief orientation. The person instigating the SBAR states who they are, where they're from, and what their role is. They confirm the identity of the person they're talking to.

The second part is a short, simple statement of the reason for the conversation, such as asking a person to come and help, asking for advice, or simply notifying someone of results or events. If the discussion is about a particular patient, the identity of the patient is explicitly confirmed.

Background

The purpose of the background statement is to relay information needed to put the situation in context. Again there are two parts to this:

first, a brief history of the patient's condition, medications, social or family issues, and clinical progress if they have been under care for any length of time;

and **second**, anything about the staff member, the team or the facility that might influence their ability to respond to the situation:

'This is my first day here and I don't know where anything is', or *'I've never used sodium nitroprusside before'*.

Assessment

A brief evaluation of what's happening has three parts.

First, a summary of recent examinations, investigations, and interventions since the current situation began—vital signs, latest pathology results, etc.;

Second, the person's provisional diagnosis—what the person believes is causing or driving the current situation, even if that diagnosis is *'I don't know'*.

Third, a projection of where things are heading: *is the situation stable, improving, or deteriorating?*

In this respect the three parts of the assessment phase match the three levels of ***situation awareness***—perception (eliciting signs), comprehension (forming a diagnosis), and projection (making a prognosis), described by Endsley.[30]

Recommendation

This is a summary of what needs to be done, usually in the form of an itemized management plan, or something as simple as '***I need you to come in***'. In an ongoing critical situation, it may be useful to state what's been done already, and then lead on to what next needs to be done.

Using SBAR

Being an overview tool, SBAR works best initially if each element is kept as brief as possible. It is useful to think of SBAR not so much as an acronym or a checklist, but rather a way of organizing thoughts not that far removed from the traditional clinical model of presenting illness, history, examination, investigations, provisional diagnosis, prognosis, and management plan. Given this, it is best where possible to take a little time to SBAR in one's own mind before picking up the phone or walking into handover. By keeping things brief and allowing the opportunity to spot, and fill gaps in one's understanding of the situation before critical conversations, this tool would be appreciated by all time-pressured colleagues.

Variations on SBAR

A variation of SBAR—iSoBAR[31]—was developed to address initial problems with SBAR:

- it was not intuitively obvious to people that they should introduce themselves;
- situations that remained unresolved due to disagreement about what plan to follow;
- occasions where a plan was discussed but not clearly understood by all parties.

The individual components of iSoBAR are **I**ntroductions, **S**ituation, **O**bservations (equivalent to 'Assessment'), **B**ackground, **A**gree (on a plan) and **R**eadback.[32] Healthcare authorities in some Australian States have adopted another variant, ISBAR[33]; and the tool has been incorporated into the national standard of clinical handover.[34] Nevertheless, high-quality research on SBAR in its various forms is still lacking.[35]

Preoperative briefings

In aviation, and in the military, briefings before and after critical missions, are standard operational requirements. Recently there has been a growing trend, toward structured briefings to try to reduce the incidence of *'wrong patient'* or *'wrong site'* surgery. A popular version of this has been the *'Time-Out'* procedure developed by the VA Hospital System in the USA, and now used across many parts of Australia.[36] Most *'Time-Outs'* constitute a brief period before surgical incision, where all members of the operating theatre team go through an itemized checklist to confirm the patient's identity, the operative procedure, the surgical site, the presence of signed consent, and other details such as the availability of X-rays and the use of antibiotics.

The World Health Organization has launched a Surgical Checklist aimed at reducing perioperative errors and adverse events.[37] Ten years on, where use of the checklist has been formally implemented and studied, there seems little doubt of its efficacy in reducing wound infections, blood loss, postoperative hypothermia, complication rates, mortality rates, and length of hospital stay.[38] Lingard *et al.*[39] have been developing a preoperative checklist for theatre teams, directed specifically at reducing specific types of communication error by using a validated assessment system. Initial studies suggest that use of the checklist halved the incidence of communication errors.

A challenge to compliance with the *'Time-Out'* tool is the differing cultural attitudes of nurses and doctors to the use of checklists. Generally, nurses view checklists as an important and reassuring safety tool, while many doctors perceive them to be a bureaucratic intrusion.[40] The truth no doubt lies somewhere in-between, and will vary according to the situation.

Anecdotally, in Australia at least, getting surgeons and anaesthetists to take responsibility for running the *'Time-Out'* has proven difficult. It is the author's view that whatever its name, a *'Time-Out'* is first and foremost a *briefing*—an opportunity for the whole team to join together for a moment, to ensure they share the same mental model of what needs to be done, to whom and by whom.

No matter how many boxes get ticked, if the surgeon is not in the room then the fundamental purpose of the briefing is frustrated. Perhaps if the exercise were 'rebranded' as a briefing rather than a checklist, better compliance could be achieved. However, it is interesting to note that in their successful study Lingard et al. secured the *a priori* cooperation of local surgeons, who took responsibility for running the checklists.

The communication roles of leadership

Leadership styles can be defined by the *authority gradient* between the leader and the rest of the team (i.e. the extent to which team leaders consult their subordinates and are prepared to accept questions, challenges, or requests for clarification of their decisions). *Autocratic* leaders tend not to consult their juniors and expect their instructions to be followed without question[41]—the authority gradient is described as *steep*.

Consultative leaders actively seek input and encourage juniors to raise questions and concerns where appropriate—the authority gradient is *shallow*. Finally, there is the '*laissez-faire*' style, where the leader eschews any authority over others and effectively offers no guidance at all—there is no authority gradient. Good leaders do not confine themselves to one leadership style, but rather adapt to the needs of the situation—a quality highly valued by other team members.[42] For example, it may well be appropriate to lead autocratically during resuscitation, and equally to lead consultatively when assessing a complex patient for an elective procedure.

As stated earlier, there are many cultural barriers to assertiveness. While there are some generational differences, generally it is common for junior members of a team to feel unsure and insecure about speaking up, even on safety issues. Implicit within the duties of being a good team leader is to make explicit the ground rules of communication between team members, and to give permission even to the most junior member of the team to speak up respectfully on matters of safety. As one fighter-pilot captain said to novices in his crew:

> '*I do not want to go out and punch holes in the sky, and commit an act of aviation with you on board, unless I am sure down to my bone marrow that you will speak up if there is anything you feel needs to be said ... Will you accept that responsibility on a co-equal basis?*'[43]

One wonders whether the prevailing medical culture will ever be ready for such a levelling of the communication gradient between trainees and consultants.

Articulating who's in command: 'handing over/taking over'

It could be observed that the likelihood of an anaesthetic adverse event seems to increase in proportion to the number of anaesthetists present at the time. When two people are sharing a vigilance role, control of the mission (i.e. '*Who's watching the patient?*') is often *implicit*—assumed and not articulated. In aviation, control and transfer of control is always *explicit*. During handovers, the pilot flying says, '*Handing over*' and does not let go of the steering column until the pilot monitoring says '*Taking over*'.

When a consultant anaesthetist is supervising a trainee, it may be useful to adopt the aviation paradigm of nominating who has the controls, and to ensure that, whenever a colleague hands over, goes on break, or needs to attend to an interruption, control of the anaesthetic is transferred explicitly using a reciprocated code phrase.

Other communication tools

The 'Below Ten' rule

The aviation industry has a 'Sterile Cockpit' or 'Below Ten' rule[10] based on the idea that whenever a passenger aircraft in flight is below 10,000 feet, it is either taking off, landing, or crashing. Thus 'Below Ten', the crew should be focused exclusively on controlling the plane; they should not be discussing non-operational matters until the critical phase has passed. When the pilot states that 'We are below ten', she is not necessarily declaring an emergency, merely that the crew need to focus on a critical task.

This technique can be used in any situation where you require the team to focus specifically—for example, during inhalational inductions of children in the operating theatre. It is useful, when dealing with an anxious child or parent, to have a neutral code phrase that is implicitly understood by the theatre team. When the anaesthetist says 'We're below ten', the scrub nurse stops clattering instruments, and everyone stops talking, quietly preparing, or standing ready to assist while the child is being anaesthetized. It is important to note that it is not the anaesthetist who is 'Below Ten'—it is the room and all the people in it. The same rule can be invoked by the surgeon during a tricky dissection or by the scrub nurse if a surgical swab is still missing after a recount. This technique requires in-servicing of all operating theatre staff, as it only works well among well-established teams where all members are cognisant of the 'Below Ten' phrase and its meaning.

'Transparent' communication

In a team environment it is useful, for at least four important reasons, to make a habit of articulating one's intentions by *transparent communication,* or what pilots call *'flying by mouth'.*

First, in general, conscious patients appreciate knowing in advance what is about to be done to them.

Second, by making one's intentions explicit to the team, it improves the team's *situation awareness* of what is being done when, and by whom.

The third reason is that it offers other team members the opportunity to notice and thereby trap an error in the making.

Finally, since experts tend to perform most of their highly skilled actions on 'autopilot'—intuitively and under minimal conscious monitoring,[44] making a habit of articulating one's intentions offers a final opportunity to bring a potentially erroneous action to one's own conscious attention before actually performing it.

There are exceptions where the overt or anticipated distress of a patient needs to be considered, but in most circumstances the routine use of transparent communication is reassuring and well-tolerated. Personnel who have worked in medical air retrieval units, where medical teams and aircrew train together, are used to this style of communication.

English language traps

Pilots worldwide undergo formal telecommunications training. Part of this training involves learning specific ways to minimize ambiguity and error during all flight communications. This is because there are many language traps, particularly in English.

The most obvious is the ambiguity of '*right*' which is used both as '*the opposite of left*' and '*the opposite of wrong*'. Another is the phonic similarity between the '**teen**' numbers and their respective '**tens**'—'*thirteen*' as opposed to '*thirty*', '*fourteen*' to '*forty*', etc. Even the similarity between hypOtension and hypERtension demonstrates that we cannot rely on Greek or Latin pedantry to help us avoid ambiguity.

Furthermore, this is compounded by a bewildering growth of acronyms, many with multiple meanings (e.g. *RA*, *OA*, *NAD*); and with over 10 years since the first edition of this chapter, there is still no internationally accepted standard for prescriber notation.[45]

Specificity in communication training

There are a number of ways individuals can train to make their everyday language less ambiguous:

◆ Use the word '*right*' only when referring to '*left*' or '*right*', and always use alternatives for its other meanings. '*The left knee is the correct knee, okay?*' as opposed to '*The left knee is the right knee, right?*'

◆ Learn the NATO phonetic alphabet, '*Alpha*', '*Bravo*', '*Charlie*', etc. to clarify the spelling of names.

◆ When giving a verbal order for a drug dose involving '*teens*' or '*tens*', spell out the digits: '*Please give 15—that's one-five—units of insulin subcutaneously stat*'.

◆ Take responsibility for the legibility of one's own handwriting.

◆ Get into the habit of following the '*five rights*' of drug prescribing—the right **drug** in the right **dose** via the right **route** at the right **time** for the right **patient**—when giving verbal or written medication orders. It is remarkable that this simple mnemonic is standard training for the nurses who administer drugs[46] but not for the doctors who prescribe them. Using the '*five rights*' will not eliminate medication errors—the causes of medication errors are complex and multi-factorial—but it's a good foundation for reducing their incidence.

Using names and numbers

It is important to know and use the names of patients, not only out of respect but also as a ready means of confirming identity. Do not accept a request to see '*a 19-year-old appendix*' but insist on the patient's name. Just as important is knowing the names of co-workers, and not just out of courtesy, but because it makes direction of instructions more effective during crises.

Many common pieces of anaesthetic equipment go by various names, and sometimes different staff use different names for the same object—for example, '*catheter mount*' or '*liquorice stick*', '*rosette clamp*', or '*armboard knob*'. It is useful over time to steer all staff, and any new staff, toward a common nomenclature for all objects, as this can minimize frustration and delay during crises.

A more difficult challenge is using '*context-independent*' language. The use of pronouns '*it*', '*them*', '*you*', pronoun adjectives '*this*', '*that*' and temporal adverbs '*soon*', '*in a moment*' is useful shorthand in everyday conversation. However, these terms are '*context dependent*' in that they rely on a person's mental context for their perceived meaning. This context changes from person to person, place to place, and over time. Where precision is required, errors may arise when these convenient, but non-specific terms are used. With training it is possible to develop a mindset where one avoids context-dependent words, specifying the names of people, objects, and drugs throughout a critical phase of a given procedure.

'*Fran, hand me the Yankauer sucker please*', as opposed to
'*Somebody give me something, I can't see a bloody thing*', or
'*I should be in theatre in 10 minutes, call me if you don't hear from me in 20*',
as opposed to '*I'll get there soon*'.

Feedback and debriefing

Healthcare involves making management plans for patients, and often these plans are conveyed verbally. Complex instructions, including drug names, dose regimens, and operative sites, are passed from one caregiver to another. Sometimes a simple error such as the transposition of a digit, mishearing a drug name, confusing an operative site, can have devastating consequences. Yet when a doctor discusses a patient's management plan with a colleague, there is no current expectation that either party will formally ensure that what was said matches what was heard.

The military use a particular technique to ensure high-fidelity transfer of meaning from one soldier to another. While those outside the military may not be familiar with its name—*challenge–response protocol*—when the technique is used just about everyone would recognize it as a form of '*military-speak*'. Soldiers are required to acknowledge that they have received an order, and for certain verbal instructions they are required to repeat the order itself.

A challenge–response protocol can be used during critical phases of a procedure, such as a MET (medical emergency team) call, or a difficult intubation. There is a convention commonly used by nurses receiving verbal orders over the telephone to ensure that the order is heard by a third person. This is done to verify that the first nurse has correctly heard the order that was given. Perhaps more important, would be to read the order back to the person giving the order, thus allowing them to verify that the order is actually what was intended.

A similar tool being used in North America is called '*Close the Loop*'.[47] When a clinician gives an order or requests information, if they get no response, she is taught to seek an acknowledgement by saying '*Close the loop*'. This is potentially a very useful way of engendering an appreciation of two-way communication during crises, and encourages staff not to assume that, just because an instruction has been given, it has been heard correctly, or even at all.

Mission debriefings are another important feedback mechanism for monitoring and improving team performance. Standard mission debriefs are conducted in three parts—viz. what was done well, what could have been done better, and a positive plan to improve future performance. This format, designed to cushion criticism between two layers of positive feedback, has become colloquially known as the *'dung sandwich'*—*'good news, bad news, good news!'*.[48] Indeed, as a training aid, routine mission debriefing, perhaps over coffee after an operating list, is useful even when there have been no overt problems in performance. In contrast, in cases of repeatedly poor, vexatious, or overtly dangerous performance, it is important to put patient safety first, and an assertive *'Level 3 or 4'* approach may become a priority. Effective debriefing, therefore is a subtle art that requires practice and reflection.

Key points

1. Good communication results from a dynamic two-way exchange between transmitter and receiver.

2. Some communication styles are more constructive than others.

3. Organizations that employ people to have a duty of care over patients, have an obligation to provide assertiveness training to all staff.

4. Graded assertiveness is one such technique, but others are available.

5. Systematic handover and briefing techniques, such as SBAR or similar, are essential to patient safety.

6. Clinical leaders and managers have the power and duty to set a constructive tone of communication for their teams and to articulate who is in control or command.

7. There are many English language traps that will lead to common communication errors, but these can often be overcome by awareness and the use of specific techniques.

8. Feedback and debriefing techniques are important not only for training and pastoral care but also to trap errors and prevent them on future occasions.

References

1. Paul M, Dueck M, Kampe S, Petzke F, Ladra A (2003). Intracranial placement of a nasotracheal tube after transnasal trans-sphenoidal surgery. *Br J Anaesth*, **91**(4), 601–4.

2. Wilson RM, Runciman WB, Gibberd RW, Harrison BT, Newby L, Hamilton JD (1995). The quality in Australian health care study. *Med J Aust*, **163**, 458–71.

3. Guttman OT, Lazzara EH, Keebler JR, et al. (2021). Dissecting communication barriers in healthcare: a path to enhancing communication. *J Patient Saf*, **17**(8), e1465–71.

4. The Joint Commission (2017). Sentinel event alert: inadequate hand-off communication. Available at https://www.jointcommission.org/-/media/tjc/newsletters/sea-58-hand-off-comm-9-6-17-final2.pdf (accessed 28 June 2024).

5. The Joint Commission (2016). Sentinel event data: root causes by event type 2004–2015. Available at: https://hcupdate.files.wordpress.com/2016/02/2016-02-se-root-causes-by-event-type-2004-2015.pdf (Accessed 31 March 2023).

6. DeVito JA (1988). *Human communication*, 2nd edition. New York, NY: Harper & Row.

7. Fletcher G, Flin R, McGeorge P, Glavin R, Maran N, Patey R (2003). Anaesthetists' non-technical skills (ANTS). Evaluation of a behavioural marker system. *Br J Anaesth*, **90**, 580–8.

8. Australian Airlines (1987). *Communication styles. Aircrew team management handbook*, pp. 73–86 (internal publication).

9. Prineas S, Wynne D. (2004). *The Caesar in Bed 12: facilitators' guide*. Sydney: ErroMed Publishers.

10. Prineas S (2005). *The Human Error and Patient Safety (HEAPS) training programme manual*. (Available through https://www.erromed.com).

11. Dunn H (2003). Horizontal violence among nurses in the operating room. *AORN J*, **78**(6), 977–88.

12. Inch J (2007). Horizontal violence: the silent destructive force. *Br J Anaest Recov Nurs*, **8**(2), 20–1.

13. Vassilopoulos T, Giordano CR, Hagan JD, Fahy BG (2018). Understanding conflict management styles in anesthesiology residents. *Anesth Analg*, **127**(4), 1028–34

14. Arriaga AF, Gawande AA, Raemer DB, et al. (2014). Pilot testing of a model for insurer-driven, large scale multicenter simulation training for operating room teams. *Ann Surg*, **259**(3), 403–10.

15. Poroch D, McIntosh W (1995). Barriers to assertive skills in nurses. *Aust N Z Ment Health Nurs*, **4**(3), 113–23.

16. Etchegaray JM, Ottosen MJ, Dancsak T, Thomas EJ (2020). Barriers to speaking up about patient safety concerns. *J Patient Saf*, **16**(4), e230–e234

17. Qantas Airways Ltd (1989). *Managing upwards: flight operations crew resource management handbook*, pp. 4.25–4.28 (internal publication).

18. Stein LI (1967). The doctor–nurse game. *Arch Gen Psychiatry*, **16**(6), 699–703.

19. Stein LI (1990) The doctor-nurse game revisited. *N Engl J Med*, **323**(3), 201–3.

20. Prineas S, Wynne N (2006). *Bertha's fall—facilitators' guide*. Sydney: ErroMed Publishers.

21. Daly Guris RJ, Duarte SS, Miller CR, Schiavi A, Toy S (2019) Training novice anaesthesiology trainees to speak up for patient safety. *Br J Anaesth*, **122**(6), 767–75.

22. Raemer DB, Kolbe M, Mineheart RD, Rudolph JW, Pian-Smith MCM (2016). Improving anesthesiologists' ability to speak up in the operating room: a randomized controlled experiment of a simulation-based intervention and a qualitative analysis of hurdles and enablers. *Acad Med*, **91**(4), 530–9.

23. US Department of Health and Human Services, AHRQ (2020). *Pocket guide: TeamSTEPPS*. Available at: https://www.ahrq.gov/teamstepps/instructor/essentials/pocketguide.html#call outhttp://teamstepps.ahrq.gov/ (Accessed 31 March 2023).

24. Wachter R, Shojania K (2004). *Internal bleeding*. New York: Rugged Land Publishers.

25. Arora V, Johnson J, et al. (2005). Communication failures in patient sign-out and suggestions for improvement: a critical incident analysis. *Qual Saf Health Care*, **14**, 401–7.

26. Pezzolesi C, Schifano F, Pickles J, et al. (2010). Clinical handover incident reporting in one UK general hospital. *Int J Qual Health Care*, **22**(5), 396–401.

27. Makary, MA, Mukherjee A, Sexton JB, et al. (2007). Operating room briefings and wrong-site surgery. *J Am Coll Surg*, **204**(2), 236–43.

28. Leonard M (2006). SBAR Tool: situation-background-assessment-recommendation. Available at: http://www.ihi.org/resources/Pages/Tools/SBARToolkit.aspx (Accessed 31 March 2023).

29. Guttman OT, Lazzara EH, Keebler JR, Webster KLW, Gisick LM, Baker AL (2021). Dissecting communication barriers in healthcare: a path to enhancing communication resiliency, reliability, and patient safety. *J Patient Saf*, **17**(8), e1465–71.

30. Endsley M, Garland D (2001). *Situation awareness: analysis and measurement*, pp. 3–29. New Jersey: Lawrence Erlbaum Associates.

31. Porteous J, Stewart-Wynne EG, Connolly M, Crommelin PF (2009). iSoBAR—a concept and handover checklist: the National Clinical Handover Initiative. *Med J Aust*, **190**(11), S152–6.

32. Department of Health [West Australia]. (2019) Clinical handover policy. Available at: https://www.health.wa.gov.au/~/media/Files/Corporate/Policy-Frameworks/Clinical-Governance-Safety-and-Quality/Policy/Clinical-Handover-Policy/Clinical-Handover-Pol icy.pdf (Accessed 31 March 2023).

33. SA Health, Safety and Quality Unit. (2016). ISBAR—a standard mnemonic to improve clinical communication. Available at: https://www.sahealth.sa.gov.au/wps/wcm/conn ect/8a8b26804896068a9cb8fc7675638bd8/15111.3-+Clinical+Handover+Fact+Sheet+ %28V1%29WebS.pdf?MOD=AJPERES&CACHEID=ROOTWORKSPACE-8a8b2 6804896068a9cb8fc7675638bd8-nwKWYoN (Accessed 1 June 2022).

34. Australian Commission for Quality and Safety in Health Care (2012). Safety and quality improvement guide—standard 6: clinical handover. Available at: https://www.safetyand quality.gov.au/sites/default/files/migrated/Standard6_Oct_2012_WEB.pdf (Accessed 31 March 2023).

35. Müller M, Jürgens J, Redaèlli M, Klingberg K, Hautz WE, Stock S (2018, August 1). Impact of the communication and patient hand-off tool SBAR on patient safety: a systematic review. BMJ Open. BMJ Publishing Group. https://doi.org/10.1136/bmjopen-2018-022202

36. NSW Health (2017). *Clinical Procedure Safety*. Available at: https://www1.health.nsw.gov. au/pds/ActivePDSDocuments/PD2017_032.pdf (Accessed 1 June 2022).

37. Haynes A, Weiser T, Berry W, et al. (2009). A surgical safety checklist to reduce morbidity and mortality in a global population. *N Engl J Med*, **360**(5), 491–9.

38. Haugen AS, Sevdalis N, Søfteland E (2019). Impact of the World Health Organisation surgical safety checklist on patient safety. *Anesthesiology*, **131**, 420–5.

39. Lingard L, Regehr G, Orser B, et al. (2008). Evaluation of a preoperative checklist and team briefing among surgeons, nurses and anaesthesiologists to reduce failures in communication. *Arch Surg*, **143**(1), 12–17.

40. Gawande A (2007). The checklist. *The New Yorker*, Dec. **10**, 86–101. Available at: https://www.newyorker.com/magazine/2007/12/10/the-checklist (Accessed 31 March 2023).

41. Sexton B, Thomas E, Helmreich R (2000). Error, stress and teamwork in medicine and aviation; cross-sectional surveys. *BMJ*, **320**, 745–9.

42. Larsson J, Holström IK (2012). How excellent anaesthetists perform in the operating theatre: a qualitative study of non-technical skills. *Br J Anaesth*, **110**(1), 115–21.

43. Nance JJ (2001). John J Nance Near-Miss Story. Video presentation by John Nance Associates. Available at: https://www.youtube.com/watch?v=hW7LGxCLauo (Accessed 31 March 2023).

44. Reason J (1990). *Human error*. Cambridge: Cambridge University Press.

45. Davis NM (2020). *Medical abbreviations: 55,000 conveniences at the expense of communication and safety*, 16th edition. Warminster, PA: Neil M Davis Publishing.

46. ASHP (1993). ASHP guidelines on preventing medication errors in hospitals. *Am J Hosp Pharm*, **50**(5), 305–14.

47. Small S, Wuerz R, Simon R, Shapiro N, Conn A, Setnik G (2008). Demonstration of high-fidelity simulation training for emergency medicine. *Acad Emerg Med*, **6**(4), 312–23.

48. Adey P (2004). Professional development for cognitive acceleration: elaboration. In: Adey P (ed.) *Professional development of teachers: practice and theory*, pp. 31–50. New York: Kluwer Academic Publishers.

Chapter 18

The theatre team

Suyin G.M. Tan

'A good surgeon deserves a good anaesthetist.
A bad surgeon needs one!'
Anon

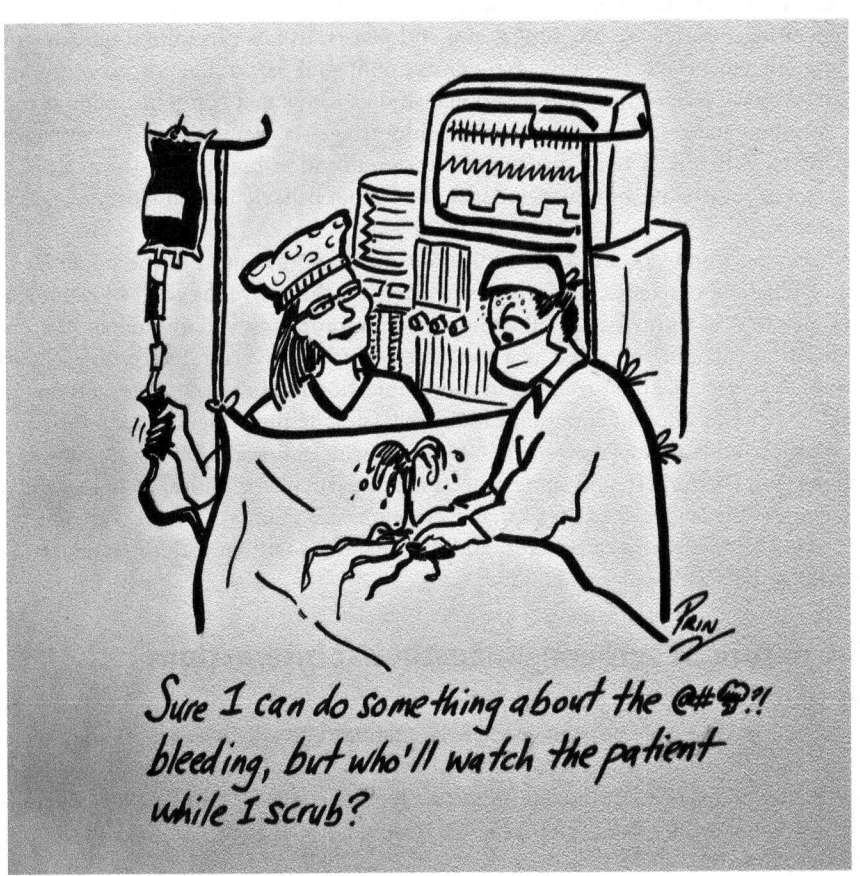

Sure I can do something about the @#$?! bleeding, but who'll watch the patient while I scrub?

What this chapter is about

A core attribute of the anaesthetist is the ability to communicate effectively in a variety of difficult situations and contexts. During the course of a theatre list the anaesthetist may interact with literally dozens of people—surgeons, patients, nurses, orderlies, radiographers, trainees, etc. Many will be complete strangers while others may be old friends, or enemies! Virtually all of them will have some part, be it big or small, to play in achieving a safe and successful outcome for patients.

Operating theatres are often busy, stressful places. Events can unfold quickly and in unpredictable ways. Tension is frequently an integral part of the process of undertaking surgical procedures.[1] Observational studies[2] show that communication errors are common and result in tension, delay, and wastage—as demonstrated by everyday experience. There is a tendency to view communication breakdowns as an inevitable fact of theatre life, however evidence shows that behaviours and attitudes can be altered.[3,4]

Improving teamwork and communication raises morale and has the potential to improve patient outcomes.[5] Most anaesthetists view themselves as good communicators, able to deal with virtually all communication problems, yet breakdown in communication is commonly cited as a root cause of medical error.[6] Interestingly, most anaesthetists feel that their training in communication has been adequate, and do not seek further education in communication skills, despite the evidence that poor communication leads to adverse events.[7,8] Much of what follows is generic to all interactions with co-workers, and some aspects are of particular significance to particular disciplines. The evidence indicates that everyone needs to improve their communication skills for the benefit of patients, and this chapter is written with the intention of providing tools with which to do this.

The nature of surgeon–anaesthetist interactions

The relationship between anaesthetist and surgeon is almost unique in medicine. In no other context, except possibly in the resuscitation room, do two or more specialists, from different disciplines, spend extended periods of time treating a single patient. The quality of this relationship has important repercussions for patient safety and outcome, professional job satisfaction, and the maintenance of good teamwork in the theatre environment.

The anaesthetist–surgeon relationship has often been described as a '*marriage*', and this may be the case, both figuratively and literally. However, in modern medicine, anaesthetist–surgeon interactions are more frequently a series of '*one-night stands!*' Good communication is the key to a successful anaesthetist–surgeon interaction—be it a '*marriage*' of 30 years or a single list.

Historically, surgeons have held the upper hand over anaesthetists. Initially anaesthetists were the most junior members of the surgical team, even the medical student, who were given the job of administering the chloroform. In more modern times anaesthetics are routinely given by non-medical practitioners in many countries. Thus, there has always been, and still is, a power and authority gradient between surgeons and anaesthetists-further exaggerated by differences in earnings, status, and gender— there are many more female anaesthetists than female surgeons.

However, the development of anaesthesia as a specialty in its own right, and the formation of anaesthetic colleges across the world has allowed anaesthetists to take their rightful place as the professional peers of surgeons. Anaesthetists can no longer be perceived as mere technicians whose job it is to serve, and service, the demands of surgeons. They are equal partners whose expertise is indispensable to patient care.

Surgeons are people, and people are infinitely varied. They are often perceived as being more outspoken, confident, and brash than their anaesthetist counterparts. The stereotype of the extrovert, bombastic surgeon and the introverted, unassuming anaesthetist still persists. Surgical training and culture tend to select individuals with no lack of self-esteem and with an ability to be the centre of attention.

The working practices of surgeons differ significantly from those of anaesthetists. Surgeons spend variable amounts of time in theatre, outpatient consultations, and ward-based care of patients. In contrast, anaesthetists are essentially theatre-based, unless they are involved in preoperative assessment clinics, pain management, or intensive care. Surgeons are often attempting to multi-task, supervising the care of patients scattered around or between hospitals, and then switching to the sustained high-level focus of an operation. Anaesthetists likewise multi-task and perform high-level focused activities, but are seldom in the position of having to care for more than one patient at a time.

Depending on surgical specialty, many surgeons work long hours with high stress levels. On a daily basis they deal with significantly higher levels of surgically related morbidity and mortality than anaesthetists. They are very often task-focused and less able to absorb the 'bigger picture'. Their lack of knowledge of the principles and practice of anaesthesia is a barrier to their understanding of what anaesthetists do, and this may lead to impatience with the time taken to perform anaesthetic tasks. These factors often underlie the tensions and conflicts that may occur in surgeon–anaesthetist interactions. It may be helpful to undertake a more detailed exploration of the factors influencing surgeons, their attitudes, and behaviours.

Surgeons and anaesthetists typically have somewhat differing views of the quality of teamwork and communication occurring in theatre,[9,10] with surgeons having a somewhat rose-tinted view of how other disciplines perceive them. They believe that teamwork and conflict resolution are good in their theatres, often contrary to the perceptions of the nurses and anaesthetists who work with them. Surgeons have a preference for steep hierarchies—that is, authority gradients.[11] They often consider themselves immune to the effects of fatigue and stress, and have a high level of confidence in their own judgement.[12] These factors combine to make surgeons often less sensitive to the nuances of communication happening in theatre, and possibly less motivated towards improving matters. Anaesthetists are fortunately in an ideal position to facilitate teamwork in the theatre for the benefit of all, especially the patient.

When one works in the theatre environment on an almost daily basis, it is sometimes difficult to recognize how abnormal or even surreal the surgical theatre setting is. To take a knife and cut a person open is an immensely challenging action requiring a great deal of skill and confidence, not always in equal measure. From the surgeons' point of view, it places an enormous burden of responsibility on them to fulfil the implicit expectation that their actions will not kill the patient. In primitive societies, and even in modern ones until fairly recently, healers, doctors and, especially, surgeons, were afforded a special status in recognition of the significance of their role. The erosion of that special status has been a mixed blessing for surgeons. To take a scalpel and cut a person open from xiphisternum to pubis requires the ability to dissociate oneself, at least momentarily, from the patient as a living individual.

When operating, particularly in difficult conditions, surgeons frequently become totally absorbed in the operation. They often fall silent, are intolerant or unresponsive to external stimuli such as background noise, and they often lose track of time. This dissociated state is what enables surgeons to do their job, but this intense focus can be a barrier to communication if the anaesthetist does not recognize what is occurring, and does not utilize the situation appropriately. Hence the importance of orientating oneself with the surgeon and the proposed surgery before the surgeon becomes engrossed in the task in hand. It is essential that the anaesthetist is, and remains, aware of the issues of '*in-flight*' communication.

Team briefing and 'time out'

In many countries, '*Time-Out*' procedures have been adopted not only to confirm correct site and patient for surgery, but also to allow information exchange within the team:

> '*This is Mr Smith, he is having a right hernia repair. Please remember he has a mitral valve replacement and is usually on warfarin.*'

The introduction of team briefing and '*time out*' procedures has been proven to decrease adverse events, and, while adoption of these practices is not yet universal, they provide a structured template to ensure that team members know each other's names and roles, have, an understanding of the procedure and, the opportunity to raise any concerns or queries. See Chapter 17.

Using 'GREAT' with surgeons

Whether the anaesthetist is meeting a surgeon for the first time or starting a list with someone known for years, '**GREAT**' helps to ensure all the important communication aspects have been covered, either informally, or within a team '*time out*' or briefing.

Greeting

Establishing and maintaining a good working relationship requires motivation, persistence, and a degree of insight. Starting off on the 'right foot' is the beginning of this process. In the theatre environment, social 'short cuts' are often taken—'*Hi there, I'm the anaesthetist*'.

Fully introducing oneself engages the surgeon's attention and gives him, or her, an idea of what to expect,

> '*Hello, I'm Dr Jones. I'm a post-fellowship registrar on rotation from St Elsewhere. I'm here for the vascular list.*'

If unsure of who the surgeon is, a brief enquiry such as,

> '*We've not met before, let me introduce myself ... and you are?*' may help ensure that when the bleeding gets out of hand you at least know the surgeon's name!

Rapport

Surgeons respect anaesthetists who take an interest in the operation and have some knowledge of the surgical anatomy. It never fails to impress if the anaesthetist knows more about the anterior triangle of the neck than the surgical registrar! Looking at the scans, having a look at the surgical field, and enquiring about how previous patients have progressed, reminds the surgeon that the anaesthetist is interested in patient management and outcome, and is not just a technician sitting by the machine doing the crossword. Surfing the internet or doing *Sudoku* sends a non-verbal message that the anaesthetist is either cool, calm and on top of everything, or completely oblivious to the four litres of blood in the sucker bottle!

An anaesthetist, as the only other doctor in theatre, is ideally placed to deal with page or phone enquiries, assuming this does not impinge on anaesthetic duties. It is far more sensible for the anaesthetist to take a message from a GP, decide if the surgeon needs to know immediately or not, and act appropriately, than a student nurse who has no experience or training to make that decision.

In facilitating the surgeon's work, the anaesthetist must be assertive but not aggressive, cooperative but not submissive. It is not necessary to love or like our surgical colleagues, but anaesthetists must be able to communicate effectively with them and be able to show professional respect, and likewise, to be shown respect. Perhaps a shared common interest in golf, fast cars, fishing, or Ukrainian folk music is helpful, but it is not a prerequisite for a successful professional relationship.

Expectations

Take the opportunity to let the surgeon know in advance, what your requirements are. For example,

> '*Mrs Jacob has bad lung disease, so I'll be putting in a thoracic epidural for her. That'll take 30 minutes but as I have a senior registrar working with me today, we'll probably be able to do this in the anaesthetic room while the previous case is being transported to recovery.*'

Letting surgeons know at the beginning of the list what time or resource constraints there are, enables them to manage their surgical time more efficiently.

'There's a department meeting at 6 pm which I'm chairing, so I will need to be out of here at 5.30 pm if at all possible.'

Not

'Damn it's 5.45 pm, I need to go now!'

Addressing concerns

The process of orientating oneself to the list may be automatic if one regularly works with a surgeon and knows exactly how long it takes her to do the case, for instance, a hysterectomy. However, if the anaesthetist is unfamiliar with the surgeon or the procedure, it is vital to obtain the relevant information.

'Dr Smith, I've not anaesthetised for a Wiseman's craniotomy before. How long will the procedure take, do you anticipate much blood loss, and are there any other specific requirements?'

Not

'Is this going to bleed?—I hope you realize there's no cross-match.'

Information exchange should be a two-way event to ensure both surgeon and anaesthetist have asked any questions they may have.

Tacit agreement

Having confirmed who you are working with, what you are all planning to do, and the special considerations of the patient, all that remains is to acknowledge that everyone is on *'the same page'* and ready to start.

'Okay, so we are all clear that we are doing a lung biopsy on the left lung and Joe will call the technician once the specimen is out . . . '

In-flight communication

The golden days of surgery, when all communication with the surgeon was conducted via the scrub nurse, are sadly gone. This leaves the anaesthetist with the, sometimes, thorny issue, of when to interrupt a surgeon who may be deeply engrossed in the procedure, or wrestling with a tricky dissection. Careful observation and an understanding of when a 'natural break' in the operation is likely to occur—for example, moving from one side of the patient to the other or adjusting their loupes—can provide an opportunity. Failing this, it is only polite to enquire if it is alright to interrupt for a second, but be specific about why you require information.

'I'm wondering if it is okay to call for the next patient.'

Not

'How much longer?' or, worse still, *'Are we there yet?'*

Recognize that a brusque or monosyllabic response from the other side of the drapes may be more a reflection of the fact that the surgeon is deeply engrossed rather than a comment on the anaesthetist's personality!

Real-life approaches to resolving conflict

Why do surgeons get upset, angry, or tetchy? Being a doctor is stressful, being a surgeon more so. Operating on a fit young person with a brain tumour, knowing that if you make a mistake, or even if you don't, the patient may die or end up hemiplegic and dysphasic, is bound to engender a degree of anxiety even in the most confident surgeon. Paradoxically, it is often elective surgery that worries surgeons more because they are playing for higher stakes. In an ideal world most surgeons want to be able to walk into theatre with a minimal amount of distraction and fuss, and get on with the focused business of operating.

However, the reality is often delays with equipment, staffing issues, and unexpected glitches. The surgeon has no direct way of controlling these events. If the autoclave is broken it is not the surgeon who can fix it, so the frustration often manifests itself in a negative outburst. At a time when they are seeking to control themselves in the process of operating, surgeons are often faced with situations they cannot control, and this leads to distress. Giving back a sense of control is often a helpful tactic:

'The endoscope you need will be ready in 40 minutes—maybe now is a good time to finish your ward round.'

or

'Would you like us to ring you ten minutes before we are ready to start?'

Not

'No, we can't start yet.'

Enlisting assistance is a useful way of occupying the impatient surgeon who is keen to start operating, and standing around breathing down the anaesthetist's neck.

'I am just going to scrub and put in a central line—perhaps you can do the arterial cannula to save time?'—assuming the surgeon knows how!

While any self-respecting anaesthetist would baulk at being a surgeon's handmaiden, there is a world of difference between being subservient, and facilitating the surgeon's job, to ensure an optimal outcome for the patient.

Although surgeons are rarely explicit in verbalizing their need for support, most will readily acknowledge that they seek and often receive the support of their theatre colleagues. This can take several forms: logistical, in terms of provision of staff and equipment to undertake operations; professional, in terms of medical advice and expertise offered by the anaesthetist and other theatre colleagues; and emotional, particularly when dealing with a difficult case or a bad outcome. See Chapter 13.

Anaesthetists are often focused on the logistical aspects of working with surgeons and can easily ignore the other important components of their relationship. Developing an appropriate professional relationship with a surgeon involves the provision of medical expertise to facilitate patient care so that the surgeon recognizes and values the anaesthetist's opinion, and seeks input, especially with difficult cases. Inevitably the development of a good professional relationship will foster a greater degree of emotional support. This should be a two-way process, but inevitably there will be different degrees of support in different contexts. All of us work at our best when we feel we are being supported logistically, professionally, and emotionally. In supporting our colleagues, we generate support for ourselves.

In the stressful theatre environment, it is inevitable that anaesthetist–surgeon conflicts will occur, and these are often perceived as personality clashes or just surgical personality! The problem frequently stems from poor communication and the failure to develop good rapport and working relationships. The issue may be chronic. For example, the surgeon recurrently arriving late or overbooking lists—or acute, as for example, the anaesthetist not sending for the next patient early enough.

There are some basic strategies which help to resolve conflicts.

1. **Recognize the emotional component.** If you feel angry, humiliated, offended etc. allow that emotion to pass before attempting to set things right. If the feeling won't go away, acknowledge it, '*I'm too angry to talk about this now*';

2. **Don't argue or fight in theatre** or anywhere in the presence of patients. Anaesthetists in a high state of emotional arousal cannot care for patients properly.

3. **Avoid the accusatory pronoun '*You*'** and take ownership of the problem using the pronoun '*I*' or sometimes '*We*'.

   '*I am concerned that the list is starting late, and we are having problems with over-runs.*'

   '*We all want to get through the cases on the list and are dependent on each other to start the list on time, so that unnecessary cancellations are avoided.*'

   Not

   '*You're always 20 minutes late!*'

4. **Use facts, not accusations, to make a point.**

   '*In the last two months 15 patients have been cancelled due to over-runs.*'

   Not

   '*You **always** overbook your list.*'

5. **Avoid blame** Seeking to attribute blame is a common behaviour when faced with a problem. If a surgeon says something like:

   '*It's not my fault that you take 40 minutes to put an epidural in. No wonder the list over-runs . . .*'

   Accept their reality either with silence or by agreeing that it isn't the surgeon's fault, without taking it personally. Having the insight to appreciate that anger or frustration is a subconscious response allows the anaesthetist to avoid escalating the situation.

6. **Focusing on the patient**

   Focusing on identifying the problem and generating potential solutions enables all parties to feel that they are making progress and can be heard. Sometimes the intervention or support of a third party, for instance the theatre manager or a senior colleague, can be useful in helping to solve a problem.

What if it just won't work?

As with marriages, not all anaesthetist–surgeon relationships work out. The frenetic workaholic, high-turnover anaesthetist will always struggle with the slow obsessive–compulsive surgeon, or vice versa. If the anaesthetist feels stuck with a surgeon that can't be reasoned with, rather than try and work out why, recognize that there are strategies available to deal with the situation, only they haven't yet been appreciated. Often there is a conflict of perceived values. Surgeons may value fast turnover, acquiescent anaesthetists, whereas anaesthetists may value attention to detail and quality patient care in a stress-free environment. Looking carefully, and objectively, at the quality of communication in the theatre, may well give clues as to how best to address the issue. For example, does the surgeon lead the theatre team or sit back as a passive consumer of theatre services?

If the best efforts at initiating and maintaining rapport and good communication are failing, then it is almost invariably due to different realities and expectations on the part of the surgeon and the anaesthetist. These conflicting realities are often dismissed as purely due to personality problems. However, it is not enough to dismiss the surgeon as an '*arrogant psychopath!*' give up, and make everybody else work with him. The 'LAURS' concept can be usefully employed in this situation. See Chapter 2. Systems issues such as poor staffing levels, inadequate theatre equipment, or inept theatre management, not infrequently contribute to the generation of a stressful environment that exacerbates communication problems. The solution often comes from a variety of approaches on both personal and institutional levels.

Crisis

The ultimate test of the quality of communication between anaesthetist and surgeon occurs in the context of crisis management. Surgeons who respect, trust and value their anaesthetic colleagues, are more likely to communicate problems, explaining them in detail.

'*I've just made a hole in the aorta—I think you'll need more blood.*'

Not

'*Whoops!*'

Surgeons may well be inhibited from communicating in detail about intraoperative problems they are encountering, due to focusing intently on controlling haemorrhage, or a sense of pride, or just sheer panic! However, encouraging dialogue helps to extract the necessary information and giving feedback helps surgeons feel more relaxed.

'*Things seem more stable at this end. Are you on top of the bleeding?*'

Likewise, when anaesthetists are having problems, 'thinking aloud' allows the surgeon to recognize a problem.

'*I can't see the larynx at all, we need a bougie.*'

Not

'*I knew I should have cancelled this one!*' (See also safety-critical communication—Chapter 17).

When things start getting out of control, anaesthetists tend to function subconsciously, and the capacity to think logically and purposefully is diminished. It is therefore important to take a step back to consider the important communication tasks involved.

In an on-table cardiac arrest situation, these might include:

- leading the resuscitation;
- calling for extra staff—for example, to take over at least every 3 minutes to give the massager a rest;
- delegating tasks to individuals by name;
- letting the surgeons know what is happening as they may not fully appreciate the severity of the situation.

The ability to communicate with others is strongly related to the ability to see others non-judgementally, to empathize and to recognize others' needs, motivations, and emotional state, even though 'putting ourselves in someone else's shoes' is not possible. However, it is possible to appreciate another's difficulty and work on a strategy that might help them through it. These are high-level cognitive and social skills which, while innate in some, can be studied, and acquired by others. In striving to improve our communication skills we inevitably improve ourselves by reflection on our own needs, motivation, and emotional state.

Communicating with nurses

Nurses often complain of the same failings in anaesthetists as anaesthetists do in surgeons. Unfortunately, very few anaesthetists are telepathic, so are condemned to communicate by the usual methods. Being aware of the capabilities of our anaesthetic nurse is the first step to establishing a safe, professional relationship.

> 'Hello, I'm Dr Jim. We've not worked together before—have you done many leg re-implantations? I'll need a size 8 tube.'

Letting nursing staff know the anaesthetist's requirements well in advance, and sometimes by means of a 'shopping list', is always helpful. Recognizing that a fellow team member is overloaded with work is an important skill, as is helping out in a busy theatre. Clear and concise instructions avoid misinterpretation, as does the use of the correct, or at least generally accepted, team member's name.

> 'Pass me the size 8 ET tube with the gum elastic bougie please.'

Not

> 'I need the white (brown or blue) thingy thing quick!'

Most people are sensitive to tone of voice. Speaking calmly, clearly, and loudly enough, helps to control the general panic when things go wrong. Shouting, sarcasm, or curses under the breath, may help to vent your spleen but do not usually improve your assistants' performance. Nurses value feedback and appreciate thanks for the assistance they provide, and this is an easy, and for most anaesthetists, effortless task to perform.

> 'Thanks for all your help today, Max. It was a great idea to try the LMA on that lady.'

The provision of teaching and practical training helps to engage nurses' attention and gives them a greater understanding of the tasks that they assist with. As an example, teaching laryngoscopy to anaesthetic nurses gives them an understanding of the anatomy and the potential problems that an anaesthetist may face. While many anaesthetists may be denied the luxury of a regular, highly-trained anaesthetic nurse, communication can easily be improved by undertaking the steps of:

- assessing the capabilities of the nurse;
- introducing ourselves;
- giving clear instructions, ideally having written your requirements in advance;
- giving and receiving feedback during and after cases;
- addressing other colleagues by name when asking for a particular task to be performed.

Handover

It is interesting to reflect that anaesthetists spend far more time communicating with surgeons and nurses than they do with their anaesthetic peers. Aside from coffee room gossip, the most common interaction between anaesthetists is handing over patients in theatre. Standardized operating procedures (SOP) for use during handovers help to ensure that the essential information is transferred in an explicit, efficient manner. See 'Safety-critical communication'—Chapter 17.

Anaesthesia handovers during surgery have been shown to be high-risk procedures and smooth transfer of responsibility is an essential factor in maintaining patient safety.[13] Despite the predictable risk of adverse events attributable to poor handover practice,[14] there is a lack of standardized practice. Guidance on what should happen lacks detail on best communication practice during handover.[15]

The Australian and New Zealand College of Anaesthetists (ANZCA) guidelines begin with the advice that assurance of competence of the relieving anaesthetist be ascertained before handover is considered. This presents significant issues. It is possible that anaesthetists may be compelled to continue cases that are beyond their perceived competence, simply by the style of communication of the transferring colleague.

'*It has been a nightmare shift. This last case has been horrendous—you're happy to take over aren't you?*'

As opposed to:

'*It has been a nightmare shift; this last case is complicated. I'll give you all the details and I am happy to wait for the consultant before completing handover.*'

The junior trainee may, or may not, be well equipped to deal with the case, but in the first instance, if then asked if he feels confident, will almost invariably acquiesce. The second example allows room for the relieving anaesthetist to take handover and assume responsibility dependent on their perception of the trainee's capabilities.

Ensuring patient safety during handover is an obvious prerequisite, therefore relative patient stability is preferred. Handover communication should be conducted under circumstances where both the receiving and transferring anaesthetist can devote their attention to the process.

A structured system for handover can be used. This should be clearly supported by written information, a well-completed anaesthetic chart and, where available, a specific handover sheet. The handover should emphasize the important details, avoiding extraneous information. No matter how well-completed charts are, spoken communication will continue to provide the *narrative*—the *unwritten feel* of anaesthetic experience to complement formal sources of knowledge contained in the chart. See Chapter 5.

Using 'GREAT' for handover

The '**GREAT**' template is a useful way of structuring a handover and facilitates quality communication.

Greeting

> **Dr Dover:** '*Hi. I'm Dr Dover but please call me Han. I'm a fourth-year registrar and am on for emergency theatre this morning. Are you able to hand over now—is the patient stable?*'
>
> **Dr Young:** '*Yes. Things have settled now, but this is only my first month of anaesthesia and the consultant is just in the coffee room. I don't think there is too much to tell you, but maybe we should get him back in. I'll get the handover sheet.*'

It is important for both anaesthetists involved in handover to understand each other's clinical experience and capacity to take over care.

Rapport

> **Dr Dover:** '*Welcome to the department. You look pretty comfortable with this case at the moment; perhaps you could give me the "heads up" before the consultant gets back from coffee.*'

Dr Dover has put the junior trainee at ease and provided him with an opportunity to make a direct contribution to the patient's care and use this as a potential teaching experience.

Expectations

> **Dr Young:** '*This 54-year-old poorly controlled asthmatic ... presented with an acute abdomen ... and her imaging showed ... We gave her ... she was a grade one intubation but on bagging her ventilation pressures were pretty high ... salbutamol seemed to settle things. She has got a 16-gauge cannula in both hands, a 4 lumen CVC in her right internal jugular ... She's had 2 litres of ... I've already arranged for Hb ... a cross-match of 4 units which should be ready in half an hour. As for*

the surgery, they've had some difficulty ... I think they are planning to do a right hemi-colectomy. We had planned to wake the patient up; however, I have spoken to critical care and they have a bed if required.'

This dialogue represents the communication required to hand over the patient's current status and plans for ongoing care.

Addressing concerns

Dr Dover: *'Okay, I just want to check what the post-op analgesia plan is?'*
Dr Young: *'I wish now I'd put an epidural in. I guess it might have been better for her chest. She hasn't been consented for one asleep.'*
Dr Dover: *'I notice she's got a sat probe on her nose—has there been a problem?'*
Dr Young: *'I've had to keep moving the saturation probe around to get a decent signal. Are you okay to take over? I'll let the consultant know.'*
Dr Dover: *'Hang on a moment. Is she a bit cold or under filled?'*
Dr Young: *'Errrrrrr ... ! I'm not sure.'*
Dr Dover: *'Well let's ask the boss ... '*

This component of the '**GREAT**' template allows clarification of aspects of the handover that need expansion before taking over the care of the patient. If there are no questions the anaesthetist *'taking over'* probably hasn't listened properly!

Tacit agreement

Dr Dover: *' ... well now that's all clear, I'm happy to let ICU know 20 minutes before we come round. Thanks for your help.'*

Interacting with anaesthesia trainees in theatre

Perhaps the most important interaction that occurs between anaesthetists is that which occurs during teaching. Part of becoming an anaesthetist involves the acquisition of *'anaesthetic culture'*—the sense of professional identity which may be either positive or negative.[16]

It is important to remember that teaching involves role-modelling as much as instruction and guidance, and creating a psychologically safe and supportive environment is key. See Chapter 19.

Communicating with secretarial staff

Most anaesthetists would acknowledge that the anaesthetic secretary is the backbone or nerve centre of any department. But there are a few rules which can help communication run smoothly:

a. If you are somewhere at variance with your planned or normal routine, let the secretaries know and ensure they have a contact number. If you don't want to be found or contacted tell them so.

b. If you require a specific task or item completed by a certain time be specific and write it down.

'*Dear Matthew, please can you sign off the attached order ASAP as I need it by next Wednesday (21st)?*'

Written communication

In contrast to the majority of our medical colleagues, anaesthetists can get away with a bare minimum of written communication. Unless working in a pain clinic, anaesthetists virtually never write letters and, with the exception of pain round entries in the notes, most anaesthetists tend to function at the level of '*fit and well*' and '*routine post-op care*' on the anaesthetic record.

When dictating letters, avoid the stream of consciousness. Think about the content and, if necessary, make notes before launching into a monologue. Indicate punctuation, new paragraphs, and side headings. Spell unusual names and check the recording has recorded properly.

The tick box format of many anaesthetic records and the accompanying computer printout are rapidly making the possession of a pen an optional extra for registrars! It does however behove the anaesthetist to ensure that documents are completed conscientiously. A brief skim through any selection of anaesthetic records inevitably reveals missing data such as start time, operator, or instructions for postoperative care. This is a source of great concern to the medical administration staff, quality controllers, and lawyers. An audit of anaesthetic record completeness often provides useful insights into any deficiencies.

Having possibly faltered at the first hurdle of the anaesthetic record, the concept of writing to another doctor may represent a further challenge to many anaesthetists. All letters need to contain the patient's full name, date of birth, and hospital ID. A heading detailing the salient problem and required action is an efficient feature for the busy GP who will not spare the time to read a two-page letter about the difficult intubation. Some departments have *pro forma* letters to deal with specific issues such as difficult intubation, post-dural puncture headache (PDPH), etc., and these are useful documents to generate and have available.

Key points

1. Quality communication in theatre is an important aspect of patient care, safety, and professional job satisfaction.

2. Understanding surgeons enables anaesthetists to optimize their working relationships.

3. There is a multitude of practical ways to improve communication with colleagues.

4. Poorly written communication is a frequent source of problems and is easily avoidable.

References

1. Lingard L, Reznick R, Espin S, Regehr G, DeVito I (2002). Team communication in the operating room: talk patterns, sites of tension, and implications for novices. *Acad Med*, 77, 232–4.

2. Lingard L, Espin S, Whyte S, et al (2004). Communication failures in the operating room: an observational classification of recurrent types and effects. *Qual Saf Health Care*, 13, 330–4.

3. Lingard L, Espin S, Rubin C, et al (2005). Getting teams to talk—development and pilot implementation of a checklist to promote inter-professional communication in the OR. *Qual Saf Health Care*, 14, 340–6.

4. Awad S, Fagan S, Bellows C, et al (2005). Bridging the communication gap in the operating room with medical team training. *Am J Surg*, 190, 770–4.

5. Sexton J, Makary M, Tersigni AR, et al (2006). Teamwork in the operating room: frontline perspectives among hospital and operating room personnel. *Anesthesiology*, 105, 877–84.

6. Gawande A, Zinner M, Studdert D, Brennan T (2003). Analysis of errors reported by surgeons at three teaching hospitals. *Surgery*, 133, 614–21.

7. Reader TW, Flin R, Cuthbertson BH (2007). Communication skills and error in the intensive care unit. *Curr Opin Crit Care*, 13, 732–6.

8. Elks KN, Riley RH (2009). A survey of anaesthetists' perspectives of communication in the operating suite. *Anaesth Intensive Care*, 37, 108–11.

9. Flin R, Yule S, McKenzie L, Paterson-Brown S, Maran N (2006). Attitudes to teamwork and safety in the operating theatre Surgeon. *Surgeon*, 4, 145–51.

10. Makary M, Sexton JB, Freischlag J, et al (2006). Teamwork in the operating room.: teamwork in the eye of the beholder. *J Am Coll Surg*, 202, 746–52.

11. Sexton JB, Thomas EJ, Helmreich R (2000). Error, stress and teamwork in medicine and aviation. A cross-sectional survey. *BMJ*, 320, 745–9.

12. Kitto S, Villaneuva E, Chesters J, Petrovic A, Waxman BP, Smith JA (2007). Surgeon's attitudes to and usage of evidence-based medicine in surgical practice: a pilot study. *ANZ J Surg*, 77, 231–6.

13. Meersch M, Weiss R, Küllmar M, et al. (2022). Effect of intraoperative handovers of anesthesia care on mortality, readmission, or postoperative complications among adults: The HandiCAP Randomized Clinical Trial. *JAMA*, 327(24), 2403–12.

14. Sun LY, Jones PM, Wijeysundera DN, Mamas MA, Bader Eddeen A, O'Connor J (2022). Association between handover of anesthesiology care and 1-year mortality among adults undergoing cardiac surgery. *JAMA Network Open*, 5(2), e2148161-e.

15. ANZCA (2013). Position statement on the handover responsibilities of the anaesthetist PS53A. Available at: https://www.anzca.edu.au/getattachment/74eae67f-3d96-4a81-a737-5b2cc9c1b261/PS53(A)-Position-statement-on-the-handover-responsibilities-of-the-anaesthetist-(PS53)

16. Lingard L, Reznick R, DeVito I, Espin S (2002). Forming professional identities on the health care team: discursive constructions of the 'other' in the operating room. *Med Educ*, 36, 728–34.

Chapter 19

Education

Sancha C. Robinson, Kirsty Forrest, and
Maurice Hennessy

'Education is the most powerful weapon which you can
use to change the world.'
Nelson Mandela

What this chapter is about

Introduction

What makes a good teacher? Which communication skills are most useful for supervision?

Communication skills are used every day by anaesthetists while *educating* trainees and others.

The term *trainee* is used to denote *colleague, medical student, learner, peer,* or *client*, and the term *educator* to denote *teacher, mentor, supervisor,* or *coach*.

By the end of this chapter readers will be able to:

◆ describe what coaching is in relation to anaesthesia education;
◆ relate education conversations to the 'LAURS' and 'GREAT' frameworks;
◆ apply 'LAURS' and 'GREAT' to education contexts, specifically the teaching list, formal supervision, and feedback conversations.

Case study questions

Consider how you might approach these situations.

Q1 There is a trainee experiencing difficulty and you are their training supervisor. The trainee's personal relationship has broken down, the trainee is a little older than other trainees, they've failed the primary exam and you've had concerning reports about a lack of vigilance on the job. How will you help them work through these issues and get their training back on track?

Q2 You are assigned a trainee to your theatre list today. They are 3 months out from their final fellowship exam and seem to know so much that you wonder if they might be on course for the prize. Not only that, but clinically they are excellent. How could you help the trainee have a useful learning experience?

What is coaching and how is it useful in education?

Coaching is a communication process for learning and development and it is a relatively new concept in medical education. It overlaps with teaching, training, supervision, and mentoring, as all these roles share a common set of communication skills encapsulated by the 'LAURS' and 'GREAT' frameworks introduced in Chapter 2.

Coaching in education may be defined as[1]:

'*A one-to-one conversation focused on the enhancement of learning and development through increasing self-awareness and a sense of personal responsibility, where the coach facilitates the self-directed learning of the coachee through questioning, active listening, and appropriate challenge in a supportive and encouraging climate.*'

The International Coaching Federation defines coaching as[2]:

'*Partnering with clients in a thought-provoking and creative process that inspires them to maximize their personal and professional potential.*'

Adopting a coaching mentality of *partnership* puts the trainee at the centre of learning. The aims of educational coaching conversations are to:

◆ define and explore the issue;

◆ broaden horizons and discover different perspectives;

◆ generate and evaluate options;

◆ create actionable goals with trainee commitment to, and accountability, for action.

All in a psychologically safe learning environment.

Think about the best educator you have encountered. What communication skills made an impression on you?

Think about the worst educator you have encountered. What communication skills made a poor impression on you?

For each of these educators consider:

How many of these points were related to their mindset—attitudes, values, beliefs, approach, ethical principles? How many of these points were related to subject knowledge, content, or format of the teaching?

Cultivating psychological safety

For a *supportive and encouraging climate*[1] it is important for the educator and trainee to communicate in a way that empowers both parties to speak up with ideas, questions, concerns, or mistakes without fear of negative consequences or embarrassment. By developing a coaching mindset, which is in essence a package of adaptive attitudes, beliefs, values, and ethical principles, educators, and trainees can co-create psychological safety.

The R of Rapport in 'GREAT' is how psychological safety happens.

Promote psychological safety by:

- building trust;
- developing a learning partnership;
- holding unconditional positive regard;
- understanding our biases;
- embracing a growth mindset.

Building trust

The Trust Triangle conceptualizes the drivers of trust as the three points of a triangle—authenticity, empathy, and logic.[3]

Authenticity is communicated through character, contribution, competency, commitment, and vulnerability. Authenticity is the educator bringing their whole self to the situation, being genuine, and acting in accordance with their own values. In other words, the trainee knows '*I experience the real you*'.[3]

Compassion and connection built through reflective listening and acceptance of the other is how **empathy** is communicated to the trainee (see Chapter 2). In other words, the trainee knows '*I believe you care about me and my success*'.[3]

Consistency, clarity, summarizing, and concurrent corrections in knowledge are all mechanisms for communicating **logic**. Educators can optimize learning by explaining, in clear terms, why they are doing something, as part of providing consistent learning experiences. In other words, the trainee knows '*I know you can do it, your reasoning and judgement are sound*'.[3]

In the book *Dare to Lead*, Brown discusses courageous conversations and leaning into **vulnerability**.[4] Much of this is about accepting emotion and discomfort. Brown describes how unease lasts on average 8 seconds, whereas if discourse is avoided, the unease can last for weeks.

So, how can educators show vulnerability? One way is to have the courage to share inner struggles, admit the possibility of being wrong and share the logic of their thinking.[5] This means providing evidence or information rather than simply saying they do something because that's what they prefer. It might also include sharing experiences that shaped the educator's thinking.

Developing a learning partnership

In the traditional learning model there is a power imbalance. The educator imparts knowledge, skills, experience, and wisdom to the trainee in a one-way transfer of information where the trainee is *taught at*.

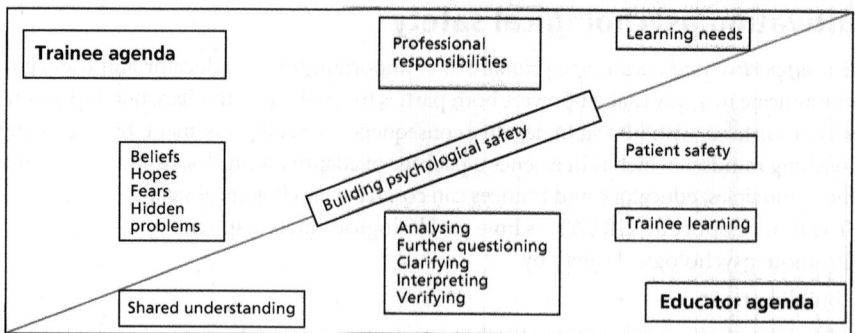

Fig. 19.1 A power-shift model of trainee and educator (adaptation of Figure 1.2. Data from Tate P. (1997). *The Doctor's Communication Handbook*, 2nd edition. Abingdon: Radcliffe Medical Press.)

In Chapter 1, Figure 1.2 details a power shift of consultation between a health practitioner and the patient. This model can also be applied to the trainee and educator relationship, where agendas may not align and may even be in conflict. Figure 19.1 shows a power shift model of trainee and educator. Moving from the right to the left side of the figure, moves from the educator agenda to the trainee agenda, and builds psychological safety.

Putting the trainee at the centre of a learning partnership is a paradigm shift from the traditional model of medical education. The partnership is co-created in a way that both educator and trainee are equal participants.

Holding unconditional positive regard

Having positive regard that is unconditional means that the educator holds a positive view of the trainee *regardless of what she might say or do during the coaching conversation*.[6] Educators assume that trainees are intelligent, well educated, want to do their best, are keen to learn, have value, and are worthy regardless of their behaviour and the situation. This requires educators to be respectful and open-minded. Believing that trainees can do more than they think they can, and more than the educator thinks they can, will optimize an educational experience.

Understanding our biases

In anaesthesia education there is sometimes tension regarding judgement. Anaesthetists are experts in anaesthesia and judge a clinical situation based on their knowledge and experience. However, expressing and receiving judgement on performance can be challenging.

Everyone has unconscious implicit biases, which unknowingly influence decisions and judgements. They are a normal part of brain processing activity and are shaped by experiences, upbringing, culture, and surrounding environment. These biases are not necessarily a bad thing. They are unintentional and when recognized, they can be addressed.

Sometimes people feel uncomfortable when biases haven't been acknowledged. As anaesthetists these biases can affect patient care, and interactions with colleagues and trainees.[7-9] The first step in managing bias is to become aware of ones' own implicit biases. Harvard University have online self-assessment tests.[10]

Embracing a growth mindset

Mindset determines how one thinks about and interprets situations, emotional reactions, decision making, and behaviour. It directly impacts the quality of relationships and interactions, including in educational environments.

Trainees and educators with a fixed mindset believe that their capabilities are innate, and difficult to change. They may avoid challenges, respond defensively and personally to feedback, and believe they are not good enough. The fixed mindset tends to be self-limiting, and often corresponds with negative self-talk (e.g. *'I'll never be any good at arterial lines'*).

Trainees and educators who embrace a growth mindset are open to learning from mistakes. They accept that *to err is human* and welcome the opportunity to learn from the experience and do something differently next time.[11] A trainee who has a growth mindset and is struggling with arterial line insertion is more likely to consider *'What do I need to do to improve?'* This makes goal-setting, feedback conversations, dealing with errors or mistakes, and managing challenges easier.

Coaching skills for conversations in education

Evidence shows that specific coaching micro-skills of active listening, asking open-ended questions, and using clarifying questions, are associated with better communication outcomes in medical education.[12]

Listening

There are several levels of listening, including cosmetic, conversational, active, and deep listening.[13]

Surface or cosmetic listening is when the listener hears words and is not thinking about what the other person is saying.

Conversational listening describes what happens when chatting in the break room. The aim is to fit in and connect with others. It keeps the conversation flowing as the listener inevitably jumps ahead to think up questions and responses, with the aim of bringing the conversation back to themselves at a socially acceptable moment.

Active listening occurs when the listener provides space, full attention, and listens, with genuine curiosity, to understand what the other person is saying.

Deep listening requires the listener to suspend judgement, remain totally present in the moment, listen for meaning in the story, the other person's understanding, and a sense of who they are.[13]

Listening for words and meaning, thereby ensuring that the trainee has been heard and understood, are essential aspects of any educational encounter. Ideally active and deep listening are employed most of the time. This requires remaining fully present in the moment, and dispensing with distractions, while also recognizing that in a busy clinical setting both educator and trainee need to maintain situational awareness.

The challenge is for educators to convey that they are listening. Silence is underrated. Timed perfectly, perhaps with the use of body language, a tilt of the head, a nod, a smile or similar, the trainee will be encouraged to expand on what they were saying.

Asking questions

The role of the educator is to encourage the trainees' development, nurture their resourcefulness, and challenge them to find other ways of thinking and doing. This is best achieved by **asking** instead of **telling**.

A powerful question is an open question asked with genuine curiosity that prompts a description to provide a complete answer and opens up possibilities for the trainee.[14] To be a powerful question, the question must be aligned with the trainee's area of interest. Powerful questions often start with '*What?*' '*When?*' '*How much?*' '*How many?*' '*How often?*' '*Who?*' '*Where?*' '*Which?*' These words are designed to elicit facts or quantify something.[15]

The tone of voice, body language and context in which the question is asked is probably more important than the exact wording of the question.

Potential pitfalls of powerful questions include:

- asking a question that is too complex[14];
- asking more than one question at once[16];
- asking a leading question[16];
- implying judgement in the way the question is asked[14];
- using '*Why?*' questions that may come across as critical, and request justification by the trainee[14,15];

> '*Telling or asking closed questions saves people from having to think. Asking open questions causes them to think for themselves.*'[15]

When stuck for how to start a conversation, consider, '*What would you like to talk about today?*'

Summarizing and clarifying questions

The aim of summarizing is twofold: to show trainees they have been listened to and to *play-back* what they have said. This encourages reflection, enhances understanding, and perhaps lead to an *Ah-ha* moment.

Educators may utilize some of the trainee's wording. New words inserted by the listener can change the meaning and project the listener's judgement onto the conversation. It is okay if the summary isn't perfect, because often the trainee's response will be '*Yes, it's sort of that and it's also ...*' leading to further discoveries or expanded thinking. Clarifying questions such as '*What I heard you say was ... Can you tell me what you meant by ... ?*' can then be used.

The educator can consider a range of options, perhaps summarizing in an iterative way, using the trainee's own words, or distilling the entire conversation to 3 to 5 bullet points. This technique may be used in a variety of educational contexts such as vivas, handover, presenting a patient and management plan, teaching a skill and preparing for job interviews. Goal directed practice can assist with learning and trainees can be encouraged to incorporate such summarizing activities into the day-to-day.

Reframing

Encouraging a **reframe** by thinking in a *positive* rather than a *negative* way can be helpful in broadening perspective. Positivity in the reframe can be summarized with the following statement[17]:

> *Focus on the future not the past. Build from success. Believe in your coachee's ability to effect positive change.*

Suggestion

Unsolicited advice—a 'seminar-for-one'[18]—is usually unhelpful and likely to be ignored. However, providing timely direction, particularly on a safety-related issue, is essential. Instructional coaching is a construct that *combines the non-directive elements of a collaborative way of working with some clearly directive elements* when this is in the best interests of the trainee and the patient.[1]

A guideline for offering information proposed by Rogers[19] is applicable for medical educators:

♦ **Seek permission**—'*Would it be okay if we went over topicalization of the airway for an awake fibreoptic?*'

♦ **Elicit what the trainee already knows**—'*What have you read about topicalizing the airway?*' '*How many cases have you done previously and what did you discover?*'

♦ **Ask how the trainee would like the information to be provided**—'*What would you like to know about topicalizing the airway?*' '*We could talk about it step by step or as an overview. What would be most helpful to you?*'

♦ **Give advice** by drawing out then adding[19] to this information—'*How would you go about starting the topicalization?... Sometimes I find it helpful to ...*'

♦ **Ask what the trainee thinks** of this advice to invite disagreement[19]—'*What are your thoughts?*'

♦ **Provide several examples of other ways** this has been done—'*There are lots of ways to topicalize an airway. For example ...*'

When there is a time-critical safety related issue it may be necessary to offer immediate advice or take corrective action since the safety of the patient is paramount.

Chapter 2 discusses the use of suggestion as part of the 'LAURS' framework. Examples of indirect suggestion in education include:

> '***Sometimes trainees find it is helpful*** *to observe for 30 minutes or so and then make a decision about what they'd like to learn based on what they've seen. How does this idea resonate with you?*'

The implication here is that the trainee can make a decision on what they'd like to learn based on what they observe.

Conversations in education

Using GREAT in the teaching list conversation

The focus is on ask, don't tell.

Greeting

Introduce the trainee, clinical team, and the patient by name. This is especially important when the educator knows the team well and does the list regularly.

Rapport

Orientate the trainee to the clinical space and equipment, including emergency trolleys and break rooms, **and** to the learning approach used in the theatre.

> *'In this operating theatre we like to promote learning by creating a safe environment and encouraging a growth mindset. How does that sound?'*

Never underestimate how little things like this can build psychological safety.

The 'LAURS' framework can be used throughout the conversation to build rapport.

Expectations

Setting expectations upfront is a key component of psychological safety. Educators may want to discuss what they want trainees to do and include any personal preferences that are non-negotiable. The trainee may also set their expectations of the educator and determine roles and responsibilities.

Educators should be explicit about what to do in situations when something appears unsafe i.e. the trainee should let them know and vice versa. For example, *'If I see something that concerns me I'll let you know. Similarly, if I do something that you are not sure about just ask me. It's all about keeping the patient safe'.*

A **needs assessment** conversation clarifying both the goals of the trainee, and the current trainee situation, is helpful in setting expectations. Some needs assessment questions include:

◆ **Goals of the trainee**

   o *'What do you want to get out of the day?'*
   o *'What would you like to focus on today?'*

◆ **General training information**

   o *'Where are you in your training?'*
   o *'What have you done so far this term?'*

◆ **Context-specific training information**

   o *'How many cases/procedures like this have you completed?'*
   o *'What went well?'*
   o *'What complications have you seen and dealt with?'*

◆ **Trainee-identified areas to work on**

   o *'How are you feeling about things today'*
   o *'Have you had any recent feedback you'd like to build on today?'*

◆ **Context-specific areas to work on**
  o *'What's stopping you being able to do this case/procedure/list on your own?'*
  o *'Which part of a case/procedure/list do you find most challenging?'*
  o *'What parts of the case/procedure/list can you do independently?'*

Having completed a **needs assessment**, the trainee and educator can then agree on the goals for learning. One way to do this is to have the needs assessment conversation early on and then at a suitable time after induction ask the trainee to have a coffee and write down their goals for learning. This gives the trainee time and space to think.

If the trainee has no idea what to get out of the list here are a few ideas to assist:

◆ *'I have some experience in this area, would it be helpful if I suggested some options?'*

◆ Relate it back to the training programme—*'I'm wondering, is there an area from the training programme we could focus on?'*—The focus might be a workplace-based assessment, a curriculum topic, or a short answer question

◆ For the trainee who is studying for exams *'What have you been studying recently?'*— the focus might then be on this topic in relation to the case/list

Addressing concerns

For each learning goal, the educator and trainee can negotiate and enact a plan. Powerful questions that might help to address concerns include:

  'What will you do?'

  'What would you like me to do?'

  'How will you let me know if you need assistance?'

  'Can you talk me through the steps?'

  'Who are you going to involve at each stage?'

  'What options are there here?'

  'What is directing you towards the option you have chosen?'

  'I'm curious to understand, what do you think about ... ?'

Summarizing and clarification are extremely important steps in this process. A good starting point is to ask trainees to reduce concepts down into 3–5 items or a three-sentence summary. For example, *'Please can you summarize the anaesthetic assessment and plan in three sentences'*.

If the trainee does not engage in the way the educator expects, it may be helpful to stay curious and accept where the trainee is at this time. and meet them there. Some questions might include:

  'I've noticed ... I'm wondering what's happening for you?'

  'I've noticed ... What is it holding you back from ... ?'

Tacit agreement

The process of feedback, and thanks for the interaction, represent not only an agreed plan of where to go from here, but also a reinforcement of the learning partnership.

Evaluation is for both the trainee and the educator. The questions below allow for reflective learning and act as a basis for ongoing development:

> '*What did you notice during the case/list?*'
>
> '*What went well? What didn't go so well?*'
>
> '*What makes that important? What have we learnt from that?*'
>
> '*Have you any further plans or goals?*'

The formal supervision conversation

Formal supervision conversations might include clinical placement meetings and reviews, assisting a trainee experiencing difficulty, yearly reviews with consultants, or term reviews with medical students. The positive impact of an unhurried conversation with someone who is really listening should not be underestimated.

Table 19.1 provides a toolbox of questions that might be useful in a supervision conversation. The intent of the question rather than the actual words used, the listening that follows, and the summary and clarifying questions, are most important.

One purpose of a supervision conversation is to establish goals. This requires the trainee to identify goals that are meaningful, relevant, doable, that they are committed to and can be held accountable for.

SMART goals (Specific, Measurable, Achievable, Realistic, Time bound) are one starting point in a supervision conversation.

Some specific examples of coaching questions for goal-setting, commitment, and accountability include:

> '*What is your goal?*' or '*Can you complete the sentence? My goal is to . . .*'
>
> '*How can you make your goal manageable and bite-sized?*'
>
> '*How can you make your goal SMART?*'
> '*How will you succeed?*'
>
> '*On a scale of 1–10 how committed are you to achieving your goal of . . . ?*' and '*What would move you up by 1 point?*'
>
> '*How will we know when you have completed your goal of . . . ?*'

It is preferable for the trainee to produce a written plan at the end of this conversation.

It is beneficial to acknowledge the hard work of the trainee and congratulate them on their progress as they strive towards their goals. Specifically acknowledge behaviour that is adaptive and explain what makes this important. For example, '*I'd like to acknowledge your honesty and vulnerability. I appreciate your openness*'.

The feedback conversation

Feedback is a non-linear process that begins the second the trainee and educator meet. Informal feedback occurs throughout the list, with non-verbal and verbal communication.

Table 19.1 Toolbox of questions

Powerful question	Rationale/Notes
'*What is the most important thing we should be discussing today?*'	These types of questions are useful in any situation and allow the trainee to direct the conversation.
'*What do you want to take-away from today's session?*'	Transfers focus onto tangible outcomes and can be used for checking-in part way through.
'*What is the significance of this for you right now?*' '*How does this relate to where you are in your training at the moment?*'	Clarify meaning and context to ensure that learning needs are relevant.
'*And what else?*'	Encourages the trainee to provide more information. Cautionary note: '*And what else?*' can turn into an unhelpful '*Guess what I'm thinking?*' question if not asked with genuine curiosity.
'*Tackling topics we've been avoiding can often help us to advance our learning. What is the one topic you are hoping I won't bring up?*' '*How can I help you tackle topics that you may have been inadvertently or even studiously avoiding?*'	This question requires good rapport and trust and assumes trainee and educator know each other well. It stretches the trainee to the edge of their knowledge or competency. **Cautionary note:** Beware stressing a potentially vulnerable trainee for example right before an exam or if high performing with low confidence.
'*You said ... Can you tell me more about that?*' '*Can you explain your thinking behind ... ?*'	Seek elaboration to understand the thinking behind a statement that the trainee provides.
'*What other options are there here?*'	Expands thinking to look at all the different opportunities available. Often trainees will not present all the options because they have ruled them out in their head prior to speaking. Provides thought processes behind decision making as well as actual decision.
'*How can you reframe that in a more positive way?*'	Thinking about it in the positive rather than negative is useful for developing a growth mindset.
'*What advice would you give another trainee in this situation?*'	Encourages summary of key learnings; useful for auditory learners; depersonalizing the conversation reduces the emotional component and assists conscientious types with a growth mindset.

The educator's intention going into the feedback conversation is vitally important as it will be revealed in their body language. Consider two different intentions for the same conversation:

1. the educator is going to provide *negative feedback* to a trainee who cannot hope to improve;

2. the educator is *facilitating* feedback conversation in *partnership* with the trainee, giving them the benefit of the doubt, with a growth mindset and focusing on the trainee's strengths when communicating, with the goal of enhancing the trainee's professional development.

The aim of the feedback conversation is that both trainee and educator come away feeling that the learning encounter has been useful. Feedback that supports learning generally comes from a place of *positive intention*, is based on an observable behaviour or fact, and is *constructive and beneficial*.[20]

Ideally, trainees and educators have feedback literacy. This is defined as[21]:

1. an appreciation of the purpose of feedback;

2. the capacity to make sound judgements;

3. the ability to manage emotions to minimize defensiveness;

4. the will to take action to continuously improve.

Solicited feedback is more likely to be accepted than unsolicited feedback. This is particularly important when the trainee has identified an area of practice on which to focus their learning.

For the educator, having a feedback conversation can be challenging.[22] Perceived challenges can be overcome by learning and practicing effective approaches to engaging in a feedback conversation. This gives the educator confidence and tangible strategies to apply to any situation.

Table 19.2 shows the key frames and actions of educators and trainees, that optimize feedback conversations. Note that during the feedback conversation it is preferable that the trainee shares their perspective first and the educator adds to it.[23] The conversation is optimized by co-creating a learning partnership based on trust, awareness of bias, belief in the trainee, and a growth mindset. The interaction requires **listening**, **asking** rather than **telling**, summarizing, clarifying, and encouraging goal-setting.

Case studies

How would you approach these situations now? Consider if and how your thinking has changed.

Table 19.2 Key frames and actions of educators and trainees in a feedback conversation using the '*GREAT*' and '*LAURS*' frameworks

Trainee	Educator
Is proactive about wanting to improve. Requests a feedback conversation, particularly if educator doesn't suggest this at the beginning of the list.	Sets the scene. Explains that the feedback conversation is part of the learning approach.
Shares mental model about feedback with educator.	Outlines options for how feedback conversation could be approached.
Stays curious. If labels or statements are unclear, asks questions for clarification.	Asks the trainee what they are hoping to learn/take away. '*What do you want to get out of today?*' Listens.
Is prepared to reflect on performance.	Stays curious. Asks the trainee questions in relation to their practice, particularly when things are done differently. Shares thoughts. Listens.
Shares thoughts, engages in discussion, and processes suggestions before accepting or rejecting them.	Invites trainee to reflect on what went well. '*What went well?*' Shares perspective about what went well. '*I liked ... because ...*' Listens.
Manages emotions to avoid becoming defensive. Shares thoughts, engages in discussion, and processes suggestions before accepting or rejecting them.	Invites trainee to reflect on areas for improvement. '*What could be done differently?*' Shares perspective on areas for improvement with **specific** ideas about how trainee might go about this. '*How about ... ?*' Listens.
Summarizes key points and actions based on the feedback.	Encourages the trainee to commit to an action for improvement. '*What are your key learning points? What will you do differently?*' Listens.
Offers educator feedback opportunity and thanks.	Considers seeking feedback from the trainee on one thing, and thanks trainee.

There is no one right way to approach these situations, and everyone will have a different answer.

Answers to case study 1

There is a trainee experiencing difficulty and you are the training supervisor.

The trainee's personal relationship has broken down; the trainee is a little older than other trainees; they've failed the primary exam; and you've had concerning reports about a lack of vigilance on the job.

How will you help them to work through these issues and get their training back on track?

As a supervisor your job is to support the trainee in meeting their educational needs. It is not the educator's role to fix or rescue them.

An older trainee can often be prejudged about how long they have been in training. Acceptance of where the trainee is, being open-minded, and establishing connection, may reveal a previous career where transferable skills can be identified.

Often trainees have significant domestic or personal issues that impact on performance at work or with study. Metaphorically and (perhaps physically!) it may be helpful to sit on your hands and listen, allowing the trainee **space** to find their own answers.

Whatever the approach, the aim is for the trainee to feel supported.

It may be helpful to suggest that the trainee brings a support person, and let them know ahead of time what the meeting is about.

Ensure they have a GP and psychologist and keep a list of other support resources to hand. Follow any protocols from the training organization you represent (e.g. trainee support processes). This is a situation commonly encountered by training supervisors and should prompt them to set time aside regularly for this trainee.

Thank the trainee for attending, build rapport, assure confidentiality, and perhaps start with a question such as: '*What is the most important thing we should be talking about today?*' Often everything will come tumbling out without much more prompting. Sitting quietly in the moment with the trainee allows time and space for emotion before cognition.

Trainees can be encouraged to choose goals that focus on bite-sized manageable tasks and pick off easy doable actions first to enhance commitment. It might be helpful to plan for accountability for example by arranging a time for your next meeting and how you might follow up.

Answers to case study 2

You are assigned a trainee to your operating theatre list today. They are 3 months out from their final specialist exam and seem to know so much that you wonder if they might be on course for the prize. Not only that, but clinically they are excellent. How could you help the trainee have a useful learning experience?

First, recognize any discomfort, for example any imposter feelings this situation may evoke in you. While the trainee may have all the knowledge and be clinically excellent, they are unlikely to manage the list as well as a consultant with real world experience and the ability to facilitate the trainee's learning. No matter how competent, no one has all the answers.

As with any interaction, the 'GREAT' 'LAURS' approach will likely help build an educational partnership and a professional collegial relationship. The Triangle of Trust can help contribute to psychological safety.

For senior trainees consider using the avoidance question, because this is likely to uncover their learning edge. *'Tackling topics we've been avoiding can often help us to advance our learning. I'm curious to know if there is such a topic you can think of?'*

Key points

Successful communication in education:

1. is about *how* things are said, rather than *what* is said;
2. depends on co-creating a learning partnership;
3. establishes a safe learning environment by giving the benefit of the doubt and building a Triangle of Trust with authenticity, empathy, and logic;
4. encourages a growth mindset;
5. focuses on listening, and asking rather than telling;
6. utilizes summaries, clarifications, and reframes.

The coaching framework is one model of how to address these points.

References

1. van Nieuwerburgh C (2018). *Coaching in education: getting better results for students, educators, and parents*, pp. 33–34. London: Routledge.
2. International Coaching Federation (2022). ICF, the gold standard in coaching: Read about ICF. [Internet]. International Coaching Federation. Available at: https://coachfederation.org/about (Accessed 27 April 2023).
3. Frei F, Morriss A (May–June 2020). Begin with Trust. The first step to becoming a genuinely empowering leader. *Harvard Business Review*. Available at: https://hbr.org/2020/05/begin-with-trust (Accessed 27 April 2023).
4. Brown B (2018). *Dare to lead: brave work. tough conversations. Whole hearts.* New York: Random House.
5. Molloy E, Bearman M (2019). Embracing the tension between vulnerability and credibility: 'intellectual candour' in Health Professions Education. *Med Educ*, **53**(1), 32–41.
6. van Nieuwerburgh C (2020). *An introduction to coaching skills. A practical guide*, 2nd edition, pp. 163–5. London: SAGE Publications.
7. FitzGerald C, Hurst S (2017). Implicit bias in healthcare professionals: a systematic review. *BMC Med Ethics*, **18**(1), 19.
8. Stiegler MP, Tung A (2014). Cognitive processes in anesthesiology decision making. *Anesthesiology*, **120**(1), 204–17.
9. Marcelin JR, Siraj DS, Victor R, Kotadia S, Maldonado YA (2019). The impact of unconscious bias in healthcare: How to recognize and mitigate it. *J Infect Dis*, **220**(Supplement 2), S62–S73.
10. Project Implicit (n.d.). Take a test. Available at: https://implicit.harvard.edu/implicit/user/demo.australia/au.static/takeatest.html (Accessed 27 April 2023).

11. Samarasekera DD, Gwee MCE (2021). *Educate, train and transform: Toolkit on medical and health professions education*. New Jersey: World Scientific.

12. Armson H, Lockyer JM, Zetkulic M, Könings KD, Sargeant J (2019). Identifying coaching skills to improve feedback use in postgraduate medical education. *Med Educ*, **53**(5), 477–93.

13. Starr J (2016). *The coaching manual: the definitive guide to the process, principles and skills of personal coaching*, 4th edition, pp. 71–83. Harlow: Pearson Education.

14. Starr J (2016). *The coaching manual: The definitive guide to the process, principles and skills of personal coaching*, 4th edition, pp. 90–104. Harlow: Pearson Education.

15. Whitmore J (2017) *Coaching for performance: The principles and practice of coaching and leadership*, 5th edition, pp. 81–8. London: Hodder & Stoughton.

16. van Nieuwerburgh C (2017). *An introduction to coaching skills. A practical guide*, 2nd edition, pp. 41–51. London: SAGE Publication.

17. Buck A (2020). *The basic coaching method*. Chapter 9. London: Cadogan Press.

18. Paice L (2013). *New coach: reflections from a learning journey*, p. 46. Maidenhead: Open University Press.

19. Rogers J (2016). *Coaching skills: the definitive guide to being a coach*, 4th edition, pp. 206–22. Maidenhead: Open University Press.

20. Starr J (2016). *The coaching manual: The definitive guide to the process, principles and skills of personal coaching*, 4th edition, pp. 107–22. Harlow: Pearson Education.

21. Carless D, Boud D (2018). The development of student feedback literacy: Enabling uptake of feedback. *Assessment & Evaluation in Higher Education*, **43**(8), 1315–25.

22. Weller JM, Jones A, Merry AF, Jolly B, Saunders D (2009). Investigation of trainee and specialist reactions to the mini-clinical evaluation exercise in anaesthesia: implications for implementation. *Br J Anaesth*, **103**(4), 524–30.

23. Whitmore J (2017). *Coaching for performance: the principles and practice of coaching and leadership*, 5th edition, pp. 145–6. London: Hodder and Stoughton.

Chapter 20

Research

Laura L. Burgoyne, Scott W. Simmons, and Allan M. Cyna

'The mind is not a vessel to be filled but a fire to be kindled.'
Plutarch

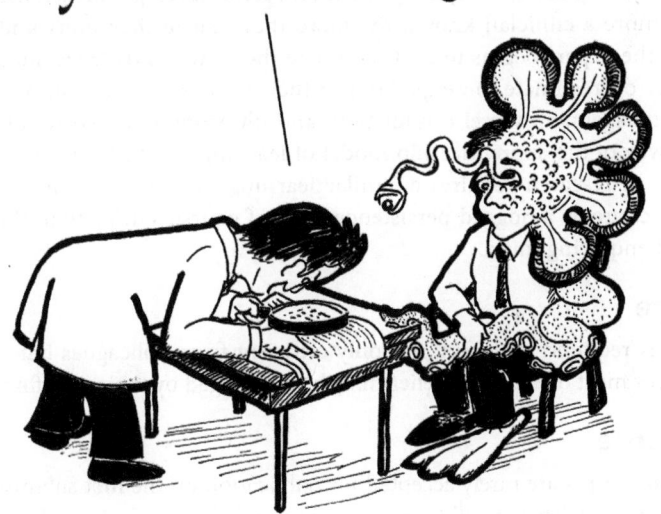

What this chapter is about

Learning and teaching how to communicate as a researcher

Anaesthetists are very familiar with the adage, '*See one, do one, teach one*'. The same approach can also be used when setting out as a prospective researcher, although educational theorists may shudder at such simplicity and demand a more sophisticated rendering of the concept. When acquiring a new skill, information is presented and understood, actions practised, and through an iterative process, there develops, confidence, efficiency, and proficiency.

Trainees move through a series of stages from novice, who doesn't know what they don't know, to a clinician at the completion of their training who thinks they know everything about everything! As their career develops further, they appreciate that the more a clinician knows, the more they realize they don't know. With experience the expert begins to underestimate their own knowledge and abilities and frequently overestimate these qualities in their trainees. For technical skills such as airway management, vessel cannulation, and ultrasound-guided needle placement, the pathway of the apprenticeship model of learning is well-trodden. Taking on the challenge of research requires a similar learning process but demands additional qualities: courage; a dogged persistence; and, of course, curiosity in the form of an open and enquiring mind.

Courage

Courage is required to accept, not only criticism from colleagues but also, that the researcher's most deeply held beliefs may be challenged by their own findings.

Persistence

Draft manuscripts are rarely accepted for publication on the first submission without revision, and persistence will be required to see the research through to publication. The authors of this chapter have been asked on occasion to provide up to eight revisions prior to final acceptance by a journal. No matter how many points need addressing, the effort to do so is usually repaid many-fold by eventual publication, ultimately justifying the hours that have already gone into the submission. Unfortunately, many papers that could have been salvaged and eventually published lie metaphorically in a researcher's drawer after a despondent author could not face the perceived time-consuming tasks required to address the editor's comments. The key to success here is to make a start, no matter how small. For example, address just one of the editor's points and write the written response. The responses to the remaining comments and edits to the revised manuscript may suddenly appear achievable.

The enquiring mind

It is essential for the prospective researcher to have curiosity and be open-minded. However, the mind needs not be so open that our brains fall out, and it is important to remain sceptical—especially when extraordinary claims are being made.[1]

Communicating with an editor of a journal as a reviewer

Journal editors rely on reviewers for a number of reasons. No editor can know his or her subject well enough to be an expert in all its aspects. It also takes a long time to establish a journal's reputation, and publishing hastily reviewed papers can lose this reputation very quickly. Expert reviewers can help spot potentially embarrassing mistakes. Lastly, most manuscripts can be improved by advice. These improvements may have nothing to do with grammar or style but may draw attention to references that are missed, conclusions which are too bold, or techniques which need further description. Many submissions are assessed and decided by one or more editors in the first instance as sending every paper out for review can cause delays and adds to the time it takes for a journal to handle the manuscript.

Most journals transmit the reviewers' comments directly to the author with the editor's decision. Usually, however, reviewers can also submit confidential comments to the editor, which are not relayed to the paper's author. Whether or not the reviewer's comments are seen by the author, one should be courteous and polite at all times. Constructive criticism is always welcome, but the review is not an opportunity to vent one's spleen, even if the paper is unspeakably bad.

Many journals operate an open peer review policy—that is, the reviewer's identity is revealed to the author. Although this is not universal practice, it is a good idea always to write as if it were. If opinions cannot be defended objectively, then they should not be expressed. There are some simple rules to being a reviewer:

1. It is important to be prompt when asked to review and the completed review submitted prior to the due date;

2. If unable to read and comment within a reasonable time, the editor will need to be informed immediately to allow another reviewer to be found;

3. If the editor is asking for replies to specific questions, these need to be addressed;

4. Do not recommend acceptance or rejection unless the editor asks for this;

5. Do not make too much of minor mistakes and problems—there is no need to share every preference;

6. Be aware that even well-known departments or famous clinicians can have their names on poor quality work;

7. Do not get in touch directly with the author during the review process.

Communicating research as an author

Every journal has some basic and universal requirements, the variations of which are enumerated in the journal's 'Instructions to Authors'. These need to be carefully followed when submitting a research article or correspondence.[2] The submitting author takes primary responsibility for communication with the journal, including manuscript submission, peer review, and the publication processes.

It is worth establishing early on who is an author, and in which order they will be placed in any publication. In addition, other contributions may need to be acknowledged. Although there is much variation, traditionally the first author is the person who writes the first draft, and the last—often the submitting author—is the senior or supervising author of the work. Unfortunately, on occasion the junior colleague, who does most of the work and initial drafting, is not placed as the first author despite being most deserving, and publication being far more important for their career.

Getting a paper accepted for publication is usually a long process and submitting a paper is merely the start of a new round of developments. Although only the authors are credited at the top of the first page of the finished product, a published paper is very much a joint effort between the authors, the reviewers, and the editor of the journal. The chances of publication are usually set at the design stage of the project. Some research papers are doomed to undergo multiple rejections simply because they report work that should never have been performed. Asking the wrong question, choosing an inappropriate methodological approach, and allowing bias to creep in because of sloppy methodology are all irretrievable problems. Poor presentation of an otherwise soundly conducted study can be corrected, but it is too late to wish the study had been done differently. Much more preferable than hearing this from the journal's reviewers is asking as many people as possible for advice on the project *before* the work begins, rather than waiting until it is completed.

First and foremost, be realistic. This is partly about science and partly about salesmanship and, although scientific writing may be specialized, it must still conform to the same principles as any other good writing. Here then is one downfall. Trainees in anaesthesia are not expected to give anaesthetics without appropriate training and supervision, yet anaesthetists are often expected to be able to write without any special preparation, training, or experience.

Follow the 'Instructions for authors' carefully. Editors are usually volunteers. Formatting references and checking spelling and grammar are tiresome, and they might be thought unnecessary tasks, but imagine having to perform such tasks on not one but 200 manuscripts per year. Remember that editors are only human. They want to publish the best, but they are also relieved when the painstaking and time-consuming work of preparing a manuscript for final publication is done for them by the author. This leaves them free to concentrate on the science and structure of the paper.

Assuming some decent work has been done and the paper has been written and submitted, the editor will send an acknowledgement. The editor will subsequently send a further communication—depending on the journal, this can be a few days or several months later. Again, depending on the journal, this may be a brief note declining publication, or a considered response accompanied by the reviewers' comments upon which the editor's verdict is based. If the editor has sent comments, authors are advised to take a deep breath and steel themselves.

Communicating with a journal editor as an author

Let us imagine that the hard yards are done: the research is complete, the manuscript is written, and the results of peer review are awaited. An email from the journal appears!

Feedback from the editor regarding a first submission is usually in the form of *Acceptance* (rare); *Provisional Acceptance*; *Minor Revision*; *Major Revision*; or *Reject*. *Revision* means that the editor wishes the corresponding author to respond to requests for changes and requires authors to either accept them or give clear reasons for not doing so.

First-time authors sometimes think a lengthy list of highly critical comments means that the paper has been rejected.

Unless the word *Reject* is written, the paper can be assumed to be provisionally *accepted*. The proviso is that the corresponding author satisfactorily responds to each and every comment from the editor in enough detail to logically and clearly answer any queries. *Rejection* is usually about basic science and methods or because it is not sufficiently aligned with the journal's objectives. The most constructive path in this situation is to use the editorial and reviewer comments as a basis for redrafting the manuscript for a different journal. This usually involves incorporating reviewer and editor comments into the Discussion. This usually entails revising the *Limitations of the study* section and avoiding opinions unrelated to the study findings. This will likely anticipate and mitigate future criticisms when the revised draft manuscript is submitted to another journal.

Responding to reviewers' comments

The reviewers' comments are usually fair and often give perspectives or requests for clarity not previously considered. On occasion, they may appear to have misunderstood the writer or be unduly picky. However, this is unusual and the editor will usually try to steer a middle course through what can sometimes appear to be conflicting comments.

It is almost unheard of for a paper—any paper—to be accepted without amendment. Most accepted papers are accepted provisionally on the understanding that the author will make certain changes. Authors need to appreciate that comments on a manuscript are not a personal criticism—especially if it is a first attempt at writing, where a considerable intellectual and emotional investment will have been made. It is all too easy to become 'precious' and possessive about the paper following constructive criticism.

The most useful sets of comments not only say what is wrong with the paper but make suggestions as to how improvements can be made. Ideally, a list of numbered points are provided for authors to respond to. The writer should then prepare a letter outlining responses to the comments and, if in agreement with a particular comment, say so and thank the reviewer. If in disagreement, then politely point out why and state the preference for leaving the text as it stands.

At this stage of the process, as at all others, it is not only courteous but also wise to highlight in the text where changes have been made, using a different colour or tracked changes. Add to that the relevant page and line numbers in the response letter so that the changes can be easily identified. In time, there will be another reply from the editor. Sometimes reviewers want to see the revised version, and sometimes not. If the writer's responses are well laid out and easy to follow, it is certain the paper will be dealt with promptly. Many papers require two or even more revisions. This is not unusual, and, like the first revision, the writer should bear in mind that the comments are designed to improve the paper and protect both the author and the journal from damage to their reputations.

If the paper is rejected, the reviewers' comments on it will still be sent. This will allow the author to decide whether it is redeemable and can be submitted to another journal, or whether it is beyond hope. Serious faults in methodology cannot be dealt with at this stage as it is too late to conduct the study again. Editorial advice is given free and is a useful source of ideas for improvement.

Using 'GREAT' and 'LAURS' to communicate a response to a review

'GREAT' and 'LAURS' can be used in responding to a request for revision but can equally be applied when reviewing for a journal or assessing a grant application. In the following section these acronyms are used to respond to the editor of a journal.

A 'GREAT' approach

Greeting

Although '*Dear Editor*', is fine, it is preferable to use the editor's proper title and name if known.

Rapport

It is important to thank the editor and reviewers for their constructive comments even if the manuscript has been rejected. Where particular comments are especially useful in improving the manuscript, it is worth stating how much these are appreciated and perhaps give examples of how they have improved the original draft.

Expectations

Every comment and question requires a point-by-point response. This is most easily done by copying and pasting the editor's and reviewers' comments and then responding to each and every phrase. Most comments and questions can be addressed by agreeing with the points raised. However, do not be afraid of acknowledging the merits of the feedback provided, and the deficiencies or points for clarification that are raised by the reviewers. This can be undertaken objectively and concisely, clarifying any issues in the response and also in the draft manuscript. A reviewer cannot possibly know your paper as well as you and may even misread, or fail to read, parts of the paper.

Addressing concerns

When responding to queries, it is probably best to do so in the order that they are written. Some authors may prefer reclassifying a response but this can be confusing.

Track all changes in the revised draft manuscript with page and line numbers for each response. Copying and pasting text changes when responding to specific questions can also be helpful in replying to the editor.

Tacit agreement

Stipulate in the letter responding to the editor how queries have been addressed and what has been changed in this revision. Then offer to address any other remaining issues.

A 'LAURS' approach

Listening and looking

Apart from following the journal's author instructions, look for the key points the editor has made, and establish some understanding of what is primarily required when responding. Prior to formulating a response, it is important to identify all queries, critical comments, and suggestions from both editor and reviewers. This will ensure a revised draft, when sent back, will have every query addressed.

Acceptance

Editors and reviewers are invariably attempting to advise how to improve the manuscript to make it suitable for publication. Editors have a vested interest in ensuring that anything appearing in their journal is relevant to the readership and of an appropriate scientific standard. This ultimately can influence key measures such as *impact factor* or the detection of plagiarism. This reality can be accommodated by considering the redrafting and further fine-tuning of the original manuscript as an active partnership, rather than an adversarial conflict. Nonetheless, on occasions, reviewer comments may seem highly critical and potentially feel like a personal attack. They are not! There are lots of ways that papers need reworking, usually involving a restating of the aim or primary research question and alignment with results and then conclusions. Authors may be required to revise the title if it is not reflective of the study that has been undertaken. A common criticism of a manuscript is *overreach* where the conclusions are inconsistent with the findings and study aims. If this is a valid criticism it may require the author to accept this and rewrite the *Discussion and Conclusions*.

Utilization

The editor and reviewers' comments can nearly always be utilized as a basis for a constructive response that will increase the likelihood of acceptance of the paper.

Reframing

Editor and reviewer comments can frequently be reframed in such a way as to provide alternative ways of dealing with perceived problems in the manuscript.

Example responses of an author to reviewer or editor comments

An editor or reviewer requests something from the authors:

> **Editor:** 'The method needs to be more clearly described.'
> **Authors' response:** '*The methods have now been more clearly described as seen with our tracked changes on Page 3, Lines 5–10.*'
> **Editor:** 'The Introduction and Discussion could be significantly shorter.'
> **Authors' response:** '*We agree, both the Introduction and Discussion have now been redrafted so that they are significantly shorter as suggested.*'

It's okay to disagree with a reviewer's comment.

> **Editor:** 'The results do not show that pain is affected by their intervention.'
> **Authors' response:** '*We disagree, pain scores are shown to have significantly decreased compared with controls (Table 2) and analgesia requirements are also significantly more in controls.*'

Both editor and reviewers' positive comments need acknowledgement and thanks and can often be used to rebut less favourable comments from other reviewers.

> **Editor:** 'Conclusions. *The authors draw a valid conclusion* that the . . . is likely to give a different assessment. *This is a clinically relevant study for clinicians*.'
> **Authors' response:** '*Thank you, we agree that our findings are clinically relevant.*'
> **Editor:** 'The authors address the limitations of the study, however, neonatal and maternal outcome may affect the perception of pain and it is important to have some indication of this in a study using obstetric patients.'
> **Authors' response:** '*Neonatal and Maternal outcome were not considered in this study. We have now included them as potential considerations in the "Future Research" section (page 19, lines 23–26).*'

The letter responding to an editor has a universal standard format (Figure 20.1). Examples of authors responses to reviewer comments are seen in Figure 20.2.

Dear Professor Critique,

Ref: FJA-2032-03554-LC05 R1 Patients versus ....– A Randomized Trial

Thank you for the opportunity to revise our previously submitted draft manuscript. We very much appreciate the reviewers' constructive comments and suggestions of our originally submitted manuscript. We believe this has helped us to significantly improve our original draft manuscript in this revision.

Please find attached:

1. A revised manuscript with tracked changes;
2. Our point-by-point response to editor and reviewer comments and queries;
3. As requested, we have also considered further published papers on this area of research in the FJA. These are now referenced and referred to in the text.

We look forward to your response.

Sincerely

Fig. 20.1 An example of a letter responding to the editor.

Conclusion

While most anaesthetists experience of structured teaching would be in the realm of technical skills, the same principles can be applied to clinical research, commencing with how to analyse a published scientific paper, through to generating and conducting a clinical trial, undertaking a peer review, journal submission, or responding to authors or editors, or research grant providers. Through an iterative process based on acquisition of core knowledge, and learning from an experienced instructor, the complete novice can break down the numerous steps of taking a basic clinical question all the way through to publication. By analogy to the technical skills domain, the anaesthetist, as seen with professional frameworks such as CANMEDs[3] seeks to best utilize the healthcare literature and perhaps further contribute to the acquisition of new knowledge. As examples, the practising clinician wishing to develop a comprehensive grounding in analysing the scientific literature can engage with the Cochrane Collaboration and undertake a systematic review.[4] It can be assured that most clinicians will never look at a published paper the same way. Similarly, and certainly more simply, reviewing a paper already published, or one planned for submission, against the established frameworks such as the CONSORT Group,[5] the STROBE Statement,[6] or the International Committee of Medical Journal Editors (ICMJE) will be highly instructive. A would-be researcher responding to seemingly complex and frustrating feedback from a journal will be better informed by having gone through the process themselves as a reviewer.

Authors' response to assessor's comments

Editor: 'Comments to the Author'

Editor: 'This study investigates ....:

1.   The assumption that .... scores are the inverse of ...scores needs more clarification and justification.'

Authors' response: '*These have been clarified and justified in more detail – see page 7 lines 22-26 in our revised draft.*'

2.   **Editor:** 'It should be made clearer and in the Methods section that informed consent was not obtained before the 'intervention', why this was done, and that this was ratified by the research committee.'

Authors' response: '*Informed consent was obtained after the intervention for reasons given in the text – see page 3 lines 8-12 . This was approved by the ethics committee as stated in the Methods section.*'

3.   **Editor:** 'A list of the questions asked in the form of a table would help as it is difficult to identify the differences between the two groups regarding what they were asked.'

Authors' response: '*A table has been added as suggested.*'

Editor: 'Specific points'

1.   **Editor:** 'Page 4; line 47-48, unnecessary comma after regarding'

Authors' response: '*Removed*'

2.   **Editor:** 'Line 52-53, There is mention of a previous study but no reference'

Authors' response: '*Reference added*'

3.   **Editor:** 'Page 2; Line 26, comma after Australia'

Authors' response: '*Done*'

4.   **Editor:** 'Line 37-38, What do the authors mean the researchers worked independently?'

Authors' response: '*When a woman was interviewed, only one of the two researchers was present in the room.*'

Fig. 20.2 Examples of detail in a response to reviewer comments.

Key points

1. Once the draft manuscript is submitted, recognize most of the work is done no matter how many comments come back from reviewers;
2. A rejection is only a rejection if explicitly stated as such;
3. The effort involved in responding and addressing editor reviewer comments not only allows the manuscript to be published but almost always improves the final paper;
4. Acting as a reviewer improves your own research and writing.

References

1. Shafer SL (2007). Did our brains fall out? *Anesth Anal*, **104**(2), 247–8.
2. BJA Author Information: Available at: https://bjanaesthesia.org.uk/content/authorinfo (Accessed Italicise BJA.
3. Frank JR, Langer B (2003). Collaboration, communication, management, and advocacy: teaching surgeons new skills through the CanMEDS project. *World J Surg*, **27**(8), 972–8.
4. Costi D, Cyna AM, Ahmed S, et al. (2014). Effects of sevoflurane versus other general anaesthesia on emergence agitation in children. *Cochrane Database Syst Rev*, **9**, Cd007084.
5. Kessler KM (2002). The CONSORT statement: explanation and elaboration. Consolidated Standards of Reporting Trials. *Ann Intern Med*, **136**(12), 926–7.
6. Vandenbroucke JP, von Elm E, Altman DG, et al. (2007). Strengthening the Reporting of Observational Studies in Epidemiology (STROBE): explanation and elaboration. *Ann Intern Med*, **147**(8), W163–94.

Chapter 21

Administrators

Scott W. Simmons

'Not everything that can be counted counts, and not everything that counts can be counted.'
William Bruce Cameron, Informal Sociology: A Casual Introduction to Sociological Thinking (1963)

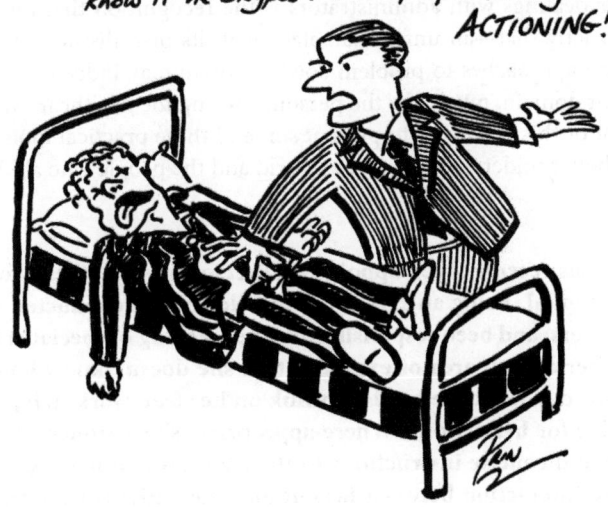

What this chapter is about

Appreciating different perspectives

In our modern healthcare systems, clinicians find themselves dealing with administrators at many levels. Unfortunately, there often appears to be a major disconnect between the two parties, and priorities may appear to be vastly different. For the busy clinical anaesthetist who encounters this in passing, there may be transient frustrations and confusion. For the anaesthetist with a designated management role, the problem doesn't go away that easily. Both, however, will better achieve their goals with a deeper insight into the nature of these interactions.

The 'LAURS' concept as presented in Chapter 2 emphasizes the generic attributes of the approach to a meaningful interaction. Of particular interest in applying this framework to our dealings with administrators is the recognition that the management 'world' is exactly that—an unfamiliar place with its own distinctive language, practical tools, and approaches to problem-solving. There may indeed be a sense of entering a different domain, much like the person entering the healthcare system as a patient. The intent of this chapter is to present some of these practical tools and perspectives to help better understand this other world and the people who abide there.

A scenario

Dr Celia Roberts has recently been appointed Director of Anaesthesia for a large public teaching hospital. Being an expert in her field she has conducted research, written several papers, and been responsible for the teaching of specialist trainees. There is little in her chosen area of expertise that she doesn't know how to deal with. In her day-to-day work she needs to think on her feet, work independently, and be accountable for her actions. Where appropriate she assumes a leadership role, giving clear and concise instructions to the team around her. Celia also excels in one-to-one interaction between herself and the patients who are seeking her help. She has a sense of achievement and satisfaction, engendering quiet self-confidence. When approached to step up to the role of Director of Anaesthesia, she reluctantly agreed.

Unfortunately, the combined effect of recent retirements and an increasing workload related to the closure of a nearby hospital is impacting seriously on the Anaesthesia Service. On taking up her appointment, Celia undertook a thorough analysis of the workload versus staffing levels and the potential impact on patient safety. The result was a 15-page document with references and appendices, resembling a research paper. The work completed, she sought a meeting with new CEO, Monika Kreutzinger, only to be told that the next available appointment was in three weeks. Despite her frustration, Celia accepted that the meeting would have to wait, and sent off her document via email.

Monika Kreutzinger was recruited 18 months previously, when significant organizational changes were being considered by the Board of Management. Her track record as a '*mover and shaker*' was well known within the health bureaucracy. She was quite unknown to the hospital's clinicians, but the Board felt she would bring no unwanted 'baggage' at a time when difficult and unpopular decisions would be necessary.

Monika has been in healthcare most of her career, starting as a radiographer. She worked to develop her management skills, acquiring several postgraduate diplomas and, ultimately, an MBA. She has natural leadership skills and has taken every opportunity for advancement. As her resumé has grown, so has her sense of achievement, engendering quiet self-confidence. It seemed a natural progression to accept the 3-year contract as CEO as a possible step up the ladder to even greater heights.

At the time of receiving Celia's email, she is extremely busy, including dealing with potential strike action by laboratory staff. Also, the Minister of Health, being under Parliamentary pressure over certain election promises, has meant everyone in the executive suite is working through a swathe of ministerial briefing notes. A log of claims from an important clinical group such as the anaesthetists is the last thing Monika needs. What's more, she receives between 500 and 600 emails per week.

Same, same but different!

Monika and Celia are both intelligent high achievers. There are many similarities between top executives and clinicians, and both will have considerable capacity for problem-solving or obfuscation. A key difference, is typically, the individual patient perspective that the clinician brings, while the manager will tend to focus more broadly. This can be interpreted by clinicians as a lack of concern about individual patient welfare.

Celia has to explain to Mrs Smith why her operation has been cancelled because theatre has over-run, while Monika has to face her Board of Management, the Health Minister, the media, or the relatives of many Mrs Smiths. The challenge is to appreciate each other's realities, strengths, and abilities and so seek opportunities for alignment. In this way solutions can be developed that build rather than sabotage each other's priorities.

The story continues ...

Three weeks have passed since the email and Celia has sat in a small waiting area for 20 minutes past the appointed meeting time. She is starting to become annoyed, used as she is to access and control over her world. Eventually she is ushered into the executive suite, and after some initial pleasantries, Monika acknowledges receipt of Celia's *'rather comprehensive'* document. While indicating a degree of sympathy for her position, no extra funding is available. Monika had also asked the Director of Medical Services to look into theatre efficiency, and the preliminary report suggested that all key performance indicators were being met. Monika had personally performed a literature search and consulted with colleagues via the health executives' e-forum. If anything, it would appear that their hospital, by benchmarking standards, was relatively overstaffed.

When Celia's attempts to draw attention to key figures in her analysis, Monika always has some counter-point that, in her view, is more significant. After a few minutes it becomes clear that the CEO just isn't *'getting it'* and doesn't care about the plight of her staff. To make matters worse, Monika expresses concern in relation to a number of recent patient complaints involving anaesthetists.

With frustration and tone of voice both rising, the discussion goes off at a tangent and there seems to be little point in continuing. Celia leaves, having undertaken to do some more homework. She can't believe what has just transpired, as she had thought that her request for extra staff was a 'slam dunk'. Not only had the CEO failed to give Celia what, in her view, was obviously required, but also Monika had left her with the frustrating impression that she believed that all that was needed was for Celia and her staff to work harder.

Solving the problem

Historically, '**communication**' has been broadly defined as, '*the imparting, conveying, or exchange of ideas and knowledge*'.[1] In its simplest form, this constitutes a simple broadcast to a passive recipient through data transfer. A more active view has been to emphasize the '*commonness*' implied within the word, which requires the parties involved coming to a shared position, based on an exchange via a set of common symbols (see Chapter 1). Recent communication research in '*improvement science*' has further developed this concept to include the importance of '*establishing, testing, and maintaining relationships*'.[2]

How can we usefully apply the principles of reflective Listening, Acceptance, Utilization, Reframing, and Suggestion as presented throughout this book to the type of interaction between Celia and Monika? What can be done, for example, to facilitate reflective listening, or use the language that the administrator best understands?

A useful starting place may be the nature of the difference between the doctor-patient relationship and that of the clinician and manager. Simplistically, clinicians go to work each day to help people and are presented with people seeking help. Does the manager, like Monika, have the same primary motivation, in this case to help Celia, or is it more that Celia's issue is a problem amongst many others that needs to be solved?

Most commonly, management in healthcare has been about making decisions around the allocation of finite resources based on **zero-sum thinking**—who gets what and who does not, from a fixed pie. By its very nature, this approach stifles opportunity for innovation. This contrasts with **positive-sum** thinking, where stakeholders are drawn to create solutions which add value, and serve to 'grow the pie'.

In attempting to shift from *zero-* to a *positive-sum* mode, there are two perspectives in the management literature worth considering. Firstly, to view each interaction as a form of conflict that must be resolved. This invokes consideration of such things as the importance of the issue to both parties, and the need for an enduring relationship. Secondly, that the process of coming to an agreement is commonly manifested as a negotiation, which has definable characteristics and agreed rules of engagement.

Conflict resolution

Greenhalgh described a conflict diagnosis model, which includes seven dimensions for consideration.[3] For each dimension, there is a continuum of possible viewpoints based on the perceived ease of resolution. Of particular importance in improving the likelihood of resolution are having long-term versus single transaction-based relationships, interdependence of the parties via seeking positive-sum solutions, involvement of a mutually trusted third party, and formulating problems as smaller divisible issues rather than matters of principle.

Assuming both parties are interested in resolving conflict as easily as possible, application of this model aims to facilitate moving parties to the *easy* side of the ledger by first appreciating their current situation, recognizing each other's reality, and then attempting, where possible, to find ways of shifting the balance. Hence, adopting this approach, and invoking some elements of reframing and suggestion, allows the following to be considered:

Celia: *'I need three extra staff which will be US$600,000 and I need them now.'*
Monika: *'We don't have that sort of money lying around and I have no hope of meeting this year's financial targets if I do this at short notice.'*

This could be reframed addressing Monika's real concerns and reducing the stakes:

Celia: *'There will be an additional cost but it can be spread over 3 years, which also allows time to develop significant cost-saving strategies that will flow from staff doing less overtime—net effect US$250,000'.*

And similarly:

> **Celia:** '*If we don't get the staff, everyone is going to leave!*'—a **negative suggestion**, as opposed to:
> '*The extra staff will enable us to implement the new day-procedure service which will not only raise more revenue but meet the Board's strategic direction*'—a **positive suggestion** facilitating a **positive-sum** solution.

Negotiating with management

A number of different approaches to negotiation have been promoted. Publications vary, from superficial guides offering advice on tactics, through to theoretical models which explore underlying personality traits and values. For the clinician manager such as Celia, the elements that may be most relevant are the personal attributes of empathy—a dominant quality of healthcare workers—and the need to develop and maintain relationships over time with different professional groups, including management. Conversely, if Monika is under substantial pressure to rein in costs, and there are no other drivers for change from the management perspective, Celia's problem will not be seen as something to take on.

The elements of any negotiation as presented by Lewicki[4] can be broken down into:

♦ preparation;

♦ determining a negotiation strategy;

♦ deciding on tactics;

♦ relationship building.

Of value at this point is to emphasize the importance of having clearly defined outcomes and boundary points for the negotiation.

♦ *Target point*—the *desired outcome*. This is exactly what you want, and why, and what you are prepared to do to get it.

♦ *Resistance point*—the *absolute boundary* beyond which you are not prepared to go. Anyone who has been involved in a real estate auction will understand this.

♦ *Settlement range*—the interval in which there is *overlap of the resistance points* of both parties.

Celia would like four extra staff but is prepared to work with two. Monika only has money for one extra but is prepared to allow two with certain provisos, such as a review of the situation in twelve months. The key to a solution lies where these ranges overlap, viz. two extra staff. Where genuine difficulty may arise is when there is no overlap. The parties then have to work at revising resistance points.

♦ *Bargaining mix*—the full range of *attributes* that totally defines the objective. Celia can have funding for three senior consultant staff if she is prepared to wait 12 months, or she can have two senior registrars next week. What does she really want in terms of timing, skill mix, etc?

♦ *Best alternative to a negotiated agreement* (BATNA)—this is the **ultimate backstop** if no solution is found.

The one-page executive summary

Much of day-to-day decision-making depends on analysing summary information to assess the impact on relevant stakeholders, only seeking greater detail for clarity in response to specific points. Anaesthetists in the midst of a busy theatre list can immediately relate to the importance of a succinct summary of the clinical problems of the next patient and the ability to quickly obtain targeted pathology results. By contrast, a lengthy dissertation with no sense of relevance to the issue at hand, is nothing but frustrating.

The one-page executive summary is the direct analogy in this context. It must tell enough of the story for the senior person, taking responsibility for the decisions, to get a satisfactory grasp of the salient features. It needs to list specific recommendations and should include likely outcomes if the recommendations are met, or not met. Further fine detail needs to be readily accessible for reference and scrutiny.

Such an executive summary is presented as Figure 21.1.

Some features to be noted:

1. How the message is sent:
   a. Use the correct medium—if the CEO prefers an organizational template to be used, get a copy and use it.
   b. The one-page summary is only one page—keep cutting to make it fit.
   c. Check for spelling errors and simple typos and ensure formatting facilitates ease of reading.

2. What is sent:
   a. Lead with the **specific decision points**—this is not a thriller with beginning, middle, and end. Making the reader search for what you really want is just a nuisance and may create the perception of hidden intent.
   b. Include **something that is likely to be agreed** to. This creates the sense of joint problem-solving and the opportunity for moving forward.
   c. Incorporate your **predetermined negotiation points**—be very clear where you are in your negotiation range, and avoid ambit claims as they rarely succeed unless you are in a very strong position.
   d. There must be **sufficient detail** to be meaningful, and 'mandatory' fields must be completed. If requests are never considered without stating the financial bottom line then this has to be included.
   e. **Directly identify respected others as contributors**—then it is not just about clinician versus manager.

3. Addressing their concerns:
   a. The language of the business world is based on money in financial statements, and cost projections. Workload is in complexity-adjusted throughput. Get the finance department to translate what you want specifically into this format.
   b. Identify the issues that concern the CEO—a request will not go far if the only concern is patient safety when there have been no serious patient incidents. Other issues like the CEO's interest in developing a new clinical service could be a source of mutual gain.

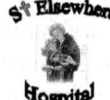

St Elsewhere Hospital

BRIEFING NOTE FOR EXECUTIVE

TO: Monika Kreutzinger, Chief Executive Officer
FROM: Dr Celia Roberts, Director of Anaesthesia
RE: Anaesthesia Staffing
DATE: 8th September 2024

RECOMMENDATIONS

It is recommended that Executive:
1. Approve the creation of one new senior registrar position as part of a strategy to reduce total cost for specialist call-backs. This is projected to save $100,000 in a full year. It will be trialled for 12 months to fully assess impact.

2. Approve the creation of three new fulltime specialist positions, each for a period of 3 years, subject to appropriate personal performance review and ongoing service needs after 12 months. This supports proposed service redesigns and will reduce uncertainty and costs related to use of casual staff. Additional cost over 3 years is $200,000.

SUMMARY OF ISSUES

a. There is currently no provision for coverage of leave: staff absences are covered by ad hoc short term arrangements dependent on availability of external staff at premium rates. Significant financial and clinical risks to the organisation exist in not being able to find suitably qualified specialist anaesthetists at short notice leading to cancellation of services and case postponements.

b. The increase in clinical activity, including total after-hours case-load, and increased patient complexity has been well-documented (Attachment 1). The impact on Specialist Anaesthetists has been increased after-hours work with resultant decreased availability for in-hours service delivery, plus increased leave-taking due to fatigue and illness (Attachment 2).

c. Certainty in staff availability, enhanced cost predictability and total cost reduction can be achieved by employing additional specialist staff on a regular basis. A Senior Registrar can perform some of the duties currently undertaken by specialists and at considerably less cost. Total overtime payments, and sick leave should fall (Attachment 3).

d. As part of planning for the proposed service redesign, modelling of the Finance Dept supports the appointment of additional staff to meet projected activity targets. Break-even points can be achieved in the range of 2-4 years dependent on actual patient numbers. (Attachment 3).

ATTACHMENTS
Attachment 1 - Patient Activity by Service Type and Complexity: Data Unit, StEH.
Attachment 2 - Annual Finance Report, Dept of Anaesthesia: Finance Dept, StEH.
Attachment 3 – Supplementary Analysis, Finance Dept, StEH.

CONSULTATION AND ADVICE FROM OTHERS
1. Jack Smith, Management Accountant, Head of Service Planning, StEH.

Fig. 21.1 Example of an executive summary—what Celia might have done differently.

c. **Know who the CEO answers to and what is of importance to them.** Solutions that address the concerns of board members and politicians will strike a chord if presented genuinely and constructively.

The communication setting

The increasing preference for using technology over direct human contact for communication, presents considerable challenges, and risks misinformation—see Chapters 1 and 22.

With the ease and familiarity of pressing **Send**, the distinction between data transfer and a two-way process, requiring active participation of both parties, can be lost. Electronic messages are hazardous! Conversations via email or SMS are typically short, asynchronous, and lack the precision of correct spelling and grammatical rules. The interacting parties do not have the considerable benefit of non-verbal cues through direct eye contact and body language.

This has become particularly significant with the widespread adoption of messaging apps, some of which allow only limited amounts of text and the added challenge of emojis and similar shorthand imagery. It is ultimately a matter of judgement as to whether an issue is suited to a quick email, a phone conversation, an informal meeting over coffee or a pre-arranged meeting with lawyers present. Simple electronic methods such as short emails and text messages are best reserved for easy-to-resolve situations when the recipient is familiar with the sender's idiosyncrasies and turns of phrase. Anything difficult requires face-to-face meetings, briefing documents, engagement of other stakeholders, accurate documentation, and opportunities for reflection.

Promoting *'win-win'* as a possible solution

A zero-sum outcome, when one party wins at the other's expense, promotes a philosophy of **winners** and **losers**. An approach based on achieving a positive-sum outcome encourages a process of constructive development. By reframing communications in the form of potential mutual gains, there is more likely to be a focus on solving the problem rather than emphasizing winning and losing.

If Celia Roberts' multi-page document ends more or less with the conclusion that management should just give her more staff, Monika will be left to make a 'Wisdom of Solomon judgement'—perhaps more anaesthesia staff but at the cost of fewer nursing staff.

Alternatively, Celia's proposals could include a range of possible system redesign initiatives alongside the extra staff. For example, the extra anaesthesia staff could be involved in multi-disciplinary pre-operative planning clinics, ultimately reducing total length of stay, or unplanned admissions. This may give Monika and perhaps other stakeholders, some ideas they can then work on, rather than seeing the issue as a matter of one group winning at another's expense.

It should also be anticipated that senior managers will not appreciate being backed into a corner. It is their job to ration resources and set strategic direction for a whole range of stakeholders, and they will generally seek solutions around negotiation.

A take-it-or-leave-it position is likely to create an impasse. A useful guide is to apply the test of what a reasonable third party would make of your stance (appreciating the 'third reality'—see Chapter 2).

Acknowledging emotions

There is always the potential for the stakes to become a matter of winning and losing and to lose sight of the original goal. It is tempting to vent feelings by picking up the phone or sending off a hastily constructed email, but this is exactly what should be avoided. Very few matters require a truly instantaneous response and it will almost always be possible to sleep on it. If you choose to respond by email, **draft the content but do not enter the addressee's name** until you have read and re-read what you have written to avoid inadvertently sending something half-baked. Placing either too much or too little importance, strikes at credibility. If possible, seek the counsel of trusted others when you are angry or the stakes are high.

There are very few instances when any one fact will have absolute dominance over all other considerations. For every fact that Celia wheels out, Monika seems able to find another. In both cases the veracity of the information is not what is in question but the relative importance being placed on them. As extensively reviewed by the members of the Harvard Negotiation Project,[5] one of the major sources of failing to move forward in a conflict situation is when the two parties descend into '*I'm right and you're wrong*'.

Energy is then expended in defending a position and attacking the other party, rather than accepting facts as facts, and coming to some agreement about their relative significance. The important insight that the other party believes it is '***right***' and has valid concerns and acceptance of this helps moving forward. The task for both parties is then to restate goals in ways that are mutually acceptable. For example, Monika's problem is commitment to the burden of recurrent expense at this time. Solutions from Celia that are less costly in the short-term, e.g. use of temporary appointments, enables an agreement to be reached.

There will be instances in difficult conversations when the emotional impact becomes the issue. A common misperception is that impact equates to intent. Hence, Celia may conclude that the rejection stems from a desire by Monika intentionally to be difficult. Failing to separate impact from intent will adversely affect Celia's capacity to remain objective and argue her case in a way that is meaningful to Monika. This will be influenced by numerous factors including personal values and previous experiences. Celia could well begin to think, '*being made to wait three weeks for an appointment, then another twenty minutes on the day; being kept in an ante-room like being back at school and then to be told you can't even get the facts straight, is not how an intelligent professional should be treated!*'

Conversation time is then spent by Celia wrestling with her emotional response to the situation and not on the substance. Monika is also likely to respond emotionally. If the conversation appears to be more about emotions, personality, and reacting, it is essential to stop, recognize the subconscious response, and revert back to substance as the most useful and likely strategy to sort this out.

Another unanticipated reason for conflict was the raising of the matter of patient complaints by the CEO. This could be perceived as a distraction, or more cynically as a deliberate ploy aimed at derailment. It can, however, be anticipated that time-poor executive managers are likely to raise further matters when the opportunity for a face-to-face meeting arises, and this should be anticipated.

There is an issue of self-image attached to any interaction like this. As explored at length in classic works by Alfie Kohn,[6] high achievers such as Celia and Monika are typically products of reward systems which have reinforced a sense of self-worth based on gold stars and public adulation. 'Failure', in the form of not getting the staff, is not only unfamiliar territory for Celia, but is likely to generate self-doubt. At least acknowledging this reaction is an important part of staying focused on the matter in hand.

Converting *'matters of principle'* to *'matters of fiscal accountability'*

Generally, problems will be broken down to a perspective based on resource allocation. Any issue that cannot be framed in terms of some form of financial bottom line will make it difficult for the manager to relate to. Although it will be easier to have a discussion which includes a financial outcome, many doctors find this conflicts with their value system. However, the patient safety initiatives in healthcare over recent years are examples of how *'matters of principle'* which may be ignored, can become *'matters of fiscal accountability'* which get implemented.[7-9]

Maintaining profile and a sense of urgency

Senior managers are time-poor, and are continually realigning job lists at short notice, depending on priorities set from competing sources. Even if the anaesthetic department issues are important today, they could easily appear less so tomorrow. Maintaining profile and a sense of urgency is required. Senior managers have a relatively short tenure compared with most medical staff. Since the 1980s, one of the major challenges identified in management thinking has been the emphasis on the capacity for change. There is abundant literature on concepts such as the *'learning organization'* and the type of executive required in this environment. Clinicians frequently interpret these behaviours as a lack of commitment or poor work quality. However, a manager operating in a corporate world where tenure is short, and job progression is based on results, has considerable motivation to achieve in a relatively short time. This should be accepted and utilized.

An alternative approach!

Communicating effectively with administration is, in principle, no different from any other interpersonal interaction. Listening to Monika, appreciating and accepting her reality at least temporarily, even if Celia doesn't agree with it, will increase rapport and facilitate trust. Utilizing Monika's language will assist in any reframes that might enhance insight and promote an alignment of possible solutions.

'GREAT' communication in the context of administration

Greeting

> **Celia:** '*Hi Monika, as stated in my email I want to discuss how we can ensure a safe working environment where lists can be covered by appropriately trained staff.*'

Early on in the interaction, common goals can be established. Once these are identified and recognized, finding a solution may be more likely. In the initial interaction, Celia did not present Monika with the goals of providing a safe working environment where lists can be covered by appropriately trained staff.

Rapport

> **Celia:** '*I appreciate that you have been here for a while and I recognize that like us you are overworked. From what you say, it appears there may be some difficulty meeting this year's financial targets given our request for your consideration at such short notice.*'

Listening, acceptance, and utilization will be the primary tools available to the anaesthetist when communicating with administration (see Chapter 2). It is particularly important to make no assumptions about the relative importance, to the other party, of the matter at hand. Planning the form and timing of the message, and creating an appropriate contextual frame, is likely to take time and effort when dealing with a senior manager whose background, biases, context, and preferred method of data presentation, may be quite different from one's own.

Expectations

> **Celia:** '*What I need is a solution to my staffing problem. Now, as can be seen from the one-page exec summary, we have a proposal that should meet our requirements regarding patient care and safety, and your requirements regarding financial constraints.*'

It is important to identify accurately and succinctly the negotiation's key issues, document meetings as soon as possible, and obtain confirmation of what was discussed, what was agreed to, and what was not. While busy managers and clinicians must juggle many different priorities, one should remember that people sometimes forget, or were actually talking about something else.

Addressing concerns

> **Celia:** '*I appreciate you taking the time to research staffing in other hospitals and acknowledge your concern that we appear to be adequately staffed. However, as*

can be seen in the summary document, this doesn't take into account long term sick leave, unexpected retirements, and the other hospital closure.'

If progress is to be made, it is essential for Celia to acknowledge and address Monika's concerns as well as voice her own. Monika could well have begun the interaction with a fairly concrete idea of how it was going to end. When it is possible for both parties to enter into reasoned debate there will be perceived opportunities for gain, and room to manoeuvre. By contrast, a difficult situation can be created when either party portrays the issue as a matter of principle. Listening reflectively, acceptance, utilization, and reframing can be useful techniques to promote rapport, develop trust, and facilitate engagement, even if an issue is initially flagged as something not open to debate. Acceptance on behalf of the anaesthetist, at least temporarily, will almost always present a way forward.

Tacit agreement

Celia: '*Okay, so we are agreed on a plan and I'll come back to you with those figures you needed—thanks for your time.*'

The buck stops with you ...

After the initial highly unsatisfactory meeting with Monika, Celia returned to the comforting home territory of her department. However, this sense of comfort quickly evaporated when two of the senior staff approached her.

'*Well, when do we get the extra staff?*' one of them asks.

It is at this point that the grim reality of the situation and the complexity of her new role sink in. As her colleagues' representative she is now carrying the responsibility for the quality of their work environment, and as a result, they are clearly seeing her differently. In her new role she is both a part of the clan, and quite separate from it.

The training and clinical life of anaesthetists is based on taking individual responsibility for one's own actions in a direct face-to-face patient encounter and then personally living with the consequences. It can be difficult to assume the role of representing others and arguing the case on their behalf.

Ultimately, the head of department or similar, is in a leadership position. He or she will be perceived by their staff as the one who directly makes decisions influencing them both professionally and personally. Decisions that do not go in favour of the staff may well attract negative emotions, a sense of betrayal, or even accusations of '*siding with the enemy*'.

The ploy of shifting responsibility to the '*evil warlords in management*' may be useful for a while but will ultimately wear thin! Similarly, adopting an adversarial advocacy posture, defending and promoting at any cost the cause of the department against administrators is difficult to sustain. This leads to missed opportunities that could otherwise flow from collaborative problem-solving.

The senior clinician manager is in a unique position to develop a hybrid leadership style with the opportunity of working with many administrative arms of the business—in finance, human resources, information technology, and medicolegal, amongst others.

Furthermore, in having to deal with numerous matters on behalf of all the departmental staff, there will be an opportunity to garner experience based on that of the many. Other clinicians may go an entire career with limited exposure to serious adverse events such as the death of one of their patients, medicolegal action, or workplace interpersonal conflict. The accumulated experience of clinician managers can be utilized to provide reassurance and to guide colleagues through what may be unfamiliar and challenging territory.

Managing a complaint

One such example is that of managing a patient complaint. The same experience that the head of department can use to support and guide staff members can equally be applied in an empathetic and constructive manner with aggrieved patients and their families. In many jurisdictions there will be codes of conduct and statutory obligations for open disclosure and/or duty of candour. Larger institutions will also have dedicated departments and trained personnel such as consumer liaison officers dealing with consumer feedback. It is important for the clinician manager to be familiar with these resources, incumbent obligations, and to ensure that affected staff are made aware of their rights and responsibilities, and what to expect as matters unfold. Hence, the department head can be seen to be in a unique position, not only as a technical expert in their own right, but as a bridge between the clinical and non-clinical worlds.

This translates to retaining a central role in the handling of these matters and to ensure that they are not simply delegated to administrative staff or chatbots. The increasing use of artificial intelligence in healthcare, to analyse text and generate responses, presents its own unique challenges.

The application of 'LAURS' principles is highly relevant. From the outset, avoid where possible language that has negative connotations, such as the word *complaint* itself.

Setting the tone by considering feedback from a patient as creating the opportunity for improvement, is more than semantic and establishes a trajectory of constructive listening rather than defensive denial. In working through such matters, the key principles are to *listen, listen, **listen** ...*

Beyond that, other major considerations include:

- timeliness of acknowledgement and follow-up with all stakeholders;
- assemble all the facts, recognizing that no single person will have a complete picture of whatever has transpired;
- use forms of communication that are appropriate for the nature of the issue and suitable and achievable for all parties;
- provide a single point of contact for the patient, which, in larger organizations, is especially critical to avoid confusion, duplication, and mixed messaging.

Summary

The characters of Celia and Monika are fictional stereotypes created to illustrate some of the principles underlying effective communication. The model proposed is based on defining communication between clinician and manager as a two-way interactive process leading to joint understanding. This necessarily requires understanding one-self as much as understanding the person with whom one is dealing. The practical approach proposed is one of resolving conflict using commonly identified negotiation skills, which can be readily reconciled with the 'LAURS' of communication.

The spectrum of encounters is wide. At one extreme there are one-off issues with little or no need to consider the impact on the relationship. At the other extreme is the clinician manager representing the interests of many, and aware of the need to preserve not only an effective relationship with management but with the people represented, and perhaps a number of other stakeholders such as patients!

Joint problem-solving is the most successful strategy when both share a desire for a good outcome and an enduring relationship. Clear target points and boundaries need to be set out before engaging. Considerable effort may be required to acknowledge emotional impact and adverse effects on self-worth. Although financial considerations are nearly always perceived as relevant, other factors such as feeling valued, being treated as a professional, and having concerns listened to and seen to be addressed, are always important.

Key points

1. Conversations in negotiation are most productive when attention is focused on the substance of the matter and mutual goals rather than on emotions.

2. Openness, honesty, and engagement within a department and with management are the mainstays enabling effective communication.

3. Planning the form and timing of the message, and an appropriate contextual frame, will take time and effort when dealing with a senior manager whose background, biases, and preferred method of data presentation, may be quite different from one's own.

4. By reframing communications in the form of potential mutual gains, there is more likely to be a focus on solving the problem rather than winning and losing.

5. Addressing the basic elements of negotiation strategy through the determination of target and resistance points, acknowledging there is a bargaining mix, and continuing to work to identify the settlement range, should facilitate mutual understanding and achieving goals.

6. Everyone is busy! One-page summaries and clear succinct information are always helpful.

References

1. Onions CT (ed.) (1973). *The Shorter Oxford English Dictionary on Historical Principles*, p. 379, 3rd edition. New York: Oxford University Press.
2. Manojlovich M, Squires JE, Davies B, Graham ID (2015). Hiding in plain sight: communication theory in implementation science. *Implement Sci*, **10**, 58.
3. Greenhalgh L (1986). Managing conflict. *Sloan Manage Rev*, Summer 1986, 45–51.
4. Lewicki RJ, Barry B, Saunders DM (2019). *Negotiation*, 8th edition. Boston: McGraw Hill.
5. Stone D, Patton B, Heen S (1999). *Difficult conversations*. New York: Penguin Books.
6. Kohn A (1993). *Punished by rewards*. New York: Houghton Mifflin.
7. Grimshaw JM, Patey AM, Kirkham KR, et al. (2020). De-implementing wisely: developing the evidence base to reduce low-value care. *BMJ Qual Saf*, **29**, 409–17.
8. Frankel A, Haraden C, Federico F, Lenoci-Edwards J (2017). *A framework for safe, reliable, and effective care. White paper*. Cambridge, MA: Institute for Healthcare Improvement.
9. Langley GL, Moen R, Nolan KM, Nolan TW, Norman CL, Provost LP (2009). *The improvement guide: a practical approach to enhancing organizational performance*, 2nd edition. San Francisco: Jossey-Bass Publishers.

Chapter 22

Media

Tanya Selak and Stavros Prineas

'Whenever you do a thing, act as if all the world were watching.'
Thomas Jefferson

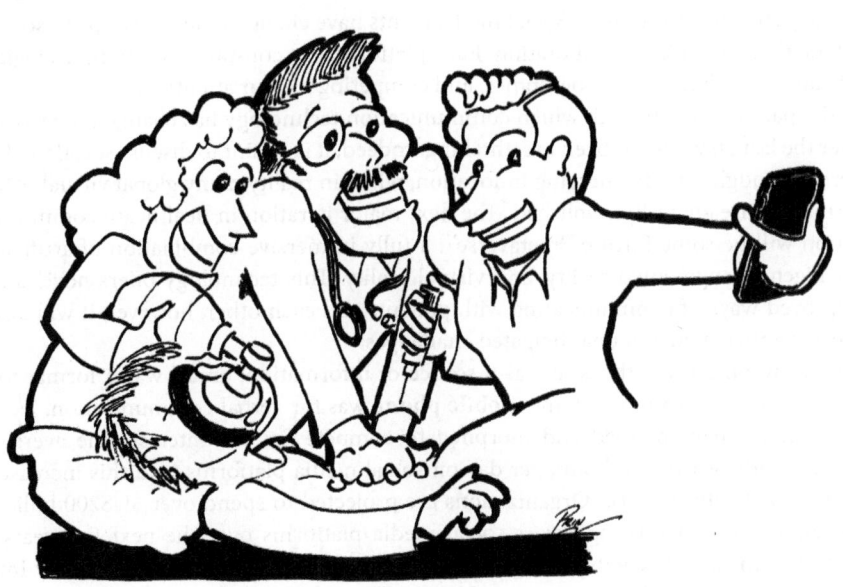

What this chapter is about

Media and healthcare

In our technologically advanced era, medical professionals increasingly use online media in their interactions with patients, and form relationships with the community in the public health setting.[1] Social media giants have changed the landscape of social interaction and online collaboration. Each platform is in constant evolution, strategically targeting different demographics, and competing for our attention.

The pace and depth with which communication technology has changed the world over the last 20 years has been breathtaking. Indeed, it is quaint to discuss social media here as though it is an emerging innovation, when in reality many global virtual platforms are already well-established. The next major iteration in healthcare communication will be some form of 'metaverse'[1]: a fully immersive combination of artificial intelligence, augmented reality, and virtual reality. This technology offers novel and improved ways of communicating with patients and each other, however, it will also present anticipated and unanticipated challenges.

Once upon a time, the **web** was a source of information, **email** was a format for written communication and, the **mobile phone** was for verbal communication. Now these media have merged and morphed to compete for our interest. The average adult spends nearly two hours per day on social media platforms, and this increases every year (statista.com).[2] Organizations are projected to spend over $US200 billion per annum on advertising across social media platforms over the next five years,[3] with the aim of influencing thoughts and behaviour. Social media has not only impacted peoples' personal lives, but it has also shaped the domain of healthcare and medical service provision. In a 3-year study involving 873 hospitals in 12 Western European countries, the use of social media increased, via YouTube from 2% to 20% and Facebook from 10% to 67%.[4] To discuss its impact on anaesthetic practice would merit a book in itself, but we attempt to cover some of the aspects in this chapter.

As members of the community, anaesthetists are present on the internet in a personal or professional capacity. These may be difficult to separate and many do not attempt to make the distinction. Anaesthetists communicate with each other, with other healthcare professionals, with decision-makers such as politicians, and with patients. When we first meet our patients in the anaesthetic bay, many have been influenced by information on the internet. The information may be accurate or inaccurate, it may be helpful or alarmist. Their information exposure and connection with healthcare workers online informs their understanding and expectations of anaesthesia, anaesthetists, and communication in the perioperative period.

Why do patients benefit?

There are many reasons patients find obtaining information via social media attractive. They may perceive their doctors as too busy to have the type of detailed discussions they seek regarding their health concerns.[5] Social media offers patients the opportunity to investigate health problems at great length and depth, which can be especially beneficial for those with chronic disease.[1,6] They can source content that closely matches their stage in the patient journey, demographics, and literacy level. The anonymity afforded by the internet may help them feel less embarrassed about seeking information or communicating with others.[7]

Sharing experiences allows patients to feel a sense of community and common purpose which may have a direct effect on healthcare outcomes.[8] Support from members of an online community may minimize stress, psychological distress, and low mood.[9] Patients with mobility issues, who live in remote or rural areas, or who care for children, disabled, or elderly family members, can benefit from the flexibility and convenience of internet-based sources of information or discourse.[5]

There is little data to suggest patients are replacing traditional sources of information with online resources,[10] but rather using it to complement sources such as face-to-face consultation. Social media use for health-related reasons can lead to more equal and active communication between patients and doctors as patients feel empowered by knowledge and preparation.[11] More than a third of patients presenting to an emergency department had searched the internet for information about their symptoms prior to presenting, with half regularly checking the internet for health information even when well.[12]

When it goes wrong

Suboptimal interactions between the patient and doctor may arise in any setting, including online. Information from online sources may not be up-to-date, accurate, or applicable, and declaring it to be misinformation may be seen as dismissive, distrusting, and patronizing.[13] Discussion of information from social media during a face-to-face consultation may be perceived by some doctors as a threat to their knowledge and experience[11]; however, in at least one study, a majority of GPs reported the pre-visit online search behaviour of patients (Dr Googling) to be beneficial to the consultation.[14]

The use of social media as a platform for doctor–patient interactions also brings its own ethical considerations, such as maintaining patient confidentiality, privacy, and the maintenance of appropriate patient–doctor boundaries.[15]

The vast majority of the impact of a conversation between two people appears to be conveyed through non-verbal cues: gestures such as facial expression, tone of voice, and pauses between responses.[16] During electronic communication there is a diminution of non-verbal cues, which can lead to misinterpretations and misunderstandings. It is not uncommon for people to respond to remote correspondence in ways that would be inappropriate face-to-face.

Cellular and internet-based modalities are not as stable as landline or face-to-face communication and are susceptible to loss of reception, buffering, and fragmentation of transmissions. This can affect the fidelity of clinical communication between parties, and increase stress and frustration in time-critical situations.

Traditional communication devices, such as the postal service, the telephone, the two-way radio, and the fax machine have over time developed conventions around their use (standard letter-writing formats, saying 'Hello', 'Over and out', fax cover pages, etc.). The uptake of newer modes of communication has been rapid, while achieving consensus on the etiquette around those modes has been comparatively slow.

When doctors post

Healthcare professionals of all craft groups have increasingly elected to post health messages online. There is a realization that despite the risks of participation, and the traditional conservative view by some that online engagement is unpalatable for a serious profession, the risks of unopposed misinformation are greater.[17] US Senator Michael Enzi said, '*If you are not at the table, you are on the menu*'. It is now routine for specialty colleges, governments, and universities, to influence the online discourse by posting their messages online and inviting dialogue. By having an online voice, and by listening carefully to others, they are more able to execute their mission, values, and purpose.

Communicating messages to a large audience will influence behaviour. Industry cleverly uses social media marketing to influence purchaser behaviour, and develop strong relationships with their consumers online.[18] The same techniques employed by industry are used in health promotion. Some medical influencers have built up large audiences with a professional, trusting, and warm demeanour, and visually pleasing, short content to influence their audience.

Many medical advocates effectively use the internet to speak directly, to decision-makers and the broader community, about issues that concern them. Climate change, vaccination, refugee issues, and health service improvements are common causes for which they advocate. There can, however, be a tension between advocating for patients and the community, and being perceived to be criticizing the healthcare system[19] and therefore violating terms of employment. Judging adherence to policies can be difficult as one person's whistle-blower is another's saboteur with some interpreting rights to freedom of speech differently.

It is not possible to completely separate personal and professional personas online, although some attempt to do this by using different accounts for different uses. Some interact using anonymous accounts or include a disclaimer such as '*personal opinions only*' or '*not a substitute for personal medical advice*'. These strategies may or may not be helpful medicolegally. There are internet sites which allow the use of enhanced privacy settings and invitation. This can paradoxically give users a false sense of freedom as they attempt to separate personal commentary from their professional persona.

An Australian healthcare worker was suspended by the Victorian Civil and Administrative Tribunal for inappropriate comments made in a small, invitation-only Facebook group.[20] The Tribunal observed that the material published encouraged manipulative, coercive, and misogynistic behaviour. Of note, the Tribunal emphasized that the social media posts were contrary to social media policy whether published to a small private group or a public site.

Communication failure can occur online just as it does during face-to-face interactions. However, internet communication can involve large numbers of people transmitting quickly, so breakdowns can escalate, and become difficult to rein in once ignited. Although online communities are usually considered to be a social support mechanism for a wide audience,[19] they can also generate anxiety and adversely affect outcomes if evidence-based care is discouraged. An example is the anti-vaccination movement.

Doctors can be targeted by trolls while posting mainstream public health messages online. More than two-thirds of scientists surveyed by *Nature* had experienced negative impacts following social media commentary about the pandemic.[21] Many had attacks on their credibility, reputational damage, and complaints to their employer. Disturbingly, some of this moved off the internet with home addresses revealed online and even subsequent physical attacks. The bullying and harassment aimed to silence their voices and was conducted in a coordinated fashion by groups such as the 'Disinformation dozen', a group of twelve individuals and organizations responsible for two-thirds of the anti-vaccination content online.[22]

Women doctors experience a double whammy online, where they are less likely to be included in scientific discourse by their peers and more likely to be harassed. While personal attacks and sexual harassment are common for all doctors online, it is more likely for women, with 1 in 6 reporting sexual harassment.[23,24] This combination of less impact and higher risk of abuse can mean online commentary is less accessible to women. Other aspects of a person's identity such as ethnicity, colour, gender identity, weight, health conditions, and sexual orientation can also make professional online interactions fraught.

Just as it is worthwhile to reflect on how to improve an interaction, it is also good to recognize when it is no longer helpful or salvageable. There are some interactions which cannot be retrieved. Each platform has tools such as muting, blocking, and reporting offensive posts to protect the user experience. There is no requirement to continue an informal online interaction if it is no longer mutually beneficial.

Privacy and documentation

It is common for departments to use email and social media platforms to discuss clinical issues. When this involves individual patients, serious issues of privacy and confidentiality can arise depending on the security of the platform used, the nature of the discussion and the size of the group. It is the responsibility of healthcare professionals to know and understand their obligations when interacting online. All large healthcare organizations such as AHPRA (Australian Health Practitioners Regulation Agency), hospitals, professional colleges and societies, and medical indemnity providers have social media policies to assist practitioners. Some are policies which are mandated by the regulator, others carry less weight as guidelines. While it may be difficult to keep up with policies which can be lengthy and complex, each document in essence directs practitioners to display the same level of professionalism online as in real life. In particular, patient confidentiality, respectful language, and not posting while providing clinical care, are important.

When doctors learn

Traditionally, scientists have communicated their work via publication of manuscripts in scientific journals. In order to be published, a manuscript has to be accepted by the editor, and pass a peer-review process. While this process is the gold standard for ensuring scientific accuracy, the peer-review process can be slow, causing delay in the communication of science. Access can also be limited to those with a personal or institutional subscription to a journal. Many scientific journals have evolved to address these limitations by rapid acceptance and peer review, and creatively disseminating paper content via social media. They do this using a number of tools such as infographics, live broadcasts, and tweet chats where anyone including patients can interact with the authors of the paper.[25] Metrics to measure the impact of research on social media are helpful, but just like traditional citation count, have flaws. Altmetric (London, UK) is the most available measure of social media impact, but other data such as impressions, likes, views, and reshares are not publicly available. While dissemination on Twitter (now known as 'X') improves citations, like traditional publications it may or may not translate to a change in behaviour at the bedside.[26]

The COVID-19 global pandemic created an urgent need to disseminate information rapidly between clinicians, resulting in an unparalleled increase in the delivery and participation of medical education online. During lockdowns, digital education was the only way to disseminate clinical learnings from those who were first experiencing the pandemic.[27] Anaesthetists from Hong Kong utilized their previous outbreak experience from the SARS pandemic to quickly create a useful airway infographic, collaborate digitally with other experts around the world, and rapidly distributed it. Papers from a scientific journal are critiqued. In contrast, information from social media must also be analysed carefully for accuracy and generalisability prior to changing patient management.[28]

Moving forward from the pandemic, there has been a realization that the virtual world has great potential for improving access to the communication of science. This is of particular importance for those who might struggle to attend conferences such as those with caring responsibilities, or those from low- and middle-income countries. There is also a rising concern about the environmental cost of flying to conferences with virtual offerings providing a more sustainable option.[29]

There are potential disadvantages. The scientific publishing industry is currently under pressure to reevaluate the free labour given by researchers to review manuscripts—the so-called *billion-dollar donation*.[30] The ease with which one can up-load and disseminate research is potentially a great advantage on the surface, however, it threatens to undermine peer-review standards. The merits of a '*just get it out there and let the scientific community be the judge*' versus traditional *peer review* are already being questioned.[31] Other issues, such as pay-for-access versus open access to scientific literature, search engine biases, and the use of technology to insinuate commercial interests, remain relatively underevaluated.

Using 'LAURS' and 'GREAT' to communicate more effectively on social media

Given that social media is ubiquitous in our community and that many patients search for health information online, communication needs to be optimized to maximize impact and minimize misunderstandings. Online interactions, however, are not like the traditional patient–doctor interaction. The advice is of a general nature and the obligations of a therapeutic relationship do not exist. Some accounts are anonymous, and it may not be known whether the account is run by a human or an automated *bot*. 'GREAT' 'LAURS' is therefore difficult to adapt in its entirety to the online world, however some elements of 'LAURS' may be useful.

Listening/Looking

Particularly in short internet posts, it can be easy to second-guess the user's intention or agenda, jump in early, and inadvertently contribute to misunderstanding. There is no possibility of observing non-verbal cues. We only have the words and images the other party elects to post. Attempts at humour using sarcasm and jokes can be poorly received. It can be hard to tell if someone is angry or amused. Others may be from a vastly different demographic from ourselves—geography, socioeconomic status, gender, ethnicity, neurodivergence. These differences contribute to the rich discussions online, but a lack of a shared understanding can sometimes prohibit the development of a respectful rapport.

The explicit use of listening reflectively and '*checking in*' can be helpful to avoid misunderstandings, and to de-escalate conflict. What seems initially a medically dubious opinion may, in fact, be perfectly acceptable practice in another healthcare setting, or in keeping with that person's particular medical issues. Asking questions improves our ability to learn and understand another person's perspective.

Acceptance

When we venture beyond our real world it is inevitable, and indeed welcome, that we encounter others who hold different views from us. Even if we scientifically disagree with a patient, we can acknowledge their view and show empathy, without endorsing medical falsehoods. Acceptance of misinformation online can be difficult, particularly when it is harmful. It is understandable that at times a strong emotional reaction can be elicited. When we notice these emotions, it is an opportunity to consider whether, to optimize the interaction, we are utilizing the most helpful communication strategy.

Adopt a 'curious not judgemental' mindset. Depending on the relationship, we can gently challenge the other party's statements, but need to learn when pursuing a disagreement is no longer helpful. There is no obligation to achieve resolution of differences online, and open conflict is rarely useful.

Utilization

Therapeutically anything the other person says online can be used to engage with a person in their preferred communication style. We can utilize the patient's sensory-perceptual language and strengths to empower them as they move forward in their health journey (see Chapter 2).

Reframing

A useful tool in online interactions is to reframe discussion. This can allow the interaction to refocus, and gently correct misinformation.

Suggestions

When interacting online, we can assist both the patient and their anaesthetist by preferencing positive suggestions over the negative to enhance the anaesthetic experience of the patient.

Conclusions

The increasing utilization of social and other media by patients and doctors over the last few decades suggest these technological platforms will continue to shape and re-model the landscape of communication in medicine.

Key points

1. Medical professionals increasingly use online media in their interactions with patients, and to form relationships with the community. This interactivity comes with substantial benefits and challenges.

2. Difficulties in separating professional and personal online personae can lead to pitfalls when posting online.

3. Clinical departments must take conscious steps to manage issues, relating to both patients and colleagues, of privacy and confidentiality that inevitably arise when discussing clinical issues through online networks.

4. Tremendous opportunities for rapid and extensive dissemination of research and educational material comes with disadvantages which we are only beginning to understand.

5. Some elements of 'LAURS' and 'GREAT' may help navigate these challenges.

References

1. Antheunis ML, Tates K, Nieboer TE (2013). Patients' and health professionals' use of social media in health care: motives, barriers and expectations. *Patient Educ Couns*, **92**(3), 426–31.

2. Statista Research Department (n.d.). Daily time spent on social networking by internet users worldwide from 2012 to 2022. Statista Inc (New York). Available at: https://www.statista.com/statistics/433871/daily-social-media-usage-worldwide/ (Accessed 23 March 2023).

3. Statista Research Department (n.d.). Social media advertising worldwide from 2021 to 2028. Available at: https://www.statista.com/statistics/271406/advertising-revenue-of-social-networks-worldwide/ (Accessed 23 March 2023).

4. Van de Belt TH, Berben SA, Samsom M, Engelen LJ, Schoonhoven L (2012). Use of social media by Western European hospitals: longitudinal study. *J Med Internet Res*, **14**(3), e61.

5. Rupert DJ, Moultrie RR, Read JG, et al. (2014). Perceived healthcare provider reactions to patient and caregiver use of online health communities. *Patient Educ Couns*, **96**(3), 320–6.

6. Griffiths F, Cave J, Boardman F, et al. (2012). Social networks—the future for health care delivery. *Soc Sci Med*, **75**(12), 2233–41.

7. Lu Y, Wu Y, Liu J, Li J, Zhang P (2017). Understanding health care social media use from different stakeholder perspectives: a content analysis of an online health community. *J Med Internet Res*, **19**(4), e109.

8. Jadad AR, Enkin MW, Glouberman S, Groff P, Stern A (2006). Are virtual communities good for our health? *BMJ*, **332**(7547), 925–6.

9. Nambisan P (2011). Information seeking and social support in online health communities: impact on patients' perceived empathy. *J Am Med Inform Assoc*, **18**(3), 298–304.

10. Powell J, Inglis N, Ronnie J, Large S (2011). The characteristics and motivations of online health information seekers: cross-sectional survey and qualitative interview study. *J Med Internet Res*, **13**(1), e20.

11. Smailhodzic E, Hooijsma W, Boonstra A, Langley DJ (2016). Social media use in healthcare: a systematic review of effects on patients and on their relationship with healthcare professionals. *BMC Health Serv Res*, **16**, 442.

12. Cocco AM, Zordan R, Taylor DM, et al. (2018). Dr Google in the ED: searching for online health information by adult emergency department patients. *Med J Aust*, **209**(8), 342–7.

13. Kata A (2010). A postmodern Pandora's box: anti-vaccination misinformation on the internet. *Vaccine*, **28**(7), 1709–16.

14. Van Riel N, Auwerx K, Debbaut P, van Hees S, Schoenmakers B. (2017) The effect of Dr Google on doctor-patient encounters in primary care: a quantitative, observational, cross-sectional study. *BJGP Open*, **1**(2), bjgpopen17X100833.

15. George DR, Rovniak LS, Kraschnewski JL (2013). Dangers and opportunities for social media in medicine. *Clin Obstet Gynecol*, **56**(3), 453–62.

16. Mehrabian A, Ferris SR (1967). Inference of attitudes from nonverbal communication in two channels. *J Cons Psychology*, **31**(3), 248–58

17. Selak T (2021). Practicing physicians should post on social media. *Am J Med*, **134** (12), e586.

18. Hanaysha JR (2022). Impact of social media marketing features on consumer's purchase decision in the fast-food industry: brand trust as a mediator. *Int J Info Man Data Insights*, **2**(2), 100102.

19. Oliver D (2020). David Oliver: Being labelled an 'activist' is a badge of honour. *BMJ*, **371**, m4186.

20. Victorian Civil and Administrative Tribunal (2021). Nursing and Midwifery Board of Australia v Palle (Review and Regulation) [2021] VCAT 1009. Available at: https://www.austlii.edu.au/cgi-bin/viewdoc/au/cases/vic/VCAT/2021/1009.html?context=1;query=%22coercive%20control%22;mask_path= (Accessed 22 March 2023)

21. Nogrady B (2021). 'I hope you die': how the COVID pandemic unleashed attacks on scientists. *Nature*, **598**(7880), 250–3.

22. Mabrey B (2021). The disinformation dozen and media misinformation on science and vaccinations. Available at: https://ir.library.oregonstate.edu/downloads/3t945z78s (Accessed 22 March 2023).

23. Pendergrast TR, Jain S, Trueger NS, Gottlieb M, Woitowich NC, Arora VM (2021). Prevalence of personal attacks and sexual harassment of physicians on social media. *JAMA Intern Med*, **181**(4), 550–2.

24. Rotenstein LS, Torre M, Cleary JL, Sen S, Guille C, Mata DA (2022). Differences in gender representation in the Altmetric Top 100. *J Gen Intern Med*, **37**(3), 590–2.

25. Johannsson H, Selak T (2020). Dissemination of medical publications on social media—is it the new standard? *Anaesthesia*, **75**(2), 155–7.

26. Luc JGY, Archer MA, Arora RC, et al. (2021). Does Tweeting improve citations? One-year results from the TSSMN prospective randomized trial. *Ann Thorac Surg*, **111**(1), 296–300.

27. Fawcett WJ, Charlesworth M, Cook TM, Klein AA (2021). Education and scientific dissemination during the COVID-19 pandemic. *Anaesthesia*, **76**(3), 301–4.

28. Chan AKM, Nickson CP, Rudolph JW, Lee A, Joynt GM (2020). Social media for rapid knowledge dissemination: early experience from the COVID-19 pandemic. *Anaesthesia*, **75**(12), 1579–82.

29. Zotova O, Petrin-Desrosiers C, Gopfert A, Van Hove M (2020). Carbon-neutral medical conferences should be the norm. *Lancet Planet Health*, **4**(2), e48–e50.

30. Aczel B, Szaszi B, Holcombe AO (2021). A billion-dollar donation: estimating the cost of researchers' time spent on peer review. *Res Integr Peer Rev*, **6**(1), 14.

31. Anonymous (2019). Quality in peer review. *Commun Biol*, **2**, 352. doi: 10.1038/s42003-019-0603-3.

Section 5

Advanced communication techniques

Chapter 23

Hypnotic techniques

Ernil Hansen, Marie-Elisabeth Faymonville,
Christel J. Bejenke, and
Audrey Vanhaudenhuyse

'You're not using hypnosis as a cure, you're using it as a
tool to develop a positive environment where you can
discover something.'
Milton H. Erickson

What this chapter is about

Anxiety, fear, tension, and apprehension are common emotions in patients undergoing surgery. Clinicians are becoming increasingly aware of the importance of patients' psychological reactions as well as their physical needs. There is an opportunity for the anaesthetist to use the preoperative assessment as a means of fostering greater rapport and providing reassurance.

Sedative and analgesic drugs are the primary means of relieving anxiety and tension prior to major anaesthesia. However, sedatives are not the only answer. Sedation can be accomplished pharmacologically, but drugs cannot empower patients in a way that enables them to respond more positively to their treatment.

For anaesthetists seeking to provide optimal anaesthetic care for their patients, the challenge is not only to become more expert in the latest state-of-the-art technology, but also to acquire the skills necessary to function effectively in the role of physician healer. Hypnosis is not a 'therapy', but a potentially valuable tool in the anaesthetist's professional armamentarium. It deserves equal consideration with other tools and skills which anaesthetists acquire. Hypnotic techniques can positively influence a patient's entire medical experience.[1-6]

Background

Hypnosis describes a non-ordinary state of consciousness characterized by focused attention, reduced awareness of the environment, a feeling of involuntariness, modulation of self-awareness, and an increased capacity to respond to suggestion.[7,8] Hypnosis has had a cyclical history of acceptance and rejection. It has been practised in one form or another for thousands of years.

In 1828 scientific publications first reported its effectiveness as an anaesthetic for surgery.[9] A few years later, decreases in the rates of surgical shock, morbidity, and mortality (from 40% to 5%) were reported in a cohort of 300 major surgical cases by using 'Mesmer's passes'.[10]

However, when volatile agents were introduced, the use of hypnosis as a sole anaesthesia technique died out. Although some authors supported the concept of combining the mind and body's abilities to alter perceptions and feelings,[11] it took until 1955 for hypnosis to be accepted by the British Medical Association in the management of acute pain.[12] Today, hypnosis is a scientifically evaluated method for psychotherapy,[13] and numerous applications, particularly in the context of anxiety and pain management[4,14] (see Chapter 9). The neurophysiological basis of hypnotic effects are becoming better understood and neuro-imaging shows that self and environmental networks are markedly changed, as are those related to pain perception during the hypnotic state.[6,15-17]

Because of its historical association with magic, hypnosis has struggled to become disentangled from faith-healing, the occult, and entertainment. It is to the credit of hypnotherapists like Milton Erickson and David Cheek to have led hypnosis from an authoritative, manipulative, and healer-centred modality to one that is permissive and patient-centred. Hypnosis allows for support and guidance of a patient-specific capability.

When and why to use hypnosis

In many hospitals around the world, hypnosis is currently used as an adjuvant to pharmacological anaesthesia.[14,18,19] For many years, pain relief and anxiolysis were the focus. Nowadays acute pain is usually well controlled with pharmacotherapy. Allergic reactions to drugs are infrequent and it is difficult now to justify the use of hypnosis as monotherapy. Nerve blocks and pharmacological sedation are recommended in therapeutic guidelines and any deviation from this approach has to be justified given the current medicolegal climate.

Hypnosis should preferentially be used to help manage numerous poorly treated problems in clinical practice such as, stress, anxiety, the feeling of helplessness, and of being left alone. Although sedatives can save the anaesthetist and surgeon from a patient's expressed distress, they usually do not really help the patient's overall experience of their clinical care. Rather, the resort to a pharmacological solution alone fails to allow patients to participate in their care. Instead, patients find themselves in a situation of prescribed passivity. It is a special strength and advantage of hypnosis to allow for and encourage the active involvement of patients in their anaesthesia care, especially in the form of self-hypnosis.

Moreover, loss of consciousness remains a horrifying idea for some patients and should be avoided whenever it is not necessary. Whatever the choice of anaesthesia, many patients need help when faced with the psychological challenge of undergoing surgery. Hypnosis offers considerable benefits as a therapeutic adjunct to local or regional anaesthesia.

Since 1992, anaesthetists at the University Hospital of Liège, Belgium, have supplemented traditional anaesthetic techniques with hypnosis. This technique, named hypnosedation, combines hypnosis with light, conscious intravenous sedation and local anaesthesia.[20]

More than 10,000 patients have comfortably undergone major head and neck or breast surgery under hypnosedation. This technique can also be used for various other procedures, including: thyroid surgery, endovascular procedures, breast and prostate biopsy, colectomy, hysteroscopic placement of implants for sterilization, tooth extraction, skin tumour removal, childbirth, glioma surgery, burn dressing changes, and uterovaginal brachytherapy.[20-23]

The most important benefit of this technique is that patients maintain consciousness and are able to communicate with the anaesthetist if required and contribute to their own treatment. During hypnosedation, in order to help patients better cope with pain and surgery, hypnosis is used for the therapeutic purpose of inducing a controlled state of dissociation. The surgical decision to operate under local anaesthesia and hypnosedation depends on the surgeon's own appreciation of feasibility, and familiarity with the technique. During the preoperative anaesthesia interview, the patient is asked about their own particular preference and motivation for this specific anaesthetic technique. Information is provided about the hypnotic state but no rehearsal is offered.

After transfer to the operating theatre, the patient is invited to choose a pleasant life experience to be 're-lived' during surgery—a 'lived-in imagination' technique. A hypnotic state is then induced. After approximately 10 minutes, the patient is usually at an adequate depth of hypnosis as evidenced by slow eye movements, a change in breathing and skin pallor. This psychological approach is supplemented by intravenous administration of remifentanil, and on occasion midazolam, in order to maintain conscious sedation, provide patient comfort, and optimize surgical conditions.

The induction is simple and straightforward, while at the same time quite complex, and illustrative of hypnotic phenomena involving, eye fixation, internal absorption, relaxation of the body, and increasing quietness of the mind. Patients are invited to relive previous pleasant autobiographical experiences without any suggestions for analgesia. As practice continues, confidence levels increase and the clinician begins to observe opportunities to tailor the hypnotic procedure to the particular needs of the moment, by utilizing what happens around the patient. This technique provides more comfort to both patient and surgeon, better perioperative pain relief and anxiolysis, more haemodynamic stability, faster recovery with less fatigue and pain, and reduced need for medication.[20–23]

What is hypnosis?

Hypnotic and imagery strategies for managing acute pain symptoms and emotional factors, associated with surgery, are described in several articles.[1–3,20,24] The construct of 'hypnosis' is used to represent both a particular state of consciousness and the technique employed to induce such a state. Like any non-ordinary state of consciousness, the hypnotic state is difficult to measure and describe objectively as it is essentially a subjective experience. In hypnosis, verbal suggestions can lead to remarkable alterations in subjective experiences. These include atypical changes in perception, memory, self-agency, dissociation, absorption, spontaneous thoughts, space and time perception, behaviour, and involuntary body functions.[6,8,15–17,25,26] Hypnotic suggestions do not ask subjects simply to 'imagine' the suggested state of affairs, rather the person under hypnosis is 'guided' to experience, as if in real life, circumstances which would permit responses consistent with the hypnotist's suggestions.

The increasing number of neurophysiological findings will help the clinician to better understand how hypnosis works as an important therapeutic technique in pain management.[16]

We now have an opportunity to explore activity in the brain during hypnotic pain modulation with neuroimaging techniques such as regional cerebral blood flow (rCBF), modification with positron emission tomography (PET)[25] and functional magnetic resonance.[26] Studies show that hypnosis influences whole brain neural connectivity, **internal** i.e. self-related, default mode, and **external**, i.e. environment-related, external control, networks activation, as well as the subjective perception of internal and external consciousness.[6,15–17]

Psychologically mediated forms of pain reduction, as shown during hypnotic procedures, modulate not only nociceptive reflexes and pain-related autonomic activity, elicited by peripheral stimulation, but also supraspinal pain control systems. Pain combines sensory, emotional, and cognitive processes, generating the activation of the pain neuromatrix, as well as some regions of the reward circuit.[27] During hypnosis, both sensory and emotional components of noxious stimuli are modulated, with specific mediation of the anterior cingulate cortex, involved in the emotional component of pain.[16]

Prerequisites and techniques for hypnosis

1. The hypnosis practitioner recognizes, accepts, and supports the patient's individuality.

2. Before the hypnotic induction procedure, the anaesthetist has asked about, and listened to, the patient's specific needs. Thereby, the patient feels respected and legitimately understood and cared about, and feels safe.

3. Hypnotic techniques rely on a harmonious trustful relationship. During the induction procedure, the anaesthetist uses specific communication skills to help guide a patient into the hypnotic state. It is a cooperative process where the hypnotist responds with verbal and non-verbal suggestions to the patient's needs.

4. To assist the patient appropriately, the anaesthetist must also accept another person's reality. Communication is adapted by integrating the patient's words and behaviours, even if these may run counter to the practitioner's own beliefs or experiences. Patients know what is good for them, and hypnosis can help them to be involved in their own recovery, and take an active role through the employment of these self-management skills.

5. Hypnotic communication skills allow anaesthetists to enhance patients' strengths and abilities to cope with the situation. Utilization techniques help anaesthetists to reframe patients' concerns into more therapeutic thoughts, perceptions, or behaviours (see Chapter 2).

6. Using hypnosis or teaching self-hypnosis techniques perioperatively, empowers patients to be their own advocate and play an active role during their care.

The challenge for anaesthetists is how best to complement their traditional anaesthesia skills to facilitate more comprehensive patient management. Anaesthetists are urged to expand their skills beyond traditional biomedical methods. and recognize language as a primary intervention in patient management. Hypnotic communication skills are effectively taught, easily learned and incorporated into routine anaesthesia practice without significantly lengthening consultations or radically changing the way medicine is practised.

Interestingly, many anaesthetists subconsciously use 'hypnotic techniques' and 'hypnotic language'—most commonly with children.[26] For example: *'getting ready for a space-flight'*, *'smelling that special astronaut air'*—the anaesthetic gas. Because these techniques work, a basic knowledge of hypnotic concepts and principles can make anaesthetic care more effective. Hypnotic concepts can help us understand more clearly why some of what we say works well, or why it doesn't. We can then develop approaches that work reliably.

Concepts of hypnosis

Hypnotic concepts and principles demonstrate the significance of nuances in language. For example, information, identical in content, can be perceived by patients as either threatening or reassuring. It all depends on how such information is formulated and transmitted—both verbally and non-verbally.[1] For example, if the anaesthetist says to a patient emerging from anaesthesia, '*It's all over!*' or '*You're finished!*' These terms could be interpreted to mean death.

What could one say instead?

> **Anaesthetist:** (cheerfully—the tone of voice is important): 'Hello! Dr Smith has just completed your operation ... You have done very well ... and you are safe ... Everything is taken care of ... and you will be going home soon ... You may even be hungry ...'

The latter two statements direct the patient's attention away from the emergency, from risks and fear, and instead direct focus on to something normal, healthy, and mundane.

Many patients in the face of pain and anxiety enter spontaneous trance states and exhibit trancelike phenomena such as: focused attention, amnesia, dissociation, and regression to a child-like level of functioning. In this state any communication can function as a suggestion and be as powerful as those given during formal hypnotic states.[1] Inadvertent negative suggestions[28] can result in unexpected and unintended detrimental effects (see Chapter 3). However, this enhanced suggestibility can also be utilized as a therapeutic opportunity. Because patients are already in a hypnosis-like state, it is not necessary to induce hypnosis, as suggestions can simply be used as if the patient is already hypnotized.

Suggestions

'Suggestions' can be one of the most useful forms of communication in anaesthetic practice (see Chapters 2–4). They can be used in most situations such as during the risk discussion when obtaining informed consent, induction of anaesthesia, or emergence in the recovery room.

While various definitions exist for this term, 'suggestion' can be understood as 'a proposal to consider a new or different view, idea or possibility'; 'to put forward for consideration'; 'to hint, imply, or intimate'. There is no expectation of 'compliance', nor is the patient 'compelled' to carry out a suggestion. Instead, the patient is offered the opportunity to entertain a different, more beneficial view or perspective, to reinterpret sensations or experiences—and most patients will choose that option.

The effect of suggestions, negative as well as positive, can not only be suspected by the hypnotherapist or subjectively reported by the patient. In the endeavour to further develop an evidence base for hypnosis and therapeutic communication, maximal arm muscle strength measured by dynamometry has been used as an objective, physiological measure when compared with individuals' baselines to test various clinical suggestions.[29,30] These included:

- remembering a negative past, as it occurs during every anamnesis, talking about an upcoming treatment with an uncertain outcome, as with any announcement of a diagnosis or treatment;

- the query of symptoms like '*Do you feel pain?*' reassurance with '*You don't need to be afraid. Don't worry!*';

- risk information for informed consent;
- non-verbal signals like watching the ceiling during a transport in a hospital, the common overhead view of the anaesthetist before induction of anaesthesia, or the view from the patient room to a parking lot.

All these suggestions led to a significant impairment of maximal arm muscle strength, i.e. a weakening of the patient. For improvement also alternative formulations were generated and tested: talking about a positive past or future without the disease, focusing on the here-and-now and asking, *'Do you feel okay?'* rather than asking about pain or nausea. Further alternative formulations avoided negations, added the benefits of the treatment to the risk information. Non-verbal suggestions included transport in an upright position, facing the patient from the front without wearing a mask, and the view to the open landscape. All these suggestions were aimed at avoiding the disempowerment of the patient and to neutralize a prior corresponding negative suggestion.

Using an objective and uniform parameter, such as maximal arm muscle strength, holds several advantages for the evaluation of suggestion effects. The quality of a suggestion, positive or negative, can be demonstrated, and the effect quantitatively assessed. Using a uniform parameter, such as arm muscle strength as a surrogate marker for general *weakening* or *strengthening* effects of suggestions, enables comparisons of the effects of different suggestions.

In contrast, the usual consideration of the specific effects (e.g. of the word *'pain'* on pain, of the term *'feeling sick'* on nausea) of a non-verbal signal on anxiety makes comparison difficult to impossible. Alternative suggestions and combinations can be evaluated, and thereby communication improved in a reproducible, scientific way.[28] Another parameter that has been used for testing suggestions was respiratory muscle strength, with high clinical relevance.[31]

Managing negative suggestions

Both nocebo effects and negative suggestions can be recognized in the working environment and should be avoided or neutralised.[29,32]

Sometimes nurses say to a patient who is just arriving in the recovery room:

'I'll put this "sick bowl" (emesis basin) *right here so you have it, when you need it',* or *'when you get sick',* or *'call me when you have to throw up.'*

In contrast, when a patient does vomit, this can be utilized and then reframed positively:

'Good! You're rid of that stale old stuff. Now you can feel so much better and already look forward to eating and drinking soon.' This is an anti-nausea suggestion.

Peristalsis can also be stimulated by the suggestion to listen for and hear, *'the churning and gurgling in your belly'.* This results in earlier resolution of postoperative ileus after intra-abdominal surgery.

Variations on the same theme:

'Do you have pain?'

'Let me know when you have pain—here is the bell.'

'Tell me when you start hurting . . .'

To patients this can mean, *'I will have pain—these people know; after all, they are experts.'*

Instead:

'Let me know how I can make you more comfortable. There are so many ways we can do that: would you like . . . ?'

The anaesthetist's communication, designed to reduce the severity of any expected postoperative pain and nausea, can include:

'Wouldn't it be nice . . . if it would be a whole lot different for you this time . . . and quite a bit easier than you might have thought?'

'You are safe' is one of the most important statements a patient can hear pre-, intra-, and postoperatively.

'Just try to relax . . .' confirms to the patient an inability to do so, and is apt to increase a sense of helplessness. In addition, *'Try'* implies doubt in the possibility of success, and therefore conveys the expectation of failure (see Chapter 4).

Alternatively consider: *'Anaesthesia has to do with comfort and safety: an anaesthetist, will care for you and make sure that you are safe. Anaesthetists watch everything very closely . . . while you are deeply relaxed and comfortable.'*

Case study

When asked how a patient expected to feel after her hysterectomy, she responded, *'My doctor says I'll feel like I've been run over by a truck!'*

> **Anaesthetist:** *'Would you mind feeling better than that?'*
> **Patient:** *'You mean . . . like being run over by a small truck?'*
> **Anaesthetist:** *'Better than that?'*
> **Patient:** *'By a car!'*
> **Anaesthetist:** *'Better than that?'*
> **Patient:** *'Maybe . . . a small car!'*
> **Anaesthetist:** *'Better than that!'*
> **Patient:** *'You mean . . . a . . . motorcycle!'*
> **Anaesthetist:** *'Better than that!'*
> **Patient:** (after thinking for a while): *'Aaaah . . . a . . . bicycle?'*
> **Anaesthetist:** *'Would you mind not feeling like being run over by anything, . . . just feeling some pressure underneath your bandages . . . and maybe some cramps . . . like when you have a period . . . and things like that?'*
> **Patient:** *'Hmm . . .'*

After the operation, when asked how she felt, the patient said, *'I feel like I've been run over by a bicycle'* and laughed! She did not suffer the expected (and suggested!) severe postoperative pain, but instead—to her surgeon's amazement—experienced minimal discomfort and recovered more rapidly than expected. This 'intervention' had taken less than one minute of suggestions as part of the anaesthetist's communication.[1]

Awake craniotomy without sedation

An extreme example demonstrating the potential of hypnosis-based communication is the support and guidance of patients having an awake craniotomy. A tumour in the vicinity of an eloquent area or motor areas of the brain may make it necessary to have the patient awake during surgery for neurological testing. This usually is achieved by an awake-sleep-awake technique where the patient receives anaesthesia or analgosedation with or without controlled ventilation.[33]

Besides pain there are a number of stress factors affecting patients. These include the noises and vibration of drilling and milling the skull, the suctioning of blood, and the knowledge of having someone working inside the brain. Pain can be managed effectively by regional anaesthesia in the form of a scalp block. At the University of Regensburg, Germany, the effects of stress are mitigated by the use of 'therapeutic communication' based on an understanding of hypnosis,[1,34] but without formal induction of hypnosis. The main constituents of the hypnotic intervention, applicable to most operations under local or regional anaesthesia, are[28]:

- Dissociation to an inner safe and comfortable place or situation;
- Reframing of disturbing noises, sensations, or conversations;
- Non-verbal suggestions such as hand-in-hand or hand-on-shoulder that are expressions of support and reassurance and mean, '*I am with you, you are not alone*';
- Specific suggestions;
- Addressing basic psychological needs to neutralize stressors;
- Therapeutic relationship.

During the preoperative visit, rapport is established, and the patient's own resources and coping strategies are evaluated by questions about family, profession, accommodation, pets, garden, favourite holiday destinations, hobbies, sport activities, experience with relaxation techniques, and preferred places of rest and recreation. One or more of these activities can be utilized later as the patient's '*Safe place*'.

To seed the option of reframing stimuli, an anecdote is told.

> '*A patient visits his dentist, who declares that he will have to drill. He asks, "What is your hobby?" "Motorcycling". "Where?" "California". "Okay, so you can close your eyes and go biking, on Highway 1". The dentist does his work, and finally asks, "How was it?" "Well, okay. But it was great when you really turned up the revs. Brrhmm, brrhmm!"*'

With only this minimal preparation, one patient, who had a 'lived-in imagination' experience of 'mountain hiking' during awake craniotomy at the time of drilling of burr holes into the skull, said: '*There's a helicopter—taking me away*', a wonderful interpretation for the noise and incidentally a metaphor for being saved.

Motivation is increased and **Safety** expressed by explaining that although all drugs are kept on standby and can be used, from mild sedation to deep anaesthesia, they will only be given if necessary. The fewer of these used, the better the testing will turn out, and the more successful the surgery.

Control is given by saying, '*Whenever you want a break or something to change, just let us know. We are with you all the time, and we can always do something helpful for you.*'

Assurance is given by placing a hand on the shoulder:

> '*This is the hand of medicine on your shoulder, representing all our experience and knowledge, all the technology and drugs we have available for you, all the good things we can do for you. This hand of medicine will stay with you to accompany you all the time, even when I take it away, until you have safely come through this therapeutic procedure, with the results that you have been looking for.*'

The awake patient is carefully positioned with his participation—a major advantage for hours fixed on the operating table. Then, the patient is guided by the anaesthetist to **dissociate** from the immediate environment and to internally focus on one of his 'safe places':

> '*We don't need you right now. You might as well go to . . . This is easy, since anywhere is nicer than in an OR.*'

Dissociation to the safe place can be deepened with questions to the different senses:

> '*How does it feel, the sun on the skin, the ground beneath the feet?*'
>
> '*Is there a smell in the air?*'
>
> '*What colours are around?*'
>
> '*Can you hear birds, or the wind?*'

Reframing of disturbing noises and sensations is offered. The noises in the operating room can be **utilized** and **reframed**. '*Everything you hear or sense can fit into your adventure. Just watch, with an open and interested mind, what comes up.*'

The suction: '*Maybe there is water running somewhere.*'

Rattle of instruments: '*There might be birds singing, or branches breaking.*'

Conversations: '*You might meet people passing by.*'

Non-verbal reassurance and support are given by handholding. At the same time, this helps to detect any tension. A **hand on the shoulder** is not only a sign of caring and a monitor of respiration, but also a tool for deepening and slowing down of breaths—by delayed pressure during expiration and delayed release with inspiration. It is not necessary nor helpful to talk to the patient all the time. As long as he is calm and relaxed there is no need to interfere. But as soon as his facial expression indicates concern or discomfort, he moves, his respiration or heart rate goes up, he opens his eyes to look around, then is the time to bring him back to his safe place or suggest another one. Actually, this intervention can be delayed a little, and if he closes his eyes again this indicates that he has checked for himself that he is more comfortable there.

As a **specific suggestion**, breathing can be used both for calming and relaxing, and as a basis for metaphors.

> '*With every breath in, you can take up fresh air and oxygen that is so essential for all the cells of the body—and with every breath out, get rid of all the used air and waste of cellular*

metabolism ... and breathe in the good oxygen ... and you may want to hold and keep it for a while—and along with expiration let it flow through your body all the way down to your toes—and take up fresh air and all the good things that can help you now—and blow away with expiration the used air and all the things that are not useful for you now or disturb you—to have the lungs ready for another deep breath to take up calmness and confidence— and exhale all stress—and take up strength and healing power ... '

These words are spoken to the rhythm of breathing, slower and slower.

The prominent role of the theatre environment as a major negative suggestion became obvious in one patient, who was fine throughout his awake craniotomy, until, at the end of surgery, he developed a vaso-vagal reaction without reporting pain. What had happened? The lights were switched back on in the OR after microscopy. The neuropsychologist responsible for neurological testing said *'good-bye'*. The patient opened his eyes to look around and noticed a monitor showing the closure of his dura mater. The neurosurgeon let him see a rivet used for closure of the craniotomy. The patient became aware of the theatre environment and then became hypotensive with a heart rate of 35/min.

This documented example demonstrates the potential for negative and disturbing effects of the theatre environment. All that this patient needed was to be taken back to the *'walk in the woods'* he had been on during the procedure.

While arousal from trance is usually expected from any disturbance, actual **utilization** of such events can be used to deepen the trance and dissociation. It is important to point out that disturbance is not a fact, but it is the patient's and the doctor's misconception and expectation that noise has to disturb relaxation.

'And whenever you feel more than you want to, you can go deeper and deeper into that wonderful, calm experience of nature, and rest. Any sensation, any noise you experience can be a signal for you that everything is proceeding well here, and that you can relax and have a good time, like going for a walk or swimming after you have given your car to the garage.'

Table 23.1 Derivation of topics for an essential, meaningful communication

Basic psychological needs	Traumatic stressors	Themes of meaning for an essential communication
Relationship and belonging	Abandonment Inability to express oneself	Accompaniment Contact
Pleasure gain and avoidance of displeasure	Pain, suffering Hopelessness	Comfort Confidence
Orientation and control	Chaos Dependence Helplessness	Information Control Instructions
Self-esteem and self-protection	Degradation Fear, threat	Respect Safety
Sense of physical integrity	Injury	Healing

Themes of meaning that should be addressed when taking care of patients, or people in need, can be derived from the basic psychological needs of humans (Table 23.1, left column).[28] When these are not fulfilled, stress is generated that can lead to post-traumatic stress disorder (PTSD). This predominantly occurs in risk populations such as refugees, combatants, accident victims, health personnel, and also in patients after burns or ICU care. Common specific triggers and stressors are listed in Table 23.1. Feelings like that are commonly found in patients.

To neutralize these stressors, it is helpful to address the '*Themes of meaning*' in Table 23.1. They have to be expressed in various formulations and in one's own words to be authentic. The assurance of support '*I am here to care for you*' can be extended to '*We are a whole team that is here for you now*', and in time: '*We will stay with you until you recover and get through this.*' Control can be given back to the patient by saying '*Whenever you want a break, tell us!*'.

Respect can be expressed by addressing the self-healing power and the valuable provision of circulation, coagulation, wound healing, immune response, etc. First rule is: No whitewashing, no concealment, no lies! Even a 'fatally' injured person can be assured of safety and healing: '*And we will do everything in our hands for your wellbeing, your safety, and healing. And you, yourself, your body is caring for and has started all its functions to improve the situation.*'

This approach can be utilized in a variety of clinical contexts, such as transporting an accident victim, caring for a conscious patient during surgery under regional anaesthesia, talking to an intensive care patient in a coma, or accompanying a dying person. Placebo effects are better described as a *meaning response*, and the communication of meaning might be the common basis for placebo effects and hypnosis.[35]

Since 2006 this approach has been established as a clinical routine at the University Hospital of Regensburg, Germany (>400 cases).[36,37] The result of the studies showed that with appropriate analgesia via nerve blocks, adequate therapeutic communication, and no sedation at all, little if any additional analgesics are necessary for such a surgical intervention with a high level of patient satisfaction. Although general anaesthesia can be replaced by this approach, it is not done to demonstrate *hypnosis instead of narcosis*. Indeed, there is an indication for avoidance of sedation, not because of *dangerous adverse effects* but of its very main effect, as even the short-acting sedatives impair the intraoperatively necessary sophisticated neurocognitive tests. Meanwhile, also formal hypnosis has been used for awake craniotomies.[38,39]

Hypnosis or hypnotic communication?

In 1962, David Cheek, an American gynaecologist and hypnotherapist drew attention to the '*Importance of recognizing that surgical patients behave as though hypnotized*'.[40] The state of consciousness called **trance** is not an artificial condition created by and for hypnosis, but a natural reaction to emergencies. In **natural trance** induced by trauma, stress, pain, and anxiety, humans are able to dissociate from life-threatening injuries and survive. Among other things it is characterized by a **focused attention** and an **increased suggestibility**, the former with the patient's peculiarity of referring everything to himself, the latter with access to strong reactions of involuntary body functions. Doctors who do not know that patients in acute medical situations enter a natural trance state, try in vain to talk to the patient rationally, unaware of the strong effects of surrounding negative suggestions. The knowledge of this non-ordinary state of consciousness in their patients is of outstanding importance for clinicians to carry out adequate and optimal treatment.

The consequence is that in acute medicine formal induction can be dispensed with in most cases. Advantages are:

- Hypnosis training can be distilled to therapeutic communication and relationship, and there is minimal if any need for psychotherapy and induction techniques.
- Instead of external experts, medical staff can be involved. The everyday source of careless potential negative suggestions can be eliminated by education, training, and motivation of healthcare personnel. They know the medical procedures and can shape hypnotic communications for maximum effect.
- The patient's active participation (self-hypnosis), and self-efficacy, comes more to the fore.
- The basis of hypnotic interventions—relationship and resonance instead of techniques—are emphasized utilizing the intrinsic conditions of medical treatment.

Combination of hypnotic approaches

Recently, a prospective multicentre study showed some remarkable effects of therapeutic suggestions given under general anaesthesia, namely a reduction in postoperative pain, pain medication,[41] nausea, and the use of antiemetics.[42] The effect sizes are similar or even higher than using traditional hypnosis,[18] possibly with the common basis of *'touching the unconscious in the unconscious'* bypassing the critical mind. This does not represent a competition but a strong call for the combination of preoperative, intraoperative, and postoperative hypnotic care of surgical patients. With the intraoperative application, the effect is expanded to a phase where the development of pain, not only its existence, can be modulated.

It turns out that the patient in acute medicine needs hypnotic communication not merely in certain phases with an expert at hand, but throughout the stay in hospital, with frequent periods of natural trance, deep anxieties, and increased suggestibility. Therefore, hypnotic principles and insights should be integrated into clinical practice and healthcare education and training.

Hypnosis is not a therapy in itself. Integration and application of hypnotic communication into a core therapeutic armamentarium, will make sense to experienced clinicians who are willing to think creatively with each new patient.

Key points

1. Attitudes regarding hypnotic communication skills need to change.
2. Be aware of inadvertent negative suggestions—'*innocent remarks*'.
3. Information and choices are empowering.
4. '*You are safe*' is important for patients to hear.
5. The therapeutic alliance is of utmost importance. The first rule is honesty—no whitewashing, no concealment, no lies.
6. Hypnosis is complementary to medical treatment, neither an alternative nor replacement.
7. Hypnotic communication permits anaesthetists to work more effectively with a wider range of patients.

Acknowledgements

This chapter was reviewed and updated by Ernil Hansen and Audrey Vanhaudenhuyse in the second edition. The chapter was originally written by Marie-Elisabeth Faymonville, Christel J. Bejenke, and Ernil Hansen in the first edition.

References

1. Bejenke CJ (1996). Painful medical procedures. In: Barber J (ed.) *Hypnosis and suggestion in the treatment of pain. A clinical guide*, pp. 209–66. New York: WW Norton.
2. Faymonville ME, Mambourg PH, Joris J, et al. (1997). Psychological approaches during conscious sedation. Hypnosis versus stress reducing strategies. A prospective randomized study. *Pain*, **73**, 361–7.
3. Lang EV, Benotsch EG, Fick LJ, et al. (2000). Adjunctive non-pharmacological analgesia for invasive medical procedures: a randomized trial. *Lancet*, **355**, 1486–90.
4. Häuser W, Hagl M, Schmierer A, Hansen E (2016): The efficacy, safety and applications of medical hypnosis—a systematic review of meta-analyses. *Dtsch Arztebl Int*, **113**(17), 289–96.
5. Thompson T, Terhune DB, Oram C, et al. (2019). The effectiveness of hypnosis for pain relief: A systematic review and metaanalysis of 85 controlled experimental trials. *Neurosci Biobehav Rev*, **99**, 298–310.
6. Vanhaudenhuyse A, Nyssen AS, Faymonville ME (2020). Recent insight on how the neuroscientific approach helps clinicians. *OBM Integrat Complement Medicine*, **5**(2), 28.
7. Elkins GR, Barabasz AF, Council JR, Spiegel D (2015). Advancing research and practice: the revised APA division 30 definition of hypnosis. *Am J Clin Hypnosis*, **57**(4), 378–85.
8. Demertzi A, Vanhaudenhuyse A, Noirhomme Q, Faymonville ME, Laureys S (2015). Hypnosis modulates behavioural measures and subjective ratings about external and internal awareness. *J Physiology-Paris*, **109**(4), 173–9.
9. Elliotson, J (1843). *Numerous cases of surgical operations without pain in the mesmeric state.* Philadelphia: Lea & Blanchard.

10. Esdaile J (1846). Mesmerism in India, and its practical application in surgery and medicine: Longman, Brown, Green, and Longmans. *Br Foreign Med Rev*, **22**, 475–87.

11. Bartolucci C, Lombardo GP (2017). The pioneering work of Enrico Morselli (1852–1929) in light of modern scientific research on hypnosis and suggestion. *Int J Clin Exp Hypn*, **65**, 398–428.

12. Subcommittee appointed by the Psychological Med Group Committee of the Br Medical Association (1955). Medical use of hypnotism. *Br Med J Supplement*, **2622**(1), S169.

13. Ahlskog G (2018). Clinical hypnosis today. *Psychoanal Rev*, **105**(4), 425–37.

14. Holler M, Koranyi S, Strauss B, Rosendahl J (2021). Efficacy of hypnosis in adults undergoing surgical procedures: a meta-analytic update. *Clin Psychol Rev*, **85**, 102001.

15. Landry M, Lifshitz M, Raz A (2017). Brain correlates of hypnosis: a systematic review and meta-analytic exploration. *Neurosci Biobehav Rev*, **81**, 75–98.

16. Vanhaudenhuyse A, Boly M, Laureys S, Faymonville ME (2009). Neuro-physiological correlates of hypnotic analgesia. *Contemp Hypn*, **26**, 15–23.

17. Vanhaudenhuyse A, Laureys S, Faymonville ME (2014). Neurophysiology of hypnosis. *Neurophysiol Clin*, **44**(4), 343–53.

18. Kekecs Z, Nagy T, Varga K (2014). The effectiveness of suggestive techniques in reducing postoperative side effects: a meta-analysis of randomized controlled trials. *Anesth Analg*, **119**(6),1407–19.

19. Zeng J, Wang L, Cai Q, Wu J, Zhou C (2022). Effect of hypnosis before general anesthesia on postoperative outcomes in patients undergoing minor surgery for breast cancer: a systematic review and meta-analysis. *Gland Surg*, **11**(3), 588–98.

20. Faymonville ME, Meurisse M, Fissette J (1999). Hypnosedation: a valuable alternative to traditional anaesthetic techniques. *Acta Chir Belg*, **99**, 141–6.

21. Gasteratos K, Papakonstantinou M, Man A, Babatsikos E, Tamalonis A, Goverman J (2022). Adjunctive nonpharmacologic interventions for the management of burn pain: A systematic review. *Plast Reconstr Surg*, **49**(5), 985e–94e.

22. Kissel M, Andraud M, Duhamel AS, et al. (2020). Hypnosedation for endocavitary uterovaginal applications: a pilot study. *Brachytherapy*, **19**(4), 462–9.

23. Chapet O, Udrescu C, Horn S, et al. (2019). Prostate brachytherapy under hypnosedation: A prospective evaluation. *Brachytherapy*, **18**, 22–8.

24. Wobst AKH (2007). Hypnosis and surgery: past, present and future. *Anesth Analg*, **104**, 1199–208.

25. Faymonville ME, Boly M, Laureys S (2006). Functional neuroanatomy of the hypnotic state. *J Physiol Paris*, **99**(4–6), 463–9.

26. Demertzi A, Soddu A, Faymonville ME, et al. (2011). Hypnotic modulation of resting state fMRI default mode and extrinsic network connectivity. *Prog Brain Res*, **193**, 309–22.

27. Bicego A, Rousseaux F, Faymonville ME, Nyssen AS, Vanhaudenhuyse A (2022). Neurophysiology of hypnosis in chronic pain: a review of recent literature. *Am J Clin Hypn*, **64**(1), 62–80.

28. Hansen E, Zech N (2019). Nocebo effects and negative suggestions in daily clinical practice—forms, impact and approaches to avoid them. *Front Pharmacol*, **10**, 77.

29. Zech N, Seemann M, Grzesiek M, Breu A, Seyfried TF, Hansen E (2019). Nocebo effects on muscular performance—an experimental study about clinical situations. *Front Pharmacol*, **10**, 219.

30. Zech N, Schrödinger M, Seemann M, Zeman F, Seyfried TF, Hansen E (2020). Time dependent negative effects of verbal and nonverbal suggestions in surgical patients—a study on arm muscle strength. *Front Psychol*, **11**, 1693.

31. Zech N, Scharl L, Seemann M, Pfeifer M, Hansen E (2022). Nocebo effects of clinical communication and placebo effects of positive suggestions on respiratory muscle strength. *Front Psychol*, **13**, 825839.

32. Häuser W, Hansen E, Enck P (2012). Nocebo phenoma in medicine: Their relevance in everyday clinical practice. *Dtsch Arztebl Int*, **109**(26), 459–65.

33. Piccioni F, Fanzio M (2008). Management of anesthesia in awake craniotomy. *Minerva Anestesiol*, **74**, 393–408.

34. Jacobs DT (1991). *Patient communication for first responders and EMS personnel.* Englewood Cliffs, NJ: Brady.

35. Moerman DE, Jonas W B (2002). Deconstructing the placebo effect and finding the meaning response. *Ann Intern Med*, **136**, 471–6.

36. Hansen E, Seemann M, Zech N, Doenitz C, Luerding R, Brawanski A (2013). Awake craniotomies without any sedation: The awake-awake-awake technique. *Acta Neurochir*, **155**(8), 1417–24.

37. Zech N, Seemann M, Seyfried TF, Lange M, Schlaier J, Hansen E (2018). Deep brain stimulation surgery without sedation. *Stereotact Functional Neurosurg*, **96**(6), 370–8.

38. Zemmoura I, Fournier E, El-Hage W, Jolly V, Destrieux C, Velut S (2016). Hypnosis for awake surgery of low-grade gliomas: description of the method and psychological assessment. *Neurosurgery*, **78**(1), 53–61.

39. Pesce A, Palmieri M, Cofano F, et al. (2020). Standard awake surgery versus hypnosis aided awake surgery for the management of highgrade gliomas: a non-randomized cohort comparison controlled trial. *J Clin Neurosci*, **77**, 41–8.

40. Cheek DB (1962). Importance of recognizing that surgical patients behave as though hypnotized. *Am J Clin Hypn*, **4**, 227–36.

41. Nowak H, Zech N, Asmussen S, et al. (2020). Effect of therapeutic suggestions during general anaesthesia on postoperative pain and opioid use—multicentre randomised controlled trial. *Brit Med J*, **371**, m4284.

42. Nowak H, Wolf A, Rahmel T, et al. (2022). Therapeutic suggestions during general anesthesia reduce postoperative nausea and vomiting in high-risk patients—a post-hoc analysis of a randomized controlled trial. *Front Pharmacol*, **13**, 898326.

Index

For the benefit of digital users, indexed terms that span two pages (e.g., 52–53) may, on occasion, appear on only one of those pages.